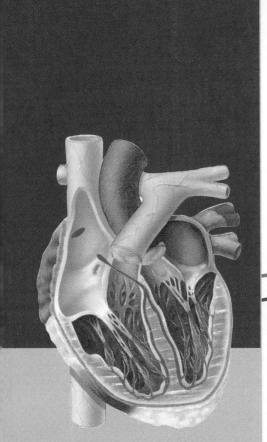

D1591969

UNDERSTANDING 12-LEAD EKGS

A PRACTICAL APPROACH

Second Edition

BRENDA BEASLEY
BS, RN, EMT-Paramedic

MICHAEL WEST
MS, RN, EMT-Paramedic

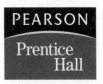

PEARSON
Prentice Hall

Upper Saddle River, New Jersey 07458

Library of Congress Cataloging-in-Publication Data
Beasley, Brenda M.
  Understanding 12-lead EKGs : a practical approach / Brenda Beasley, Michael West.—2nd ed.
    p. ; cm.
  Companion v. to: Understanding EKGs. 2nd ed. c2003.
  Includes bibliographical references and index.
  ISBN 0-13-170789-2 (alk. paper)
  1. Electrocardiography.
  [DNLM: 1. Electrocardiography. 2. Arrhythmia—diagnosis. 3. Heart Conduction System—
physiology. 4. Myocardial Infarction—diagnosis. WG 140 B3676ua 2006] I. West, Mike,
(date) II. Beasley, Brenda M. Understanding EKGs. III. Title.
  RC683.5.E5B374 2006
  616.1′207547—dc22

2005005893

Publisher: Julie Levin Alexander
Publisher's Assistant: Regina Bruno
Executive Editor: Marlene McHugh Pratt
Senior Managing Editor for Development: Lois Berlowitz
Project Manager: Josephine Cepeda
Editorial Assistant: Matthew Sirinides
Director of Marketing: Karen Allman
Executive Marketing Manager: Katrin Beacom
Senior Channel Marketing Manager: Rachele Strober
Marketing Coordinator: Michael Sirinides
Director of Production and Manufacturing: Bruce Johnson
Managing Editor for Production: Patrick Walsh
Production Liaison: Faye Gemmellaro
Production Editor: Emily Bush, Carlisle Publishers Services
Manufacturing Manager: Ilene Sanford
Manufacturing Buyer: Pat Brown
Senior Design Coordinator: Christopher Weigand
Cover Design: Solid State Graphics
Composition: Carlisle Publishers Services
Printing and Binding: Banta Menasha
Cover Printer: Phoenix Color

Notice: The author and the publisher of this book have taken care to make certain that the information given is correct and compatible with the standards generally accepted at the time of publication. Nevertheless, as new information becomes available, changes in treatment and in the use of equipment and procedures become necessary. The reader is advised to carefully consult the instruction and information material included in each piece of equipment or device before administration. Students are warned that the use of any techniques must be authorized by their medical advisor, where appropriate, in accordance with local laws and regulations. The author and the publisher disclaim any liability, loss, injury, or damage incurred as a consequence, directly or indirectly, of the use and application of any of the contents of this book.

Studentaid.ed.gov, The U.S. Department of Education's website on college planning assistance, is a valuable tool for anyone intending to pursue higher education. Designed to help students at all stages of schooling, including international students, returning students, and parents, it is a guide to the financial aid process. The website presents information on applying to and attending college as well as on funding your education and repaying loans. It also provides links to useful resources, such as state education agency contact information, assistance in filling out financial aid forms, and an introduction to various forms of student aid.

Pearson Prentice Hall™ is a trademark of Pearson Education, Inc.
Pearson® is a registered trademark of Pearson plc
Prentice Hall® is a registered trademark of Pearson Education, Inc.

Pearson Education Ltd.
Pearson Education Singapore, Pte. Ltd.
Pearson Education Canada, Ltd.
Pearson Education—Japan
Pearson Education Australia Pty. Limited

Pearson Education North Asia Ltd.
Pearson Educación de Mexico, S.A. de C.V.
Pearson Education Malaysia, Pte. Ltd.
Pearson Education, Upper Saddle River, New Jersey

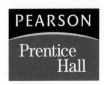

10 9 8 7 6 5 4 3 2 1
ISBN 0-13-170789-2

Dedication

This book is dedicated to the memory of a special man who was a revered friend, a mentor, and an enthusiastic educator for Emergency Medical Services.

His passion for quality patient care was a driving force in his role as a physician who helped to develop excellence in EMS education. He was a consummate professional and a wonderful human being.

Dr. Willis D. C. Israel

Dr. I., we miss you!

B. M. B.

Brief Contents

Contents

Foreword

The value of over 30 years of combined EMS educational experience enables Brenda Beasley and Michael West to bring a unique and insightful approach to the topic of 12-lead EKGs and their interpretation. The authors have presented a complex yet vitally important subject in a comprehensive, straightforward, and easy-to-understand format.

The text serves a wide audience of health-care providers, including prehospital providers, nurses, physician assistants, respiratory therapists, and anyone requiring a thorough understanding of electrocardiography. I believe that this book fills a void in the subject matter of EKG interpretation. It demonstrates the ability to educate medical personnel who are new to the subject matter while providing a review to those who are more experienced.

Using a reader-friendly writing style, the authors create a text that begins with the basics of EKG interpretation and then introduces a building-block approach to a more detailed discussion of this topic. Many illustrations, tables, and graphs are used to help highlight the important issues of each topic. Also, the reader will find the review questions at the end of each chapter useful in helping to solidify knowledge of salient issues.

Ms. Beasley has played a vital role in EMS education throughout the state of Alabama. She has made a difference in the lives of many people as well as influenced many career decisions. It was her commitment to education in and excitement about emergency medicine that was a significant factor in my choice of medicine as a career and, later, emergency medicine as a profession. The nursing background of both Ms. Beasley and Mr. West and their experience as EMS educators give them the wisdom to continue their roles of educating and influencing others through this text.

The importance of the communication and understanding of EKG changes among all medical personnel cannot be overemphasized. As an emergency medicine physician, I congratulate both Ms. Beasley and Mr. West on a book that provides common ground for physicians, nurses, and prehospital personnel.

Benjamin J. Camp, MD
Emergency Medicine Physician

Preface

Our purpose in writing the first edition of *Understanding 12-Lead EKGs: A Practical Approach* was to create a learning resource that was reader-friendly yet comprehensive in its approach to the interpretation of the 12-lead electrocardiogram. Remaining true to that original purpose, we have revised the text in order to update the content as applicable. This text continues to serve as a companion text to the second edition of *Understanding EKGs: A Practical Approach*.

The second edition of this text consists of 18 chapters that are designed to provide the user with a practical approach to the skill of 12-lead EKG interpretation. The original chapters have been updated and new artwork has been added. As from its inception, the goal of this text continues to be to provide a useful and understandable learning tool for health-care providers in their provision of optimum patient care.

We continue to believe that an essential prerequisite to understanding 12-lead EKG interpretation is a thorough understanding of basic EKG interpretation. With this thought in mind, we began this book with a series of chapters that review basic dysrhythmia interpretation. This book includes rhythm strip examples within each applicable chapter, as well as an entire chapter devoted to 12-lead EKG review strips. In addition, there are updated chapters devoted to cardiovascular pharmacology and therapeutic modalities.

It has been our intent to present the material in a logical order. In order to enable students to work comfortably through the technical information, the content is presented in short, succinct chapters in a building-block format. Students thereby achieve understanding of each chapter before proceeding to the next chapter. At the end of each chapter, we have expanded the section of multiple-choice questions to be used for self-assessment and review. In addition, we have included a practice EKG review strip at the end of the type-specific MI chapters.

An overview of major updates and additions to this revision may be helpful to you. These changes are summarized in the "What's New" list below.

WHAT'S NEW IN THE SECOND EDITION

➤ Information has been updated to reflect current standards of care.
➤ Current treatment regimens for AMI and fibrinolytics (formerly referred to as thrombolytics) and new, updated pharmacologic agents are addressed.
➤ Enhanced, up-to-date graphics accompany each chapter.
➤ Numerous examples of 12-lead EKGs are presented, and new EKG review strips have been added at the end of each applicable chapter.
➤ Margin glossaries appear throughout the text.
➤ Each chapter features a Summary as a wrap-up of chapter content.
➤ The feature Key Points to Remember has been added at the end of each chapter.
➤ Each chapter has additional review questions (30% more review questions).

➤ An Instructor's Resource CD consists of
  ➤ PowerPoint Slides—updated and revised to include new artwork and all Chapter 18 review strips.
  ➤ Lesson Plans for each chapter.
  ➤ Test Bank with more than 250 questions.

Since the late 1980s, the use of thrombolytics (now referred to as fibrinolytics) in the treatment of acute myocardial infarctions has become an expanding, dynamic component of the health-care profession. As a direct result of this, more and more health-care providers are required to interpret, understand, and apply their knowledge of 12-lead EKGs in the clinical setting. We sincerely hope that this logical, comprehensive approach to 12-lead EKG interpretation will provide the student, as well as other health-care providers, with a substantial foundation to understand and interpret electrocardiology. Ultimately, it is our wish that your future patients will benefit from the knowledge that you attain from this text.

Brenda M. Beasley
e-mail: bjm18@aol.com

Michael C. West
e-mail: MWest44266@aol.com

Acknowledgments

The first edition of *Understanding 12-Lead EKGs: A Practical Approach* was created as a result of our collective experiences in EMS education as well as in the clinical practice of emergency medicine. As we embarked on the revision of this text, we called on the advice of our graduates and colleagues as well as professional reviewers. We wish to recognize the following individuals who were instrumental, each in his or her own unique way, in making this textbook a reality.

We offer our sincere appreciation to the professional and competent team at Brady! The support of Marlene Pratt has been unwavering and much appreciated. Lois Berlowitz (a real angel) has skillfully guided us through completion of this project, and Jo Cepeda patiently steered us through the tedious process of making the book look good! We'd like to recognize Monica Moosang, who has been involved with every phase of the review process and has done a remarkable job. The numerous demands of production have been in the very competent and efficient hands of Patrick Walsh, Production Manager, and Faye Gemmellaro, Production Liaison, Emily Bush, Production Editor (CPS), and we are appreciative of their efforts. We also thank Katrin Beacom for marketing expertise during the promotion of this book revision.

Thanks are also due to Dr. Ben Camp for writing the Foreword for this book as well as for lending his advice and expertise to us throughout the entire project. Our expert reviewers, John Beckman, Danny Bercher, Merlin Curry, James P. Medeiros, Jeff Mitchell, Rick Slaven, Scott Snyder, and Robert Vroman, deserve much thanks for providing excellent suggestions and ideas for improving the text.

And last but not least, we gratefully acknowledge our families, friends and colleagues for their support, encouragement, and acceptance of our long absences during this textbook revision. Without the strength and love we received from each of you this task would have not been possible. Thank you so much for your continuing support.

INSTRUCTOR REVIEWERS

John Beckman, FF/PM
EMS Instructor
Good Samaritan Hospital; Addison Fire Department
Addison, IL

Danny Bercher
University of Arkansas for Medical Sciences
Little Rock, AR

Merlin Curry, EMT-P
EMT Program Director
Clackamas Community College
Oregon City, OR

James P. Medeiros, MFA, NREMT-P
Lecturer, Division of Emergency Services
Community and Technical College of Shepherd
Martinsburg, WV

Jeff Mitchell
EMS Program Director
Calhoun Community College
Athens, AL

Rick Slaven, NREMT-P, CC, AAS
Walters State Community College
Morristown, TN

Scott Snyder, BS, CCEMTP
Folsom, CA

Robert Vroman, BS, NREMT-P
EMS Instructor
HealthONE EMS
Englewood, CO

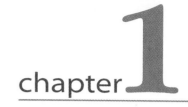

chapter 1

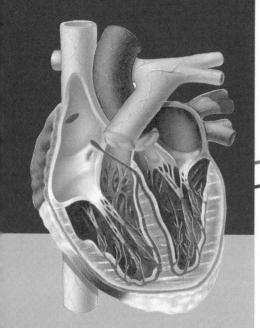

The Anatomy of the Heart
(Structure)

objectives

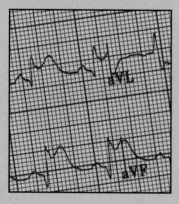

Upon completion of this chapter, the student will be able to:

➤ Identify the location, shape, and size of the heart

➤ Describe the chambers of the heart

  a. Atria

  b. Ventricles

➤ Name and locate the layers of the heart

➤ Name and locate the valves of the heart

➤ Describe the structure and function of the blood vessels

  a. Arteries

  b. Coronary arteries

  c. Veins

  d. Capillaries

INTRODUCTION

It is our belief that in order to properly master the art of 12-lead EKG interpretation, you must first have a thorough understanding of the structure of the heart. Therefore, this chapter provides you with a foundation upon which to review the fundamental knowledge of basic **dysrhythmia** interpretation. The focus of this chapter is thus to provide you with a simple yet comprehensive reassessment of cardiac anatomy. After you have reviewed the knowledge of basic cardiac anatomy (structure), you will be prepared to move into the next chapter, which reexamines the basic physiology (function) of the heart.

dysrhythmia
abnormal rhythm

ANATOMY OF THE HEART

As you will recall, the heart is a muscle. Although we don't usually think of exercising our heart muscle when we go to the gym, the fact is that the heart muscle (myocardium) is constantly in the *exercise mode*. At times of rest, the exercise is more sedate. However, think of the vigor with which your heart muscle must exercise when you walk (or run) up six flights of stairs. Now as you feel your heart pumping, you can easily understand that your heart muscle is indeed exercising.

We often hear the heart referred to as a *two-sided pump*. This analogy works well in our understanding of the basics of cardiac anatomy. Indeed, one can visualize this pump as having a right side and a left side. On each side of the pump, there is an upper chamber, which is referred to as the **atrium** (*atria*, plural) and a lower chamber known as the **ventricle** (Figure 1–1). There is a total of four hollow chambers in the normal

atrium upper
chamber of the heart

ventricle lower
chamber of the heart

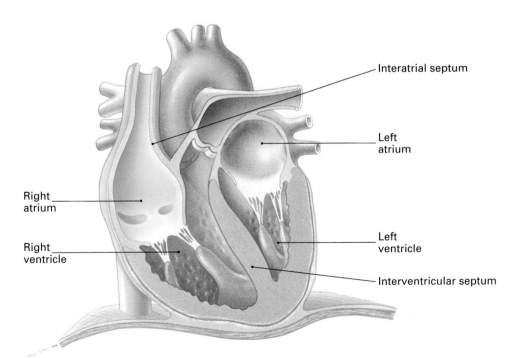

Figure 1–1. The chambers of the heart

heart. Again, the two upper chambers of the heart are called atria and the two lower chambers are called ventricles.

Separating the upper chambers is the interatrial septum, and the interventricular septum separates the lower, inferior chambers. Externally, the atrioventricular groove divides the atria from the ventricles. The anterior and posterior interventricular grooves separate the ventricles externally. The muscle fibers of the ventricles are continuous, as are the atrial muscle fibers.

The two upper chambers of the heart are located at the base, or top, of the heart whereas the lower chambers are located at the bottom, or apex of the heart. The upper chambers of the heart are thin-walled and receive blood as it returns to the heart. The lower chambers of the heart have thicker walls and pump blood away from the heart. The right ventricle pumps blood to the pulmonary circulation and the left ventricle pumps blood throughout the systemic circulation.

LOCATION, SIZE, AND SHAPE OF THE HEART

It is important for you to understand the location of the heart in that the effectiveness of one of our most basic, yet most important skills—namely, CPR—depends on reasonable knowledge of this position. The proper placement of electrodes to record an electrocardiogram, either 3-lead or 12-lead, depends upon the proper understanding of the location of the heart.

The central section of the thorax (chest cavity) is called the **mediastinum.** It is in this area that the heart is housed, lying in front of the spinal column, behind the sternum and between the lungs (Figures 1–2 and 1–3). When thinking of the heart muscle in

mediastinum
central section of the thorax (chest cavity)

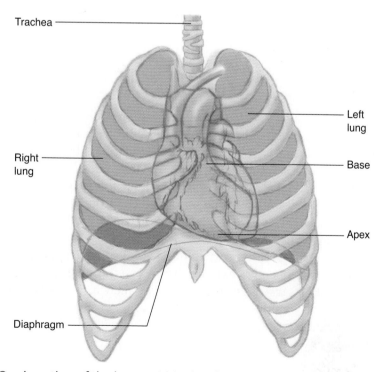

Figure 1–2.   Location of the heart within the chest

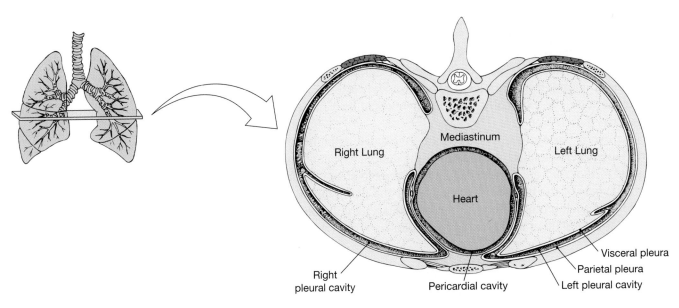

Figure 1–3. Anatomical relationships in the thoracic cavity

terms of its mass, one should realize that two-thirds of the heart lies to the left of the midline. The apex of the heart lies just above the diaphragm, and the base of the heart lies at approximately the level of the third rib.

The exact size of the heart varies somewhat among individuals, but on average it is approximately 5 inches (10 to 12 centimeters) in length and 3 inches (9 centimeters) wide. The shape of the heart is somewhat cone-like in appearance. It is appropriate to visualize the heart as approximately the size of the owner's closed fist.

LAYERS OF THE HEART

Pericardium

pericardium
closed, two-layered sac that surrounds the heart. Also called pericardial sac

Surrounding the heart is a closed, two-layered sac referred to as the **pericardium,** also known as the *pericardial sac.* In direct contact with the pleura is the outer layer or the parietal pericardium. This layer consists of tough, nonelastic, fibrous connective tissue and serves to prevent overdistention of the heart. The thin, serous inner layer of the pericardium is called the visceral pericardium and is contiguous with the epicardium, which surrounds the heart. A space filled with a scant amount of fluid (approximately 10 cc) separates the two pericardial layers. This fluid helps to reduce friction as the heart moves within the pericardial sac by acting as a lubricant.

pericarditis
inflammation of the serous pericardium

An inflammation of the serous pericardium is called **pericarditis.** Although the cause of this disease is frequently unknown, it may result from infection or disease of the connective tissue. This disease can cause severe pain, which may be confused with the pain of myocardial infarction. Pericarditis can cause changes in the 12-lead EKG and can mimic an acute myocardial infarction, which will be addressed later in the text. This can make physical assessment of the cardiac patient a real challenge for the clinician.

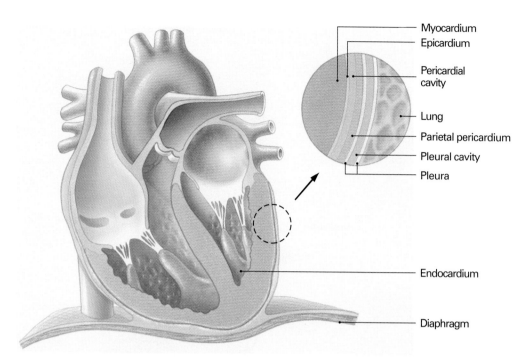

Myocardium
Epicardium
Pericardial cavity
Lung
Parietal pericardium
Pleural cavity
Pleura
Endocardium
Diaphragm

Figure 1–4.   Layers of the heart

The heart wall

Three layers of tissue compose the heart wall: the **epicardium,** the **myocardium,** and the **endocardium** (Figure 1–4). This specialized cardiac muscle tissue is unique to the heart. The epicardium accounts for the smooth outer surface of the heart. The thick, middle layer of the heart is called the myocardium and is the thickest of the three layers of the heart wall. The myocardium is composed primarily of cardiac muscle cells and is responsible for the heart's ability to contract. The innermost layer, the endocardium, is comprised of thin connective tissue. This smooth inner surface of the heart and heart valves serves to allow blood to flow more easily throughout the heart.

VALVES OF THE HEART

The four valves of the heart allow blood to flow in only one direction. There are two sets of valves: the *atrioventricular valves* and the *semilunar valves* (Figure 1–5).

Atrioventricular valves

As indicated by their name, the **atrioventricular valves (AV)** are located between the atria and the ventricles. These valves allow blood to flow from the atria into the ventricles. They are also effective in preventing the blood from flowing backward from the ventricles into the atria. The **tricuspid valve** is named for its three cusps and is located between the right atrium and the right ventricle. Free edges of each of the three cusps extend into the ventricles where they attach to the **chordae tendineae.** Chordae tendineae are fine chords of dense connective tissue that attach to papillary muscles in the wall of the ventricles. Chordae tendineae and papillary muscles work in concert to

epicardium
smooth outer surface of the heart

myocardium
thick middle layer of the heart composed primarily of cardiac muscle cells; responsible for the heart's ability to contract

endocardium
innermost layer of the heart; composed of thin connective tissue

atrioventricular valves the valves through which the blood passes from the atria to the ventricles

tricuspid valve named for its three cusps; located between the right atrium and right ventricle

chordae tendineae fine chords of dense connective tissue that attach to papillary muscles in the wall of the ventricles

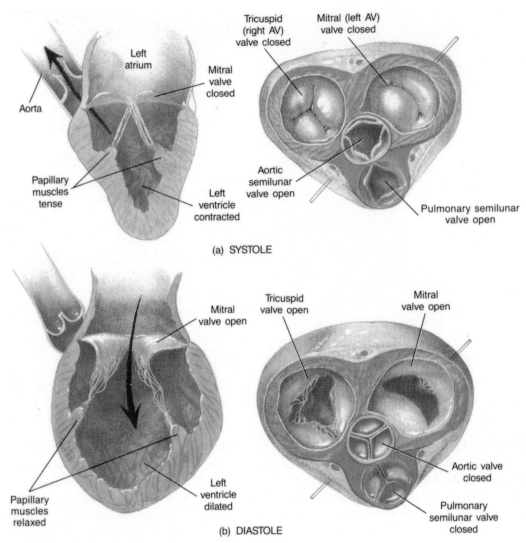

(a) SYSTOLE

(b) DIASTOLE

Figure 1–5. Valves of the heart

mitral valve
similar in structure to the tricuspid valve but has only two cusps; located between the left atrium and the left ventricle. Also called bicuspid valve

semilunar valves prevent the backflow of blood into the ventricles; each valve contains three semilunar (or moon-shaped) cusps

pulmonic valve
semilunar valve located between the right ventricle and the pulmonary artery

aortic valve
semilunar valve located between the left ventricle and the trunk of the aorta

prevent the cusps from fluttering back into the atrium, allowing disruption of blood flow through the heart. The **mitral valve** (or bicuspid valve) is similar in structure to the tricuspid valve but has only two cusps. The mitral valve is located between the left atrium and the left ventricle.

Semilunar valves

In much the same manner as the atrioventricular valves prevent backflow of blood into the atria, the **semilunar valves** serve to prevent the backflow of blood into the ventricles. Each semilunar valve contains three semilunar (or moon-shaped) cusps. The semilunar valves are the pulmonic and aortic valves. The semilunar valve located between the right ventricle and the pulmonary artery is called the **pulmonic valve.** The semilunar valve located between the left ventricle and the trunk of the aorta is called the **aortic valve.**

Changes in chamber pressure govern the opening and closing of the heart valves. During ventricular systole (contraction of the ventricles), the atrioventricular valves close and the semilunar valves open. During ventricular diastole (relaxation of the ven-

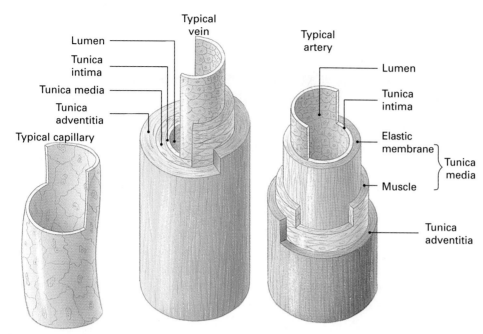

Figure 1–6.   Arterial wall layers

tricles), the aortic and pulmonic valves are closed and the mitral and tricuspid valves are open. Passive filling of the coronary arteries occurs during ventricular diastole.

ARTERIES, VEINS, AND CAPILLARIES

Because we tend to refer to the heart as the body's pump, we can similarly consider the vasculature, or the blood vessels, as the container for the fluid, or blood. When considering the purpose of this text, it is appropriate to discuss three commonly accepted groups of blood vessels: arteries, veins, and capillaries.

Arteries

Arteries, by virtue of their primary function, are relatively thick-walled and muscular. These blood vessels function under high pressure in order to convey blood from the heart out to the rest of the body. One definition of the prefix *a* is *away from,* so a helpful hint is to remember that the word *artery* also begins with the letter *a,* and thus arteries carry blood *away from* the heart. The larger arterial blood vessels are called arteries, which branch off into smaller blood vessels known as *arterioles.* Arteries carry oxygenated blood, with the exception of the pulmonary and umbilical arteries.

Arteries also operate in the regulation of blood pressure through functional changes in peripheral vascular resistance (the amount of opposition to blood flow offered by the arterioles). Arterial walls consist of three distinct layers: the intima, media, and adventitia (Figure 1–6). These layers are also called *tunics* (coats or coverings). The *tunica intima* is the innermost layer and consists of endothelium and an inner elastic membrane. This inner elastic membrane separates the intimal layer from the next layer, the *tunica media.* The *tunica media* is the middle layer and consists of smooth muscle cells. In this middle layer, blood flow through the vessel is regulated by constriction or dilation. Vasoconstriction, or a decrease in the diameter of the blood vessel, produces a

arteries thick-walled and muscular blood vessels that function under high pressure to convey blood from the heart out to the rest of the body

Table 1–1

Arterial wall layers		
Name	**Layer**	**Tissue Type**
Tunica intima	Innermost	Connective and elastic
Tunica media	Middle	Smooth muscle, elastic, and collagen
Tunica adventitia	Outermost	Connective

decrease in blood flow. In contrast, vasodilation, or an increase in the diameter of the blood vessel, produces an increase in blood flow. The *tunica adventitia,* or outermost layer, is composed of various connective tissue that anchor the blood vessels to adjacent tissues. (See Table 1–1.)

Coronary arteries and the coronary sinus

The primary structures of importance in this section are the coronary arteries and the coronary sinus.

coronary arteries the two arteries—right and left—that supply blood to the myocardium

Two Main Coronary Arteries   The two main **coronary arteries,** the right and left, arise from the trunk of the aorta and function to carry oxygenated blood throughout the myocardium. These arteries branch off into smaller vessels to supply the heart with oxygen. Because the left side of the heart is more muscular than the right side, the left coronary artery branches are more muscular than the right coronary artery branches. Oxygenated blood is distributed throughout the heart muscle through the process known as *coronary circulation* (discussed in detail in Chapter 7).

As the left coronary artery leaves the aorta, it immediately divides into the left anterior descending artery and the circumflex artery. The anterior descending artery is the major branch of the left coronary artery and supplies blood to most of the anterior part of the heart. A marginal branch of the left coronary artery supplies blood to the lateral wall of the left ventricle. The circumflex branch of the left coronary artery extends around to the posterior side of the heart, and its branches supply blood to much of the posterior wall of the heart. Each of these divisions has numerous branches that form a network of blood vessels, which in turn serve to provide oxygenation of designated portions of the myocardium.

The right coronary artery extends from the aorta around to the posterior portion of the heart. Branches of the right coronary artery supply blood to the lateral wall of the right ventricle. A branch of the right coronary artery called the posterior interventricular artery or posterior descending artery lies in the posterior interventricular region and supplies blood to the posterior and inferior part of the heart's left ventricle. The right coronary artery branches also supply oxygen-rich blood to a portion of the electrical conduction system.

coronary sinus passage that receives deoxygenated blood from the veins of the myocardium

Coronary Sinus   The **coronary sinus** is a short trunk that serves to receive deoxygenated blood from the veins of the myocardium. This trunk empties into the right atrium. (See Figure 1–7.)

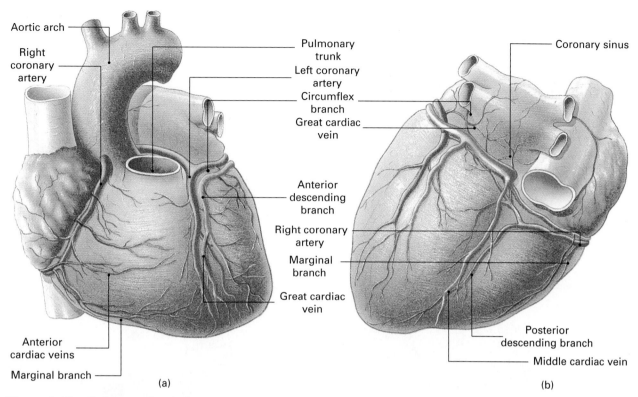

Figure 1–7.   Coronary circulation

Veins

Veins are blood vessels that carry blood back to the heart. Veins branch off into smaller vessels known as *venules.* With the exception of venules, veins are structurally similar to arteries in that they also have three layers. Unlike arteries, however, veins operate under low pressure, and are relatively thin-walled and contain one-way valves. With the exception of the pulmonary vein, the veins convey deoxygenated blood. The larger veins of the body ultimately empty into the two largest veins, the **superior vena cava** and the **inferior vena cava,** which empty deoxygenated blood into the heart's right atrium. The superior vena cava drains blood from the head and neck while the inferior vena cava collects blood from the rest of the body.

Capillaries

Capillaries are tiny blood vessels whose walls are the thinnest of all blood vessels. There is a greater number of capillaries in the human body than any other blood vessel. In fact, capillaries are so tiny that red blood cells must pass through them in single file. From the arterioles, blood flows into the capillaries, where the vast majority of gas exchange occurs.

      In summary, arterioles transport oxygenated blood into the capillaries. Capillaries allow for the exchange of oxygen, nutrients, and waste products between the blood and body tissues and are viewed as "connectors" between arteries and veins. The smallest of the veins, the venules, then receive the deoxygenated blood, which travels back to the heart via the venous system. (Refer to Figure 1–8 for the major veins and arteries of the circulatory system.)

veins blood vessels that carry blood back to the heart, operate under low pressure, and are relatively thin-walled

superior vena cava drains blood from the head and neck

inferior vena cava collects blood from the lower portion of the body

capillaries tiny blood vessels that allow for the exchange of oxygen, nutrients, and waste products between the blood and body tissues; connectors between arteries and veins

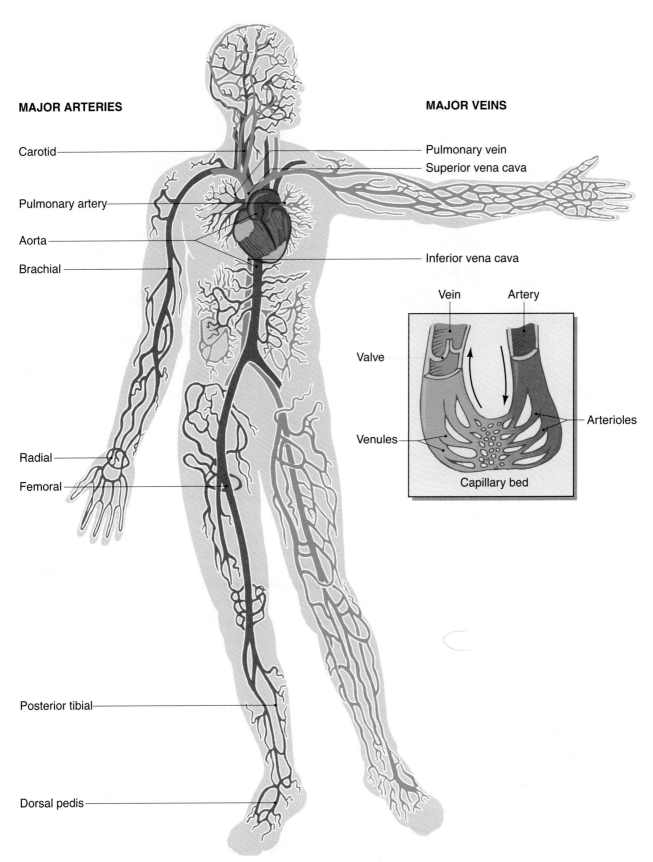

Figure 1–8.   Circulatory system

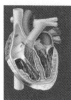

Summary
CHAPTER 1

This chapter has provided you the student with a simple yet comprehensive look at cardiac anatomy. A thorough understanding of cardiovascular anatomy is integral to appropriate dysrhythmia recognition.

Key Points to Remember
CHAPTER 1

1. The heart is located in the mediastinum.

2. The heart lies in front of the spinal column behind the sternum and between the lungs.

3. In terms of its mass, two-thirds of the heart lies to the left of the midline.

4. The apex (bottom) of the heart lies just above the diaphragm.

5. The base of the heart lies at approximately the level of the third rib.

6. The shape of the heart is cone-like in appearance.

7. It is appropriate to visualize the heart as approximately the size of the owner's closed fist.

8. There are a total of four hollow chambers in the normal heart.

9. On each side of the heart, there is an upper chamber, which is referred to as the *atrium* (*atria,* plural) and a lower chamber known as the *ventricle.*

10. Surrounding the heart is a closed, two-layered sac referred to as the *pericardium,* which is also known as the *pericardial sac.*

11. The epicardium accounts for the smooth outer surface of the heart.

12. The thick, middle layer of the heart is the myocardium and is the thickest of the three layers of the heart wall.

13. The innermost layer, the endocardium, is comprised of thin connective tissue.

14. The four valves of the heart allow blood to flow in only one direction.

15. The atrioventricular valves are located between the atria and the ventricles.

16. The AV valves allow blood to flow from the atria into the ventricles.

17. The semilunar valves serve to prevent the backflow of blood into the ventricles.

18. Each semilunar valve contains three semilunar (or moon-shaped) cusps. The semilunar valves are the pulmonic and aortic valves.

19. Arteries are relatively thick-walled and muscular in structure.

20. Arteries function under high pressure in order to convey blood from the heart out to the rest of the body.

21. Veins are defined as blood vessels that carry blood back to the heart.

22. Veins operate under low pressure, are relatively thin-walled, and contain one-way valves.

23. Capillaries are tiny blood vessels whose walls are the thinnest of all blood vessels.

24. Capillaries allow for the exchange of oxygen, nutrients, and waste products between the blood and body tissues and are viewed as connectors between arteries and veins.

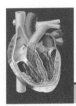

Review Questions
CHAPTER 1

1. When reviewing the layers of the heart, you will recall that the fibrous sac covering the heart, which is in contact with the pleura, is called the:

   a. epicardium.

   b. myocardium.

   c. pericardium.

   d. endocardium.

2. The heart chamber with the thickest myocardium is the:

   a. right ventricle.

   b. left ventricle.

   c. right atrium.

   d. left atrium.

3. The pulmonic and aortic valves are open during:

   a. systole.

   b. diastole.

   c. cardiac cycle.

   d. systole and diastole.

4. The large blood vessel that returns unoxygenated blood from the head and neck to the right atrium is called the:

   a. jugular vein.

   b. carotid artery.

   c. superior vena cava.

   d. inferior vena cava.

5. The innermost layer of the arterial wall is called the:

   a. tunica intima.

   b. tunica media.

   c. myocardium.

   d. tunica adventitia.

6. The most numerous blood vessels in the body are the:

   a. arteries.

   b. capillaries.

   c. venules.

   d. veins.

7. Blood flow between the heart and lungs comprises the:

   a. systemic circulation.

   b. venous circulation.

   c. myocardial circulation.

   d. pulmonary circulation.

8. Blood vessels that function under high pressure in order to convey blood from the heart out to the rest of the body are called:

   a. venules

   b. veins

   c. arteries

   d. capillaries

9. The blood vessel that returns unoxygenated blood from the myocardium to the right atrium is called the great cardiac vein or the:

   a. jugular vein.

   b. carotid artery.

   c. coronary sinus.

   d. inferior vena cava.

10. ___ ___ are fine chords of dense connective tissue that attach to papillary muscles in the wall of the ventricles.

    a. Coronary arteries

    b. Coronary sinuses

    c. Chordae tendineae

    d. Purkinje fibers

11. The right and left coronary arteries branch off of the:

    a. coronary sinus.

    b. right atrium.

    c. left atrium.

    d. trunk of the aorta.

12. The central section of the thorax is called the:

    a. costal margin.

    b. mediastinum.

    c. diaphragm.

    d. xiphoid.

13. The smooth outer surface of the heart is called the:

    a. myocardium.

    b. epicardium.

    c. endocardium.

    d. pericardium.

14. An inflammation of the serous pericardium is called:

    a. myocarditis.

    b. pericarditis.

    c. pulmonitis.

    d. tendonitis.

15. The coronary ___ is the short trunk that serves to receive deoxygenated blood from the veins of the myocardium.

    a. artery

    b. fiber

    c. sinus

    d. tissue

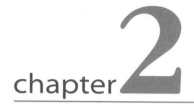

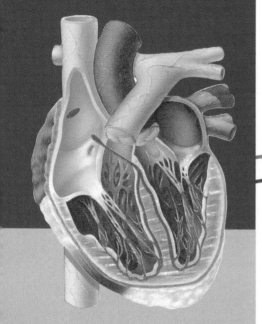

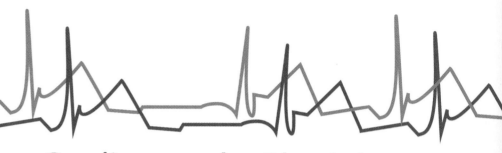

Cardiovascular Physiology
(Function)

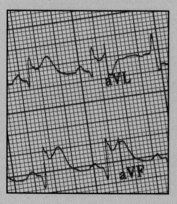

objectives

Upon completion of this chapter, the student will be able to:

➤ Describe the sequence of blood flow through the heart

➤ Describe the cardiac cycle, including

   a. Definition

   b. Systole

   c. Diastole

➤ Discuss the term *stroke volume*

➤ Discuss cardiac output, preload, Starling's Law, and afterload

➤ Describe the autonomic nervous system

➤ Discuss the two major divisions of the autonomic nervous system

INTRODUCTION

Now that you have reviewed the structure of the heart, it is time to address the basic function (or physiology) of the cardiovascular system. The focus of this chapter is to provide you with an uncomplicated yet inclusive review of cardiac physiology. After you have mastered it, you will be prepared to move into the next chapter, which addresses the basic electrophysiology of the heart.

NOTE: Now is the perfect time to look back at the review questions from Chapter 1. Then proceed on through the objectives and contents of this chapter.

BLOOD FLOW THROUGH THE HEART

The path of blood flow through the heart is our first consideration in reviewing the knowledge of the physiology of circulation (Figure 2–1). Imagine that the right atrium is a receptacle that functions, in part, to receive unoxygenated blood from the head, neck, and trunk. The right ventricle receives blood from the right atrium and pumps it to the pulmonary system. The left atrium receives oxygenated blood from the pulmonary system. The left ventricle receives this oxygenated blood from the left atrium and pumps it to the body system.

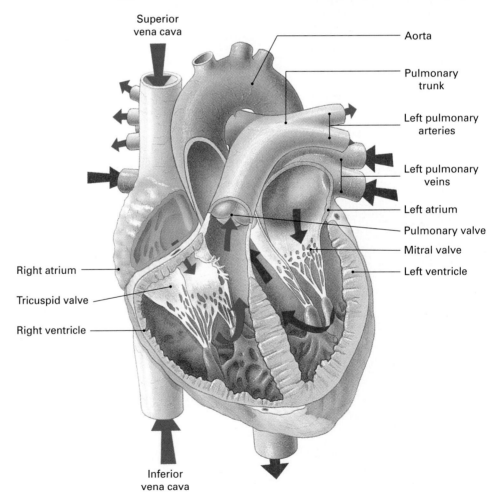

Figure 2–1. Blood flow through the heart

In order to simplify the route of circulation, you may choose to divide this concept into three components. The first component would consist of blood flow through the right heart. That is, unoxygenated blood flows from the inferior and superior vena cavae into the:

Right atrium	Through the tricuspid valve	Into the right ventricle	Through the pulmonic valve

The second component of blood flow through the pulmonary circulation continues when the blood travels from the pulmonic valve into the:

Pulmonary arteries	Into the lungs	Through the pulmonary alveolar-capillary network	Into the pulmonary veins

The third and final component of blood flow through the pulmonary circulation continues when the blood travels from the pulmonary veins into the:

Left atrium	Through the mitral valve	Into the left ventricles	Through the aortic valve into the aorta and out to the systemic circulation

It should be noted that the freshly oxygenated blood traveling through the aortic valve also enters into the coronary arteries in order to accomplish myocardial oxygenation. The vital function of gas exchange occurs in the second or middle component of pulmonary circulation when carbon dioxide is exchanged for oxygen in the pulmonary alveolar-capillary network.

CARDIAC CYCLE

The heart functions as a unit in that both atria contract simultaneously, and then both ventricles contract. When the atria contract, the ventricles are filled to their limits. Blood is ejected into both the pulmonary and systemic circulations when the simultaneous contraction of the ventricles occurs. At the time of ventricular contraction, the mitral and tricuspid valves are closed by the pressure of the contraction and the pull of the papillary muscles, while the pulmonic and aortic valve are opened. The **cardiac cycle** represents the actual time sequence from initiation of ventricular contraction through to initiation of the next ventricular contraction.

Systole, also referred to as *ventricular systole,* is consistent with the simultaneous contraction of the ventricles, while **diastole** is synonymous with *ventricular relaxation.* The ventricles fill passively with approximately 70% of the blood that has collected in

cardiac cycle
actual time sequence between ventricular contraction and ventricular relaxation

systole contraction of the chambers of the heart. Also called ventricular systole

diastole
synonymous with ventricular relaxation

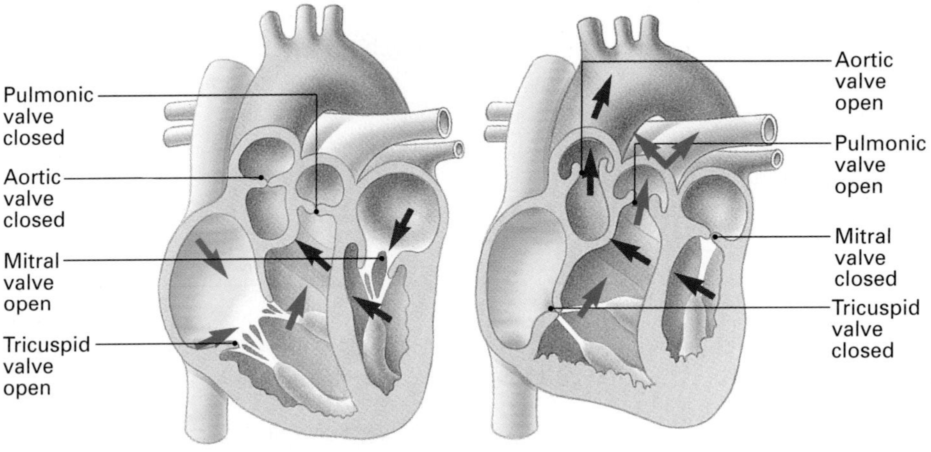

Figure 2–2. Relation of blood flow to cardiac contraction

the atria during ventricular diastole. Then the active contraction of the atria propels the remaining 30% of the blood into the ventricles. This is known as *atrial kick.* Atrial contraction represents only a minimal role in filling; consequently, even if the atria do not contract effectively, ventricular filling still ensues. During periods of ventricular relaxation, cardiac filling and coronary perfusion occur passively.

One cardiac cycle occurs every 0.8 seconds. Systole lasts about 0.28 second while diastole lasts about 0.52 second. Thus, the period of diastole is substantially longer than the period of systole. (See Figure 2–2.)

STROKE VOLUME

stroke volume volume of blood pumped out of one ventricle of the heart in a single beat or contraction

Stroke volume may be defined as the volume of blood pumped out of one ventricle of the heart in a single beat or contraction. Stroke volume is estimated at approximately 70 cc per beat. The number of contractions, or beats per minute, is known as the **heart rate.** The normal heart rate is 60 to 100 beats per minute.

CARDIAC OUTPUT

heart rate number of contractions, or beats, per minute

cardiac output amount of blood pumped by the left ventricle in 1 minute

Cardiac output is the amount of blood pumped by the left ventricle in 1 minute. The output of the right ventricle is normally equal to the left, because these two chambers contract simultaneously. By remembering the following formula, you can determine the cardiac output:

Cardiac output (CO) =	Stroke volume (SV) × heart rate (HR)

Consequently, if a patient has a heart rate of 80 beats per minute (BPM) and a stroke volume of 70 cc per beat, the resulting cardiac output will be approximately 5,600 cc per minute (or 5.6 liters per minute). When, for a variety of reasons, the patient's cardiac output is outside the normal range, the heart will try to balance it by changes in either the stroke volume or the heart rate. Inadequate cardiac output may be indicated by a combination of any of the following signs and symptoms: shortness of breath, dizziness, decreased blood pressure, chest pains, and cool and clammy skin.

Commonly called *end-diastolic pressure,* **preload** is the pressure in the ventricles at the end of diastole and **afterload** is the resistance against which the heart must pump. This pressure also affects stroke volume and cardiac output.

When the volume of blood in the ventricles is increased, stretching the ventricular myocardial fibers and consequently causing a more forceful contraction, a concept known as **Starling's Law of the heart** is the result. This law of physiology basically states: The more the myocardial fibers are stretched, up to a certain point, the more forceful the subsequent contraction will be. Thus we can assume that if the volume of blood filling the ventricle increases significantly, so will the force of the cardiac contraction. This law is thought of as analogous to the stretching of a rubber band—the farther you stretch a rubber band, the harder it snaps back to its original size.

The amount of opposition to blood flow offered by the arterioles is known as the peripheral (or systemic) vascular resistance. If the peripheral vascular resistance remains uniform, a patient's blood pressure may increase or decrease if the cardiac output changes significantly. Vasoconstriction and vasodilation determine **peripheral vascular resistance (PVR).** Blood pressure is subject to change if the cardiac output or peripheral vascular resistance changes.

Therefore it may be helpful to remember the following formula:

Blood pressure (BP) =	Cardiac output (CO) × peripheral vascular resistance (PVR)

AUTONOMIC NERVOUS SYSTEM

The **autonomic nervous system** regulates functions of the body that are involuntary or are not under conscious control. Thus, we do not have to consciously think about our heartbeat or about regulating our blood pressure. Heart rate and blood pressure are regulated by this component of the nervous system (Figure 2–3).

There are two major divisions of the autonomic nervous system: the **sympathetic nervous system** and the **parasympathetic nervous system.** The sympathetic nervous system is responsible for preparation of the body for physical activity ("fight or flight") and the parasympathetic nervous system regulates the calmer functions of our existence ("rest and digest"). The majority of organs in the body, including the heart, are innervated by both systems. It is important to note that blood vessels are only innervated by the sympathetic nervous system.

RECEPTORS AND NEUROTRANSMITTERS

Nerve endings of the sympathetic nervous system and the parasympathetic nervous system secrete neurotransmitters. The sympathetic nervous system has two types of receptor fibers at the nerve endings: the alpha and beta receptors. The chemical neurotransmitter for the sympathetic nervous system is **norepinephrine.** These nerve endings are called *adrenergic.* When norepinephrine is released, an increase in heart rate and contractile force of cardiac fibers and vasoconstriction will result.

preload pressure in the ventricles at the end of diastole

afterload resistance against which the heart must pump

Starling's Law of the heart the more the myocardial fibers are stretched, up to a certain point, the more forceful the subsequent contraction will be

peripheral vascular resistance (PVR) amount of opposition to blood flow offered by the arterioles

autonomic nervous system regulates functions of the body that are involuntary or not under conscious control

sympathetic nervous system responsible for preparation of the body for physical activity ("fight or flight")

parasympathetic nervous system regulates the calmer ("rest and digest") functions

norepinephrine chemical neurotransmitter for the sympathetic nervous system

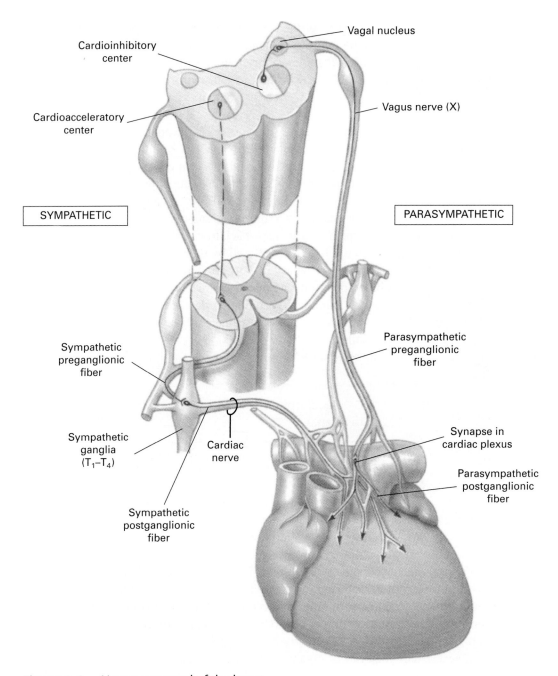

Figure 2–3.   Nervous control of the heart

acetylcholine
chemical
neurotransmitter for
the parasympathetic
system

The chemical neurotransmitter for the parasympathetic nervous system is **acetylcholine,** and the nerve endings are known as *cholinergic.* When acetylcholine is released, the heart rate slows, as does atrioventricular conduction rates. With the exception of capillaries, all of the body's blood vessels have alpha-adrenergic receptors whereas the heart and lungs have beta-adrenergic receptors.

For further details regarding receptors and neurotransmitters, refer to Chapter 2 of *Understanding EKGs: A Practical Approach,* 2nd Edition, the companion book to this text.

Summary

CHAPTER 2

It is important to understand not only the structure of the cardiovascular system, but also the function of the various structures. Indeed, it would be difficult to understand just why a particular component of the heart has ceased to function properly unless you were familiar with the proper (or normal) function of that component. Thus, this chapter has focused on simplifying a very complicated subject, cardiovascular physiology.

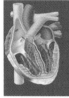

Key Points to Remember

CHAPTER 2

1. The right atrium functions in part to receive unoxygenated blood from the head, neck, and trunk.

2. The right ventricle receives blood from the right atrium and pumps it to the pulmonary system.

3. The left atrium receives oxygenated blood from the pulmonary system.

4. The left ventricle receives this oxygenated blood from the left atrium and pumps it to the body system.

5. The cardiac cycle represents the time from initiation of ventricular contraction to initiation of the next ventricular contraction.

6. Systole (ventricular systole) is consistent with simultaneous contraction of the ventricles.

7. Diastole is synonymous with ventricular relaxation.

8. Stroke volume refers to the volume of blood pumped out of one ventricle of the heart in a single beat or contraction.

9. Stroke volume is estimated at 70 cc per beat.

10. Cardiac output is the amount of blood pumped by the left ventricle in 1 minute.

11. Also called end-diastolic pressure, preload is the pressure in the ventricles at the end of diastole.

12. Afterload is the resistance against which the heart must pump.

13. When the volume of blood in the ventricles is increased, stretching the ventricular myocardial fibers and consequently causing a more forceful contraction, a concept known as Starling's Law of the heart is the result.

14. The autonomic nervous system regulates functions of the body that are involuntary or are not under conscious control. Heart rate and blood pressure are regulated by this component of the nervous system.

15. There are two major divisions of the autonomic nervous system: the sympathetic nervous system and the parasympathetic nervous system.

16. The sympathetic nervous system is responsible for preparation of the body for physical activity ("fight or flight").

17. The parasympathetic nervous system regulates the calmer ("rest and digest") functions of our existence.

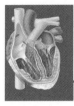

Review Questions
CHAPTER 2

1. The left side of the heart is referred to as a low-pressure pump.
   a. True
   b. False

2. The major blood vessel that receives blood from the head and upper extremities and transports it to the heart is the:
   a. aorta.
   b. superior vena cava.
   c. inferior vena cava.
   d. pulmonary artery.

3. The course of blood flow through the heart and lungs is referred to as ___ circulation.
   a. aortic
   b. pulmonary
   c. systemic
   d. collateral

4. Cardiac output is a product of which of the elements listed below?
   a. heart rate
   b. stroke volume
   c. partial vascular resistance
   d. a and b

5. The chief chemical neurotransmitter for the parasympathetic nervous system is:
   a. acetylcholine.
   b. norepinephrine.
   c. epinephrine.
   d. atropine.

6. The heart has ___ chambers.

   a. two

   b. three

   c. four

   d. six

7. The chief chemical neurotransmitter for the sympathetic nervous system is:

   a. acetylcholine.

   b. norepinephrine.

   c. ephedrine.

   d. atropine.

8. Unoxygenated blood flows from the inferior and superior vena cavae into the:

   a. left atrium.

   b. left ventricle.

   c. right ventricle.

   d. right atrium.

9. One cardiac cycle occurs every ___ seconds.

   a. 0.8

   b. 0.5

   c. 0.52

   d. 1.2

10. With the exception of ___, all of the body's blood vessels have alpha-adrenergic receptors, whereas the heart and lungs have beta-adrenergic receptors.

    a. arterioles

    b. capillaries

    c. venules

    d. aorta

11. The autonomic nervous system is divided into the sympathetic nervous system and the ___ nervous system.

    a. adrenergic

    b. cholinergic

    c. parasympathetic

    d. neurosympathetic

12. The pressure in the ventricles during diastole is called:

    a. preload.

    b. afterload.

    c. postload.

    d. endload.

13. Starling's Law of the heart states that the more the myocardial fibers are stretched (to a point), the more forceful the cardiac contraction will be.

   a. True

   b. False

14. The nerve endings of the sympathetic nervous system are called:

   a. cholinergic.

   b. adrenergic.

   c. dopaminergic.

   d. acetylilnergic.

15. Stroke volume is estimated as ___ cubic centimeters per beat.

   a. 60

   b. 70

   c. 80

   d. 90

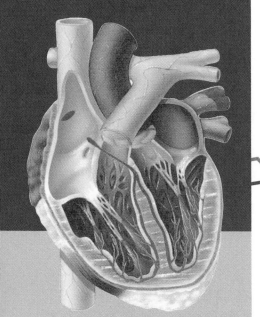

Basic Electrophysiology

objectives

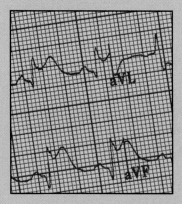

Upon completion of this chapter, the student will be able to:

➤ State the two basic myocardial cell groups

➤ Describe the function of each myocardial cell group

➤ Discuss the four primary properties of cardiac cells

➤ List the three major electrolytes that affect cardiac function

➤ Describe the movement of ions across cell membranes

➤ Describe cardiac depolarization

➤ Describe cardiac repolarization

➤ Define refractory period

➤ Describe the absolute refractory period

➤ Describe the relative refractory period

INTRODUCTION

Although the in-depth study of cardiac electrophysiology can be quite complicated and baffling to the novice student, the intent of this text is to concentrate on a review of the *basics* of dysrhythmia interpretation. Thus, this discussion of electrophysiology will center on rudimentary but very important concepts.

In the Chapter 1 discussion of cardiac anatomy, it was established that the heart is indeed a very unique and distinctive organ, unlike any other organ in the human body. The heart is composed of cardiac muscle, which is made up of thousands of myocardial cells. For purposes of discussion, consider that there are two basic myocardial cell groups: the **myocardial working cells** and the specialized pacemaker cells of the electrical conduction system.

myocardial working cells responsible for generating the physical contraction of the heart muscle

BASIC CELL GROUPS

Myocardial working cells

The myocardial working cells are responsible for generating the physical contraction of the heart muscle. The muscular layer of the wall of the atria, as well as the thicker muscular layer of the ventricular walls, are constructed by the myocardial working cells. Myocardial working cells are permeated by contractile filaments that, when electrically stimulated, produce myocardial contraction. Thus, the primary functions of the myocardial working cells include both contraction and relaxation.

It should be noted that this physical contraction of myocardial tissue actually generates blood flow; however, organized electrical activity is required in order to produce the physical contraction. As the myocardial tissue contracts, the size of the atria and ventricles decrease, producing the ejection of blood from the chambers.

Specialized pacemaker cells

specialized pacemaker cells responsible for controlling the rate and rhythm of the heart by coordinating regular depolarization; found in the electrical conduction system of the heart

Unlike the myocardial working cells, the **specialized pacemaker cells** of the electrical conduction system do not contain contractile filaments and thus do not have the ability to contract. Rather, this specialized group of cells is responsible for controlling the rate and rhythm of the heart by coordinating regular depolarization (see the section on cardiac depolarization later in this chapter). These cells are found in the electrical conduction system of the heart. Thus, the generation and conduction of electrical impulses are the primary functions of the specialized myocardial pacemaker cells.

Cardiac muscle cells have the ability to contract in response to thermal, chemical, electrical, or mechanical stimuli. All atrial muscle cells contract simultaneously; comparably, all ventricular muscle cells contract together.

threshold refers to the point at which a stimulus will produce a cell response

The term **threshold** refers to the point at which a stimulus will produce a cell response. When a stimulus is strong enough for cardiac cells to reach threshold, all cells will respond to this stimulus and will thus contract. This action is known as the all-or-none phenomenon of cardiac muscle cells; that is, either all cells will respond or none will respond. Hence, cardiac muscle functions on an all-or-none principle.

PRIMARY CARDIAC CELL CHARACTERISTICS

Cardiac cells possess four primary cell characteristics (Table 3–1). These properties are automaticity, excitability (or irritability), conductivity, and contractility (or rhythmicity). Only one of these characteristics—contractility—is considered a mechanical function of the heart. The other three characteristics—automaticity, excitability, and conductivity—are electrical functions of the heart.

Automaticity is the ability of cardiac pacemaker cells to spontaneously generate their own electrical impulses without external (or nervous) stimulation. This intrinsic spontaneous depolarization frequency produces contraction of myocardial muscle cells. This characteristic is specific to the pacemaker cell sites of the electrical conduction system (the SA node, the AV junction, and the Purkinje network fibers).

Excitability is the ability of cardiac cells to respond to an electrical stimulus. This characteristic is shared by all cardiac cells and is also referred to as *irritability*. A weaker stimulus is required to cause a contraction when a cardiac cell is highly irritable.

Conductivity is the ability of cardiac cells to receive an electrical stimulus and to then transmit the stimulus to other cardiac cells. This characteristic is shared by all cardiac cells because these cells are connected together to form a syncytium (they function collectively as a unit).

Contractility is also referred to as *rhythmicity* and is the ability of cardiac cells to shorten and cause cardiac muscle contraction in response to an electrical stimulus. Contractility can be thought of as the coordination of contractions of cardiac muscle cells to produce a regular heart beat. Through the administration of certain medications, such as dopamine and epinephrine, cardiac contractility can be strengthened.

MAJOR ELECTROLYTES THAT AFFECT CARDIAC FUNCTION

Because myocardial cells are bathed in **electrolyte** solutions, both mechanical and electrical cardiac function is influenced by electrolyte imbalances. An electrolyte is a substance or compound whose molecules dissociate into charged components, or ions, when placed in water, producing positively and negatively charged ions. An ion with a positive charge is called a **cation** and an ion with a negative charge is called an **anion.**

The three major cations that affect cardiac function are potassium (K), sodium (Na) and calcium (Ca). Magnesium (Mg) is also an important cation. Potassium (K), magnesium (Mg), and calcium (Ca) are intracellular (inside the cell) cations, whereas sodium (Na) is an extracellular (outside the cell) cation.

automaticity ability of cardiac pacemaker cells to generate their own electrical impulses spontaneously without external (or nervous) stimulation

excitability ability of all cardiac cells to respond to an electrical stimulus. Also called irritability

conductivity ability of cardiac cells to receive an electrical stimulus and then transmit it to other cardiac cells

contractility ability of cardiac cells to shorten and cause cardiac muscle contraction in response to an electrical stimulus. Also called rhythmicity

electrolyte substance or compound whose molecules dissociate into charged components when placed in water, producing positively and negatively charged ions

cation ion with a positive charge

anion ion with a negative charge

Table 3–1

Primary cardiac cell characteristics

Characteristic	Location	Function
Automaticity	SA node, AV junction, Purkinje network fibers	Electrical
Excitability	All cardiac cells	Electrical
Conductivity	All cardiac cells	Electrical
Contractility	Myocardial muscle cells	Mechanical

Potassium performs a major function in cardiac depolarization and repolarization. An increase in potassium blood levels is known as *hyperkalemia;* a potassium deficit is defined as *hypokalemia.* Sodium plays a vital part in depolarization of the myocardium. An increase in sodium blood levels is known as *hypernatremia;* a sodium deficit is defined as *hyponatremia.* Calcium renders an important function in myocardial depolarization and myocardial contraction. An increase in calcium blood levels is known as *hypercalcemia;* a calcium deficit is defined as *hypocalcemia.*

MOVEMENT OF IONS

Think now about the cardiac cell at rest or in its resting state. Normally, there exists an ionic difference on the two sides of the cell membrane. In this state, potassium ion concentration is greater inside the cell than outside, and sodium ion concentration is greater outside, the cell than inside. Potassium ions can diffuse through the membrane more readily than can sodium ions. By means of an active (or energized) mechanism of transport called the *sodium-potassium exchange pump,* potassium and sodium ions are moved in and out of the cell through the cell membrane. During the polarized or resting state, the inside of the cell is electrically negative relative to the outside of the cell. For purposes of discussions in the upcoming chapter of this text, it should be noted that during this resting period, a baseline or **isoelectric line** is recorded on the EKG strip.

isoelectric line the line created on an EKG strip when no electrical current is flowing. Also called baseline

CARDIAC DEPOLARIZATION

When an impulse develops and spreads throughout the myocardium, certain changes occur in the heart muscle fibers. These changes are referred to as *cardiac depolarization* and *cardiac repolarization.* In order to accurately and reasonably understand EKG interpretation, one must understand the concept of cardiac depolarization and repolarization.

First, here are some terms (with definitions) that will be used in this discussion:

➤ **Resting membrane potential** — the state of a cardiac cell in which the inside of the cell membrane is negative when compared to the outside of the cell membrane; exists when cardiac cells are in the resting state.

➤ **Action potential** — a change in polarity; a five-phase cycle that produces changes in the cell membrane's electrical charge; caused by stimulation of myocardial cells that extends across the myocardium; propagated in an all-or-none fashion.

➤ **Syncytium** — cardiac muscle cell groups that are connected together and function collectively as a unit.

➤ **Polarized state** — the resting state of a cardiac cell wherein the inside of the cell is electrically negative relative to the outside of the cell.

➤ **Depolarization** — an electrical occurrence normally expected to result in myocardial contraction; involves the movement of ions across cardiac cell membranes, resulting in positive polarity inside the cell membrane.

➤ **Repolarization** — process whereby the depolarized cell is polarized and positive charges are again on the outside and negative charges on the inside of the cell; a return to the resting state.

For the sake of clarity, cardiac depolarization may be thought of as the period during which sodium ions rush into the cell, changing the interior charge to positive, after a myocardial cell has been stimulated. Recall that this change of polarity is referred to as the *action potential.* In an effort to change the interior cell polarity to positive, calcium also slowly enters into the cell. This activated state of the myocardial cells now spreads through the syncytium, followed closely by myocardial muscle contraction. This difference in the electric charge or polarity on the outside of the cell membrane results in the flow of electric current, which is recorded as waveforms on the EKG.

CARDIAC REPOLARIZATION

At the end of cardiac depolarization, the sodium actively returns to the outside of the cell and potassium returns to the inside of the cell (Figure 3–1). This exchange takes place via the sodium-potassium exchange pump. The cell has now returned to the recovered

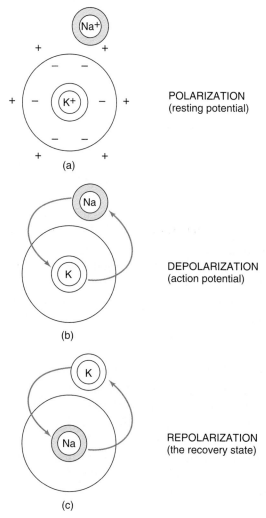

POLARIZATION
(resting potential)

(a)

DEPOLARIZATION
(action potential)

(b)

REPOLARIZATION
(the recovery state)

(c)

Figure 3–1.   Ion shifts during depolarization and repolarization

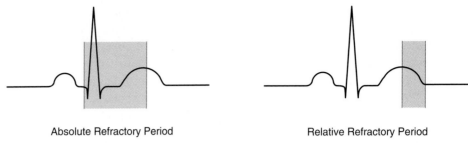

Absolute Refractory Period   Relative Refractory Period

Figure 3–2.   Refractory periods

or repolarized state. The cardiac cell is now ready to be stimulated again. Repolarization is a slower process than depolarization.

It may be helpful to recall that the polarized cell is in the resting state; the depolarization of the cell is utilizing its action potential; and the repolarized cell is in the recovery phase. Note that the last area to be depolarized is the first area to be repolarized in the normal, healthy cardiac muscle.

REFRACTORY PERIODS

Like all other excitable tissue, cardiac muscle tissue has a refractory period that attempts to ensure that the muscle is totally relaxed before another action potential or depolarization can be initiated. The refractory period of atrial muscle is much shorter (approximately 0.15 sec) than that of ventricular muscle refractory period (approximately 0.25 to 0.3 sec). Thus, the rate of atrial contractions can potentially be much faster than that of the ventricles.

After electrical impulse stimulation and myocardial contraction, the cardiac cells enjoy a brief resting period. As you read earlier in this discussion, this period of rest is referred to as *cardiac repolarization*. During this state of repolarization, the heart goes through two stages: the absolute refractory period and the relative refractory period (Figure 3–2).

During the majority of the process of repolarization, the cardiac cell is unable to respond to a new electrical stimulus. In addition, the cardiac cell cannot spontaneously depolarize. This stage of the cell is referred to as the **absolute refractory period.** Remember that regardless of the strength of the stimulus, the cardiac cell cannot be stimulated to depolarize during this time. The absolute refractory period corresponds with the beginning of the QRS complex to the peak of the T wave on the EKG strip.

The second part of the refractory period follows the absolute refractory period and is referred to as the **relative refractory period.** The relative refractory period is the period when repolarization is almost complete and the cardiac cell can be stimulated to contract prematurely if the stimulus is much stronger than normal. On the EKG strip, the relative refractory period corresponds with the downslope of the T wave. The relative refractory period is also known as the vulnerable period of the cardiac cells during repolarization.

absolute refractory period stage of cell activity in which the cardiac cell cannot spontaneously depolarize

relative refractory period period when repolarization is almost complete, and the cardiac cell can be stimulated to contract prematurely if the stimulus is much stronger than normal

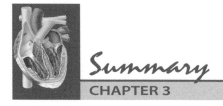

Summary
CHAPTER 3

The heart is a unique organ, unlike any other in the human body. You should now understand that it is composed of cardiac muscle made up of thousands of myocardial cell groups: the myocardial working cells and the specialized pacemaker cells of the electrical conduction system.

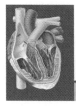

Key Points to Remember
CHAPTER 3

1.   The myocardial working cells are responsible for generating the physical contraction of the heart muscle.

2.   The specialized pacemaker cells are responsible for controlling the rate and rhythm of the heart by coordinating regular depolarization. These cells are found in the electrical conduction system of the heart.

3.   Automaticity is the ability of cardiac pacemaker cells to spontaneously generate their own electrical impulses without external (or nervous) stimulation.

4.   Excitability is the ability of cardiac cells to respond to an electrical stimulus. This characteristic is shared by all cardiac cells and is also referred to as irritability.

5.   Conductivity is the ability of cardiac cells to receive an electrical stimulus and to then transmit the stimulus to other cardiac cells.

6.   Contractility is also referred to as rhythmicity and is the ability of cardiac cells to shorten and cause cardiac muscle contraction in response to an electrical stimulus.

7.   Potassium performs a major function in cardiac depolarization and repolarization.

8.   Sodium plays a vital part in depolarization of the myocardium.

9.   Calcium renders an important function in myocardial depolarization and myocardial contraction.

10.   When the cardiac cell is at rest, the potassium ion concentration is greater inside the cell than outside and sodium ion concentration is greater outside the cell than inside.

11.   By means of an active mechanism of transport called the sodium-potassium exchange pump, potassium and sodium ions are moved in and out of the cell through the cell membrane.

12. Depolarization is an electrical occurrence resulting in myocardial contraction involving the movement of ions across cardiac cell membranes, resulting in positive polarity inside the cell membrane.

13. Repolarization is a process whereby the depolarized cell is polarized and positive charges are again on the outside and negative charges on the inside of the cell. It is a return to the resting state.

14. During the majority of the process of repolarization, the cardiac cell is unable to respond to a new electrical stimulus; the cardiac cell cannot spontaneously depolarize and is referred to as the absolute refractory period.

15. The relative refractory period is the period when repolarization is almost complete and the cardiac cell can be stimulated to contract prematurely if the stimulus is much stronger than normal.

16. On the EKG strip, the relative refractory period corresponds with the downslope of the T wave and is called the vulnerable period of repolarization.

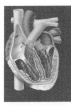

Review Questions
CHAPTER 3

1. The primary functions of the myocardial working cells include:
   a. automaticity.
   b. regeneration.
   c. contraction and relaxation.
   d. impulse propagation.

2. The ability of cardiac pacemaker cells to spontaneously generate their own electrical impulses without external (or nervous) stimulation is known as:
   a. automaticity.
   b. contractility.
   c. conductility.
   d. action potential.

3. Which one of the following characteristics is specific to the pacemaker cell sites of the electrical conduction system (the SA node, the AV junction, and the Purkinje network fibers)?
   a. automaticity
   b. contractility
   c. conductility
   d. excitability

4. The ability of cardiac cells to respond to an electrical stimulus is referred to as:
    a. automaticity.
    b. contractility.
    c. conductility.
    d. excitability.

5. Excitability is also referred to as:
    a. irritability.
    b. automaticity.
    c. contractility.
    d. conductility.

6. The ability of cardiac cells to receive an electrical stimulus and to then transmit the stimulus to other cardiac cells is known as:
    a. irritability.
    b. automaticity.
    c. contractility.
    d. conductivity.

7. Conductivity is a characteristic shared by all cardiac cells.
    a. True
    b. False

8. Cardiac muscle cell groups that function collectively as a unit are known as:
    a. syncytia.
    b. refractory.
    c. electrical.
    d. bundles.

9. Repolarization is a slower process than depolarization.
    a. True
    b. False

10. The period during which repolarization is almost complete and the cardiac cell can be stimulated to contract prematurely if the stimulus is stronger than normal is known as the:
    a. relative refractory period.
    b. absolute refractory period.
    c. action potential phase.
    d. active depolarization.

11. The relative refractory period is also known as the ___ period.

a. action

b. vulnerable

c. potential

d. absolute

12. A decrease in sodium blood levels is called:

a. hypernatremia.

b. hyponatremia.

c. hyperkalemia.

d. hypocalcemia.

13. A increase in calcium blood level is called:

a. hypercalcemia

b. hypocalcemia

c. hyponatremia

d. hyperkalemia

14. The resting state of a cardiac cell, wherein the inside of the cell is electrically negative relative to the outside of the cell, is called:

a. active state.

b. polarized state.

c. depolarization.

d. repolarization.

15. The point at which a stimulus will produce a cell response is called the:

a. threshold.

b. J point.

c. action potential.

d. refractory period.

The Electrical Conduction System

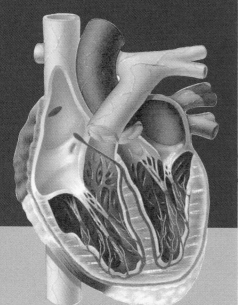

objectives

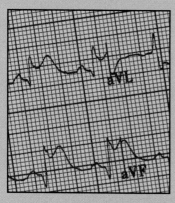

Upon completion of this chapter, the student will be able to:

➤ Identify the location of the following

   a. SA node

   b. Internodal pathways

   c. AV node

   d. Bundle of His

   e. AV junction

   f. Bundle branches

   g. Purkinje's network

➤ Describe the function of the following

   a. SA node

   b. Internodal pathways

   c. AV node

   d. Bundle of His

   e. AV junction

   f. Bundle branches

   g. Purkinje's network

➤ Relate the normal path of an impulse traveling through the electrical conduction system

INTRODUCTION

The heart's pacing (or conducting) system is responsible for the electrical activity that controls each normal heartbeat (Figure 4–1). This unique system consists of specialized cells and fibers that are collectively known as *nodes* and *bundles*. These nodes and bundles are relatively small and are located primarily beneath the endocardium (the innermost lining of the chambers of the heart). Specialized parts of this system are capable of initiating electrical activity automatically and can act as pacemakers for the heart.

A thorough understanding of the electrical conduction system of the heart is an essential component of learning and understanding an EKG strip. It is important to note that the 3-lead EKG strip is representative of *only* the electrical activity of the heart, but you must also understand that the clinician cannot determine the mechanical activity of the patient's heart by merely looking at a 3-lead EKG strip. However, by incorporating the basic knowledge of 12-lead EKG interpretation, you will gain more knowledge about the changes occurring in the myocardium when a patient is experiencing a myocardial infarction, specifically regarding the area of myocardial tissue involvement, as well as which coronary artery is most likely involved.

In order to begin to determine that an EKG strip is abnormal, you must first understand the normal parameters for the graphic representation of the electrical activity of the heart. It is to that end that this chapter is presented. In this chapter, you will recall the locations of the pacemakers and conducting fibers, as well as how they function during a normal heart beat.

Table 4–1 gives an overview of the electrical conduction system of the heart. Also refer to Figure 4–2.

sinoatrial (SA) node commonly referred to as the primary pacemaker of the heart because it normally depolarizes more rapidly than any other part of the conduction system

SA NODE

The **sinoatrial (SA) node** is located in the upper posterior portion of the right atrial wall of the heart, near the opening of the superior vena cava. The node is made up of a clus-

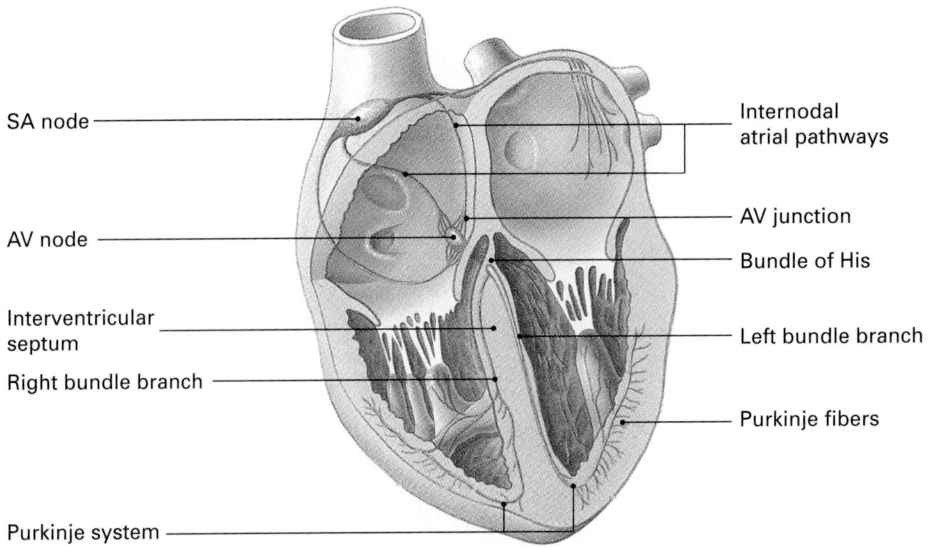

Figure 4–1. The cardiac conduction system

Table 4–1

Review of the electrical conduction system of the heart

SA Node	Internodal Pathways	AV Junction (AV Node and Bundle)	Bundle Branches	Purkinje's Network
Firing rate 60–100 BPM	Transfer impulse from the SA node throughout the atria to the AV junction	Slows impulse; intrinsic firing rate of 40–60 BPM	Two main branches (left and right) transmit impulse to ventricles	Spreads impulse throughout the ventricles; intrinsic firing rate of 20–40 BPM

ter of hundreds of cells that comprise a knot of modified heart muscle that is capable of generating impulses that travel throughout the muscle fibers of both atria, resulting in depolarization. The SA node primarily receives its blood supply from the SA artery.

The SA node is commonly referred to as the primary pacemaker of the heart because it normally depolarizes more rapidly than any other part of the conduction system. The normal range or firing rate of the heart's primary pacemaker—the SA node—is 60 to 100 beats per minute (BPM).

If, for any number of reasons, the dominant pacemaker fails to fire within the normal range, another group of specialized tissues, such as the atrioventricular tissue or the Purkinje network of fibers, will assume the duties of the pacemaker. These "back-up" pacemakers are arranged in a waterfall fashion. Depolarization and resultant myocardial contraction occurs as the impulse leaves the SA node and travels further down the path of the electrical conduction system.

INTERNODAL PATHWAYS

Three **internodal tracts** or pathways receive the electrical impulse as it exits the SA node. These tracts distribute the electrical impulse throughout the atria and transmit the impulse from the SA node to the AV node. The internodal tracts consist of anterior, middle, and posterior divisions. A group of interatrial fibers contained in the left atrium are referred to as **Bachmann's Bundle.** Bachmann's Bundle is a subdivision of the anterior internodal tract. This specialized group of cardiac fibers conducts electrical activity from the SA node to the left atrium.

AV NODE

The **atrioventricular (AV) node** is located on the floor of the right atrium just above the tricuspid valve. At the level of the AV node the electrical activity is delayed approximately 0.05 second. This delay allows for atrial contraction and a more complete filling of the ventricles. The AV node includes three regions: the AV junctional tissue between the atria and node, the nodal area, and the AV junctional tissue between the node and the bundle of His. In the normal heart, the AV node is the only pathway for conduction of atrial electrical impulses to the ventricles.

internodal tracts distribute the electrical impulse throughout the atria and transmit the impulse from the SA node to the AV node

Bachmann's Bundle subdivision of the anterior internodel tract; conducts electrical activity from the SA node to the left atrium

atrioventricular (AV) node located on the floor of the right atrium near the opening of the coronary sinus and just above the tricuspid valve; at the level of the AV node, the electrical activity is delayed approximately 0.05 second

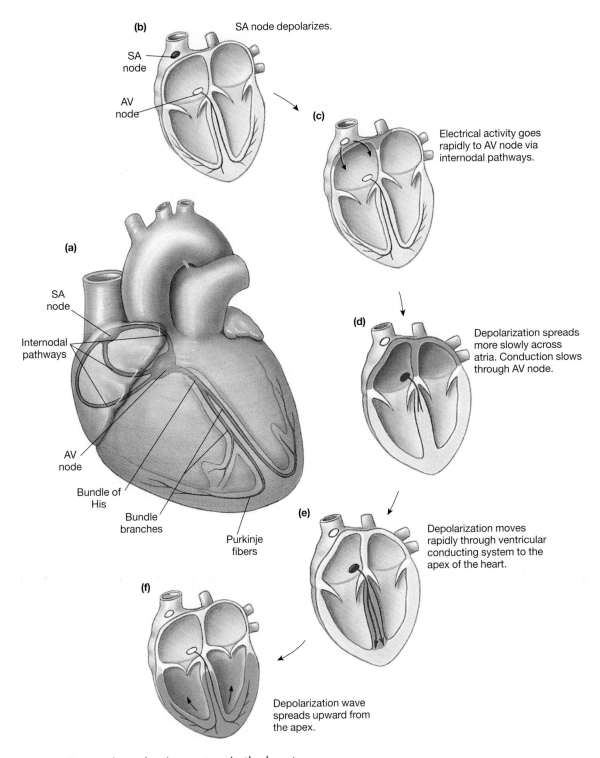

(b) SA node depolarizes.

SA node

AV node

(c) Electrical activity goes rapidly to AV node via internodal pathways.

(a)

SA node

Internodal pathways

AV node

Bundle of His

Bundle branches

Purkinje fibers

(d) Depolarization spreads more slowly across atria. Conduction slows through AV node.

(e) Depolarization moves rapidly through ventricular conducting system to the apex of the heart.

(f) Depolarization wave spreads upward from the apex.

Figure 4–2.   Electrical conduction system in the heart

AV JUNCTION

The region where the internodal pathways leading from the SA node join the bundle of His is called the **AV junction.** Similar to the SA node, the AV junctional tissue contains fibers that can depolarize spontaneously, forming an electrical impulse that can spread to the heart chambers. Therefore, if the SA node fails or slows below its normal range, the AV junctional tissues can initiate electrical activity and thus assume the role of a secondary pacemaker.

BUNDLE OF HIS

The conduction pathway that leads out of the AV node was described by a German physician, Wilhelm His, in 1893 and has subsequently been referred to as the **bundle of His.** The bundle of His is approximately 15 millimeters long and lies at the top of the interventricular septum. The interventricular septum is the wall between the right and left ventricles.

The bundle of His is also traditionally referred to as the *common bundle.* This bundle of specialized cells contains pacemaker cells that have the ability to self-initiate electrical activity at an intrinsic firing rate of 40 to 60 beats per minute.

BUNDLE BRANCHES

The bundle of His divides into two main branches at the top of the interventricular septum. These **bundle branches** are the right bundle branch and the left bundle branch. The primary function of the bundle branches is to conduct electrical activity from the bundle of His down to the Purkinje network. A long, thin structure lying beneath the endocardium, the right bundle branch runs down the right side of the interventricular septum and terminates at the papillary muscles in the right ventricle. This bundle branch functions to carry electrical impulses to the right ventricle. Shorter than the right bundle branch, the left bundle branch divides into pathways that spread from the left side of the interventricular septum and throughout the left ventricle. The two main divisions of the left bundle branch are called *fascicles.* Whereas the anterior fascicle carries electrical impulses to the anterior wall of the left ventricle, the posterior fascicle spreads the impulses to the posterior ventricular wall. The bundle branches continue to divide until they finally terminate in the Purkinje fibers.

PURKINJE'S NETWORK

Bundle branches lead to a network of small conduction fibers that spread throughout the ventricles. These fibers were first described in 1787 by Johannes E. Purkinje, a Czechoslovakian physiologist. This network of fibers carries electrical impulses directly to ventricular muscle cells. The fibers that connect with Purkinje's fibers start in the atrioventricular node in the right atrium of the heart.

Purkinje's network can only be identified with the aid of a microscope but are larger in diameter than ordinary cardiac muscle fibers. Ventricular contraction is facilitated by the rapid spread of the electrical impulse through the left and right bundle branches and Purkinje fibers into the ventricular muscle. Purkinje's network fibers possess the intrinsic ability to serve as a pacemaker. The firing rate of the Purkinje pacemaker fibers is normally within the range of 20 to 40 beats per minute.

AV junction region where the AV node joins the bundle of His

bundle of His conduction pathway that leads out of the AV node. Also called the common bundle

bundle branches two main branches, the right bundle branch and the left bundle branch, conduct electrical activity from the bundle of His down to the Purkinje network

Purkinje's network network of fibers that carries electrical impulses directly to ventricular muscle cells

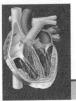

Summary
CHAPTER 4

A thorough understanding of the heart's normal electrical conduction system is vital to your understanding of the various heart rhythms. In order to understand the causes of dysrhythmias, it is imperative that you have a working knowledge of the underlying concepts of normal sinus rhythm. As you now understand, the electrical impulse arises in the SA node and terminates in the Purkinje network.

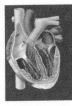

Key Points to Remember
CHAPTER 4

1. The SA (or sinoatrial) node is located in the upper posterior portion of the right atrial wall of the heart and serves as the primary pacemaker of the heart.

2. The SA node generates impulses that travel throughout the muscle fibers of both atria, resulting in depolarization.

3. Three internodal tracts or pathways receive the electrical impulse as it exits the SA node.

4. The internodal pathways distribute the electrical impulse throughout the atria and transmit the impulse from the SA node to the AV node.

5. The AV (or atrioventricular) node is located on the floor of the right atrium just above the tricuspid valve.

6. The AV junction is where the internodal pathways leading from the SA node join the bundle of His.

7. The bundle of His leads out of the AV node.

8. The bundle of His may be referred to as the common bundle.

9. The bundle of His divides into two main branches at the top of the interventricular septum. Those branches are the right bundle branch and the left bundle branch.

10. The primary function of the bundle branches is to conduct electrical activity from the bundle of His down to the Purkinje network.

11. Purkinje fibers make up a network of small conduction fibers that spread throughout the ventricles.

12. The Purkinje fibers carry electrical impulses directly to ventricular muscle cells.

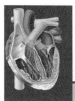

Review Questions

CHAPTER 4

1. The sinoatrial node is located in the:
    a. right atrium.
    b. right ventricle.
    c. Purkinje fiber tract.
    d. atrioventricular septum.

2. The AV node is located in the:
    a. right atrium.
    b. left ventricle.
    c. Purkinje fiber tract.
    d. atrioventricular septum

3. The intrinsic firing rate of the AV junction is ___ beats per minute.
    a. 15–25
    b. 25–35
    c. 35–45
    d. 40–60

4. The intrinsic rate of the SA node in the adult is ___ beats per minute.
    a. 20–60
    b. 40–80
    c. 60–100
    d. 80–100

5. The electrocardiogram is used to:
    a. determine pulse rate.
    b. detect valvular dysfunction.
    c. evaluate electrical activity in the heart.
    d. determine whether the heart is beating.

6. The normal conduction pattern of the heart follows:

    1. SA node
    2. Purkinje fibers
    3. bundle of His
    4. AV node
    5. bundle branches
    6. internodal pathways

    a. 1, 2, 3, 5, 6, 4
    b. 1, 6, 4, 3, 5, 2
    c. 1, 6, 4, 2, 3, 5
    d. 6, 1, 5, 4, 6, 2

7. The primary pacemaker of the heart is the:
   a. AV node.
   b. SA node.
   c. Purkinje.
   d. SV node.

8. The bundle of His is also traditionally referred to as the:
   a. lesser bundle.
   b. chordae tendinea.
   c. common bundle.
   d. coronary sinus.

9. The fibers of the Purkinje network can only be identified with the aid of a microscope.
   a. True
   b. False

10. The region where the internodal pathways leading from the SA node joins the bundle of His is called the:
    a. Bachmann's bundle.
    b. AV junction.
    c. SA junction.
    d. common bundle.

11. The intrinsic rate of the Purkinje fibers is ___ beats per minute.
    a. 50–60
    b. 60–70
    c. 10–20
    d. 20–40

12. A group of interatrial fibers contained in the left atrium is referred to as:
    a. Bachmann's bundle.
    b. AV junction.
    c. SA junction.
    d. common bundle.

13. The interventricular septum is the wall between the:
    a. right and left atrium.
    b. right and left ventricle.
    c. inferior and superior chambers.
    d. inferior and superior vena cavae.

14. Purkinje's network fibers are smaller in diameter than ordinary cardiac muscle fibers.

    a. True

    b. False

15. The SA node receives its blood supply primarily from the:

    a. coronary artery.

    b. great cardiac vein.

    c. SA artery.

    d. aorta.

chapter **5**

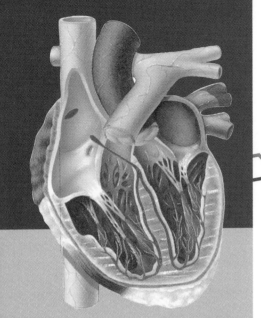

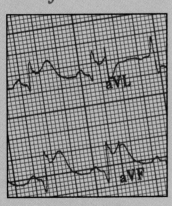

The Electrocardiogram

objectives

Upon completion of this chapter, the student will be able to:

➤ Describe the types of EKG leads

➤ Identify and explain the grids and markings on a representative strip of EKG graph paper

➤ Discuss the electrical basis of the electrocardiogram

➤ Describe the relationship of the following EKG waveforms to the electrical events in the heart

   a. P wave

   b. PR interval

   c. QRS complex

   d. J point

   e. ST segment

   f. T wave

INTRODUCTION

The medical use of the electrocardiogram dates back less than a century ago to around the year 1900. Modern technology has brought us very far in the past 100 years to the point where almost every emergency department and pre-hospital advanced life support (ALS) unit has equipment suitable for obtaining either a 3-lead or a 12-lead EKG on a patient whenever and wherever indicated. The most significant lesson that you will learn from this textbook centers not on the EKG tracing, but on the clinical picture of your patient. You must continually ask yourself, "How is this rhythm clinically significant to the patient?" Regardless of the pattern observed on the oscilloscope or EKG static strip, your patient's condition is and must be your primary concern. Keep this important fact in mind, and your patient's best interest will always be served.

ELECTRICAL BASIS OF THE EKG

Chapter 4 explored the components and functions of the heart's electrical conduction system. Based on that knowledge, you should understand that the heart generates electrical activity in the body; thus, the body can be thought of as a major conductor of electrical activity. This electrical activity can be sensed by electrodes placed on the skin surface and can be recorded in the form of an **electrocardiogram (EKG).** Cardiac monitors depict the heart's electrical impulses as patterns of waves on the monitor screen or oscilloscope. Because electrical impulses present on the skin surface are very low voltage, the impulses must be amplified by the EKG machine. The printed record of the electrical activity of the heart is called a **rhythm strip** or an EKG strip. (See Figures 5–1 and 5–2.)

**electrocardio-
gram (EKG)**
graphic
representation of the
electrical activity of
the heart

rhythm strip
printed record of the
electrical activity of
the heart. Also called
EKG strip

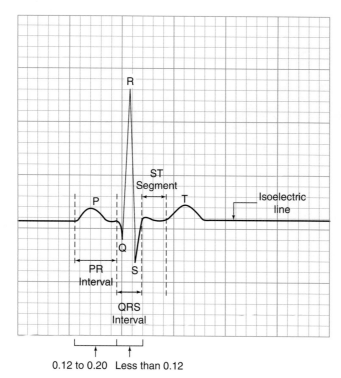

Figure 5–1.   The EKG

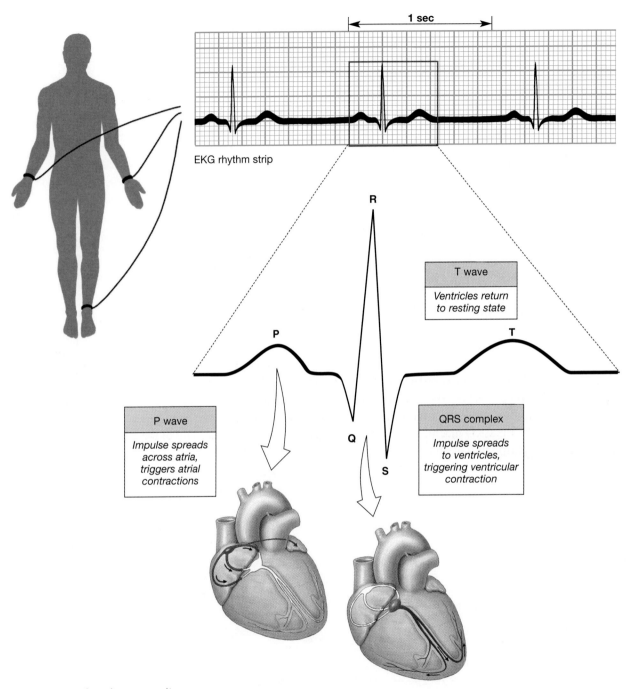

Figure 5–2. The electrocardiogram

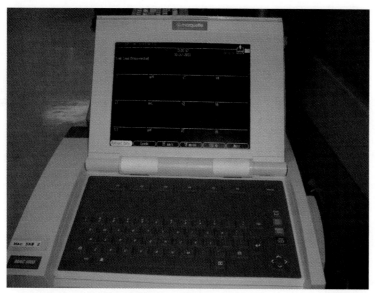

Figure 5–3. In-hospital 12-lead EKG machine

EKG LEADS

As discussed earlier, the cardiac monitor receives electrical impulses from the patient's heart through electrodes placed on particular areas of the body. An **electrode** is an adhesive pad that contains conductive gel and is designed to be attached to the patient's skin. The electrodes are then connected to the monitor or EKG machine by wires called **leads.** These wires are generally color-coded in order to be user-friendly.

In EKG monitoring, the term *lead* is sometimes used in two different contexts. Another meaning of this term is referenced when speaking of a pair of electrodes, such as chest Lead I, II, MCL, and so on. In the latter usage, the term is generally capitalized.

In order for the monitor or EKG machine to receive a clear picture of the electrical impulses generated by the heart's electrical conduction system, there must be a positive, a negative, and a ground lead. You should remember that the electrical current of the heart flows from right to left. The ground lead serves to minimize outside electrical interference.

The exact portion of the heart being visualized depends, in large part, on the placement of electrodes. It may be helpful to envision the heart as an object placed on a pedestal around which a person can move, while taking photographs from all angles (different views). This analogy would describe the 12-lead EKG, whereas only one snapshot or view of the heart would represent the 3-lead EKG.

The 12-lead EKG is commonly used in hospitals and clinics (Figure 5–3), whereas the 3-lead EKG is typically used in the field. In some areas of the country, 12-lead EKGs are being utilized in the prehospital setting regularly to aid in screening patients who are potential candidates for fibrinolytic therapy (Figure 5–4). It is important to note that the 3-lead EKG is sufficient for detecting life-threatening dysrhythmias.

electrode
adhesive pad that contains conductive gel and is designed to be attached to the patient's skin

leads electrodes connected to the monitor or EKG machine by wires; also, may refer to a pair of electrodes

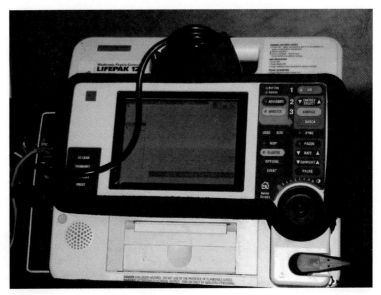

Figure 5–4. Prehospital 12-lead EKG machine

Table 5–1

Bipolar lead placement		
Lead	**Positive Electrode**	**Negative Electrode**
I	Left arm	Right arm
II	Left leg	Right arm
III	Left leg	Left arm

bipolar leads
leads that have one positive electrode and one negative electrode

Lead II and the modified chest lead (MCL) are the most common leads used for cardiac monitoring because of their ability to visualize P waves. Leads I, II, and III are known as **bipolar leads,** which means that they each have one positive electrode and one negative electrode. Bipolar leads are sometimes referred to as *limb leads.* Table 5–1 represents the placement of electrodes of the three bipolar leads on certain areas of the body.

An imaginary inverted triangle is formed around the heart by proper placement of the bipolar leads. This triangle is referred to as *Einthoven's triangle* (Figure 5–5). The top of the triangle is formed by Lead I, the right side of the triangle is formed by Lead II, and the left side of the triangle is formed by Lead III. Each lead represents a different look or view of the heart.

You may recall from discussions of topographic anatomy in your basic anatomy courses that the term *plane* refers to an imaginary surface. You should be aware that the 12-lead EKG views the heart in two distinct planes. These planes include the horizontal and frontal planes (Figure 5–6). The vector (V) leads look at the horizontal plane and the limb leads look at the frontal plane.

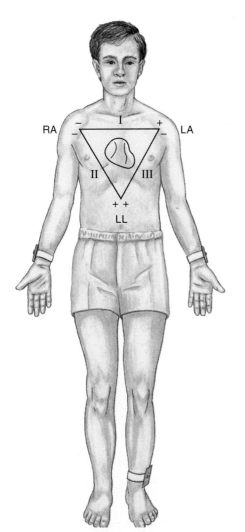
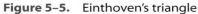

Figure 5–5.   Einthoven's triangle

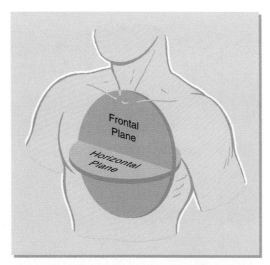

Figure 5–6.   Frontal and horizontal planes

Standard limb leads

The **standard limb leads,** Leads I, II, and III, comprise the first leads of a 12-lead EKG. At this point, it is important to emphasize the significance of the specific placement of leads (Figure 5–7). The left arm lead should be placed at a location between the left shoulder and wrist, away from bony prominences, as bone is a poor conductor of electricity. Also, the right lead should be placed between the right shoulder and wrist. The left leg lead should be placed between the left hip and ankle, also away from bony prominences. The right leg lead is placed between the right hip and ankle and sometimes utilized as an additional ground lead.

If you feel obligated or if local protocol dictates that you place the limb leads on the trunk, rather than the extremities, you should make note of this action on the 12-lead strip, as further evaluation may be affected by this decision. In other words, if placement of the limb leads deviates from the normal position (extremities), then this positioning may effect the direction of the axis. (Axis deviation will be discussed in detail in Chapter 14.)

standard limb leads Leads I, II, and III; current flows from the limbs through the heart

Limb Lead Placement

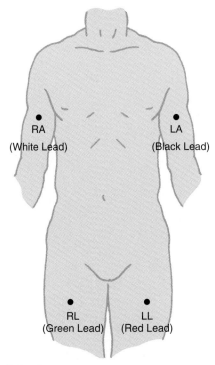

Figure 5–7.   Standard limb leads

Table 5–2

Augmented leads	
Augmented Leads	**Position of Flow**
aVR—augmented voltage, right arm	From the heart to the right arm
aVL—augmented voltage, left arm	From the heart to the left arm
aVF—augmented voltage, left foot	From the heart to the left foot

Augmented limb leads

augmented limb leads Leads aVR, aVL, and aVF; current flows from the heart outward to the extremities. Also called unipolar leads

In order to simplify the explanation of the **augmented limb leads,** we suggest that you begin by viewing the heart as the focal point of this discussion. In the first three leads (standard), the negative-to-positive current flows from the limbs through the heart. However, in the augmented leads, the current flows from the heart outward to the extremities; hence the name *augmented* or *extended from the heart* (Table 5–2). Augmented leads are also referred to as *unipolar* (having only one true pole) leads. It may also be valuable for you to understand that the EKG machine must boost (or raise) amplification due to the position of these leads.

Chest leads

chest leads Leads V₁ through V₆; unipolar leads. Also called precordial or vector leads

The **chest leads** are also unipolar and comprise the last six leads on the 12-lead EKG (Figure 5–8). These leads look at the heart via the horizontal (or transverse) plane. These

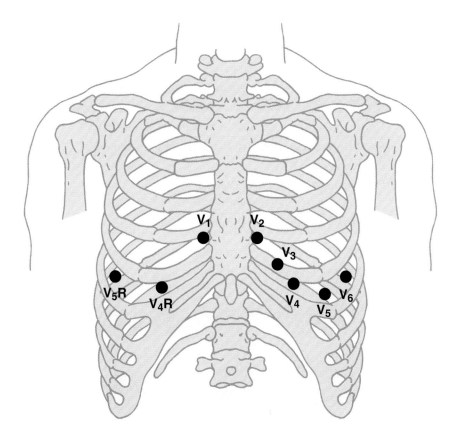

V₁—4th intercostal space, right of the sternum
V₂—4th intercostal space, left of the sternum
V₃—5th intercostal space, halfway between V₂ and V₄
V₄—5th intercostal space, left midclavicular line
V₅—5th intercostal space, left anterior axillary line
V₆—5th intercostal space, left midaxillary line
V₄R—5th intercostal space, right midclavicular line
V₅R—5th intercostal space, right anterior axillary line

Figure 5–8.   Chest lead placement

leads are also called *precordial* or *vector (V) leads.* Proper placement of the V leads is critically important to the correct interpretation of the 12-lead EKG strip (Table 5–3). Specific guidelines should be established and followed each time a 12-lead EKG is obtained—merely guessing about placement is not allowed!

You should become proficient in correct lead placement in order to assure that 12-lead EKG interpretation is consistent with each patient. It is important that the patient's skin be properly prepared before attaching the leads. You should complete the following steps:

1. Clean the area with an alcohol swab and allow the area to dry.
2. Shave excess hair as indicated.
3. If the patient is diaphoretic, attempt to dry the area or use spray antiperspirant to the area to induce drying.
4. Proper placement, including measuring each lead, is imperative. Improper lead placement can affect R wave progression through the V leads. (R wave progression is discussed later in this chapter.)
5. Make sure that the conductive gel is pliable in order to ensure proper conduction.

Table 5–3

Lead	Placement
V_1	Fourth intercostal space just to the right of the sternum
V_2	Fourth intercostal space just to the left of the sternum
V_3	Between V_2 and V_4
V_4	Fifth intercostal space midclavicular line
V_5	Anterior axillary line, level with V_4
V_6	Midaxillary line, level with V_4 and V_5

Chest lead placement

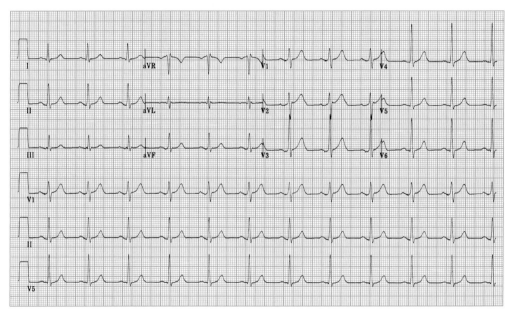

Figure 5–9.   12-lead EKG

Note that although we refer to the 12-lead EKG, only 10 cardiac monitor leads are required (4 limb leads and 6 chest leads) to obtain the tracing. Only by completing steps 1–5 in an efficient and timely manner can you ensure that each 12-lead EKG strip is done consistently.

EKG GRAPH PAPER

Electrocardiographic paper is arranged as a series of horizontal and vertical lines printed on graph paper. It provides a printed record of cardiac electrical activity (Figure 5–9). This paper is standardized to allow for consistency in EKG rhythm strip analysis. EKG paper leaves the machine at a constant speed of 25 millimeters per second (mm/sec) for a standard 12-lead EKG. Speed may be varied on some machines to assist with interpretation.

Both time and amplitude (or voltage) are measured on graph paper. Time is measured on the horizontal line; amplitude, or voltage, is measured on the vertical line. The vertical axis reflects millivolts (two large squares = 1 mV and 1 mV = 10 mm). The millivolt (mV) is the standard calibration for 12-lead EKGs. EKG graph paper is divided into small squares, each of which is 1 millimeter (mm) in height and width and represents a time interval of 0.04 second.

Darker lines further divide the paper every fifth square, both vertically and horizontally. Each of these large squares measures 5 millimeters in height and 5 millimeters in width and represents a time interval of 0.20 second. There are five small squares in each large square; therefore, 5 (small squares) × 0.04 second = 0.20 second. The squares on the EKG paper represent the measurement of the length of time required for the electrical impulse to traverse a specific part of the heart (Figure 5–10). Proper interpretation

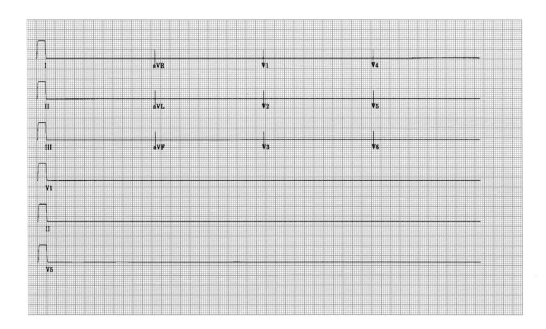

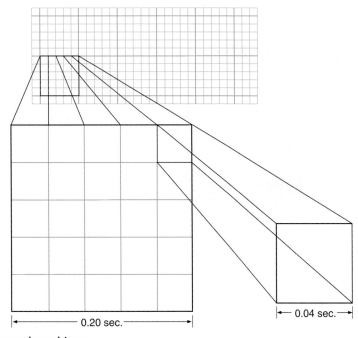

Figure 5–10.   EKG paper and markings

of EKG rhythms is dependent, in part, on understanding the time increments as represented on EKG paper.

EKG WAVEFORMS

EKG waveform wave recorded on an EKG strip; refers to movement away from the baseline or isoelectric line and is represented as a positive deflection (above the isoelectric line) or as a negative deflection (below the isoelectric line)

baseline straight line seen on an EKG strip; represents the beginning and end point of all waves. Also called isoelectric line

P wave represents depolarization of the left and right atria

PR interval represents the time interval needed for the impulse to travel from the SA node through the internodal pathways in the atria and downward to the ventricles. Sometimes referred to as PRI

An **EKG waveform,** or wave, recorded on an EKG strip refers to movement away from the **baseline,** or isoelectric line, and is represented as a positive deflection (above the isoelectric line) or as a negative deflection (below the isoelectric line). The baseline is the straight line seen on an EKG strip and represents the beginning and ending point of all waves.

As the electrical impulse leaves the SA node, waveforms are produced on the graph paper. One complete cardiac cycle is represented on graph paper by five major waves: the P, Q, R, and S waves (normally referred to as the *QRS complex*) and the T wave.

P wave

As discussed in Chapter 4, the SA node fires first during a normal cardiac cycle. This firing event sends the electrical impulse outward to stimulate both atria and manifests as the **P wave** (Figure 5–11). When observed on a Lead II EKG strip, the P wave is a smooth, rounded upward deflection. The P wave represents depolarization of both the left and right atria and is approximately 0.10 second in length.

PR interval

Sometimes abbreviated as the PRI, the **PR interval** represents the time interval necessary for the impulse to travel from the SA node through the internodal pathways in the

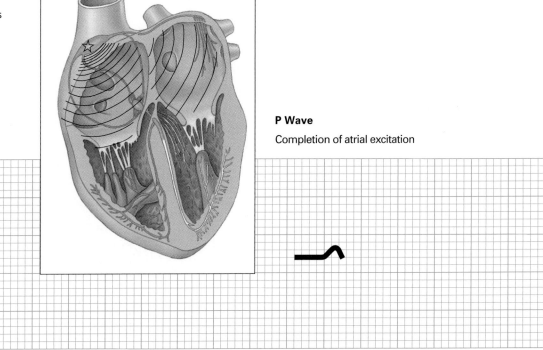

P Wave

Completion of atrial excitation

Figure 5–11. The P wave

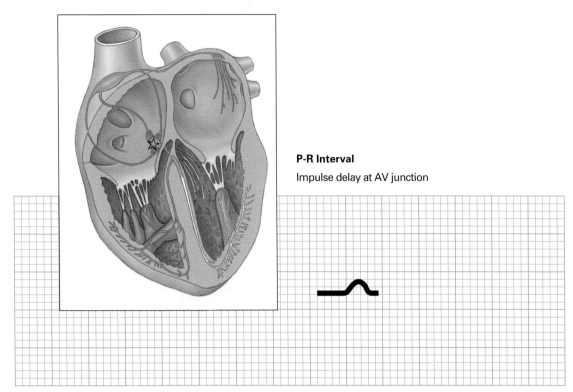

P-R Interval

Impulse delay at AV junction

Figure 5–12. The PR interval

atria and downward to the ventricles. In simpler terms, the PRI is said to be representative of the distance from the beginning of the P wave to the beginning of the QRS complex. The normal PR interval is measured as three to five small squares of the EKG graph paper and is 0.12 to 0.20 second in length (Figure 5–12).

QRS complex

The **QRS complex** (Figure 5–13) consists of the Q, R, and S waves and represents the conduction of the electrical impulse from the bundle of His throughout the ventricular muscle, or ventricular depolarization. The Q wave is seen as the first downward deflection following the PRI. The R wave is the first upward deflection of the QRS complex and is normally the largest deflection seen in chest Leads I and II. Immediately following the R wave, there is a downward deflection called the *S wave.*

The QRS complex is measured from the beginning of the Q wave to the point where the S wave meets the baseline. Normally, the QRS complex measures less than 0.12 second or less than three small squares on the EKG graph paper. It should be noted that the shape of the QRS complex will vary from individual to individual and all three waves are not always present.

J point

The point at which the QRS complex meets the ST segment is known as the **J point** (Figure 5–14) and is an important landmark in 12-lead EKG interpretation. Generally, an elevation or depression of 1 millimeter or more (above or below the isoelectric line) may be indicative of myocardial injury or ischemia. Consideration of ST segment elevation or depression begins with the analysis of the J point.

QRS complex consists of the Q, R, and S waves and represents the conduction of the electrical impulse from the bundle of His throughout the ventricular muscle, or ventricular depolarization

J point the point on the EKG strip where the QRS complex meets the ST segment

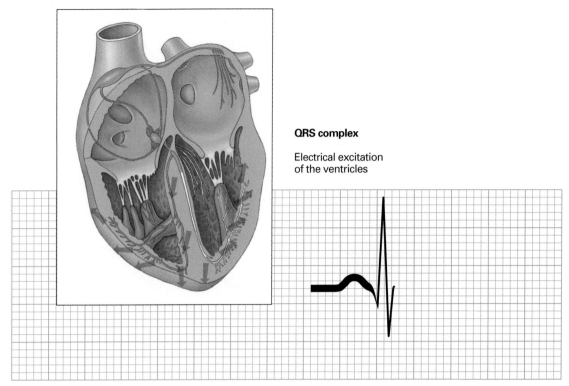

QRS complex

Electrical excitation
of the ventricles

Figure 5–13. The QRS complex

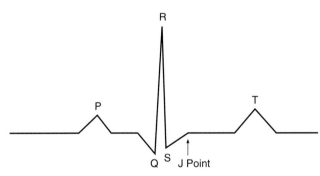

Figure 5–14. The J point

ST segment

ST segment time interval during which the ventricles are depolarized and ventricular depolarization begins

The time interval during which the ventricles are depolarized and ventricular repolarization begins is called the **ST segment.** Normally, the ST segment is isoelectric, or consistent with the baseline. In certain cardiac disease processes, the ST segment may be elevated or depressed due to ischemia and/or infarction. Elevation of the ST segment is one of the major EKG changes noted in an acute myocardial infarction.

T wave

T wave represents ventricular repolarization; follows the ST segment

Following the ST segment is the **T wave** (Figure 5–15), which represents ventricular repolarization. The T wave is normally seen as a slightly asymmetrical, slightly rounded, positive deflection. Recall now that ventricular repolarization is an electrical event with

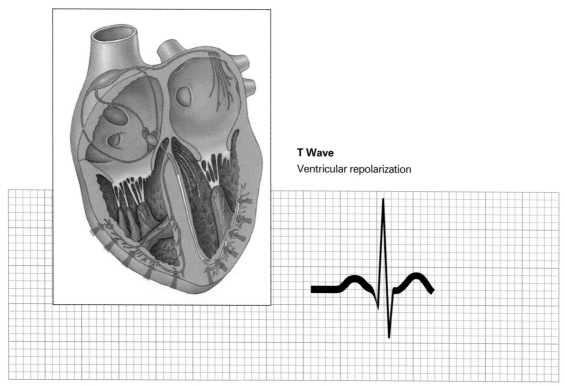

T Wave
Ventricular repolarization

Figure 5–15. The T wave

Table 5–4

Summary of EKG waveforms and correlating cardiac events

P wave represents	Atrial depolarization
QRS complex represents	Ventricular depolarization; atrial repolarization (hidden in QRS complex)
T wave represents	Ventricular repolarization

no associated activity of the ventricular musculature. The T wave is often referred to as the *resting phase* of the cardiac cycle.

Recall also that the refractory periods, both absolute and relative, are in place during the EKG representation of the T wave, and thus the heart may be vulnerable to strong impulses that may lead to ventricular dysrhythmias. The T wave may be either elevated or depressed in the presence of current or previous cardiac ischemia. Normally, one complete cardiac cycle is represented by the P-QRS-T pattern (Table 5–4).

STANDARD 12-LEAD EKG WAVEFORMS

The understanding of normal 12-lead EKG waveform configurations is imperative in the correct interpretation of the 12-lead EKG (Figure 5–16). Specifically, you should remember that in limb Leads I, II, and III, all waveforms should be positively deflected (upright). In the augmented leads (aVR, aVL, aVF) the deflection of waveforms varies. In the aVR lead, all waveforms are negatively deflected; however, in aVL, the P wave

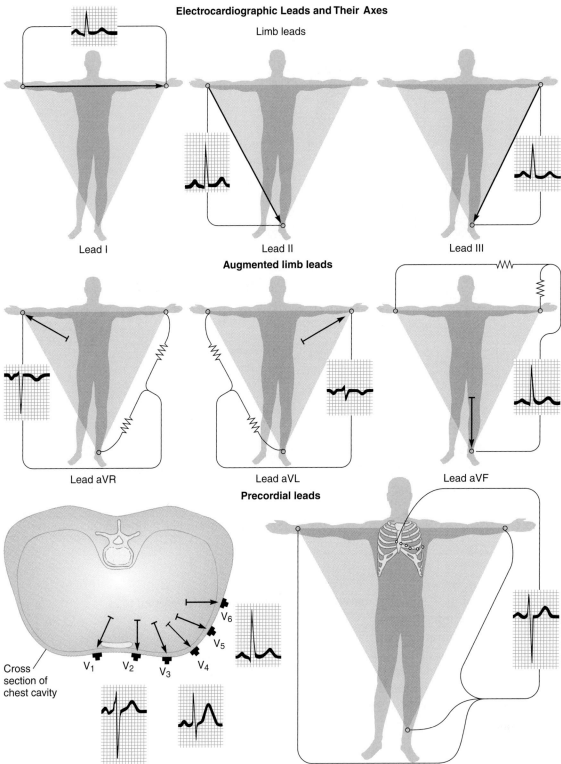

Electrocardiographic Leads and Their Axes

Limb leads

Lead I

Lead II

Lead III

Augmented limb leads

Lead aVR

Lead aVL

Lead aVF

Precordial leads

Cross section of chest cavity

V₁ V₂ V₃ V₄ V₅ V₆

When current flows toward arrowheads (axes), upward deflection occurs in EKG
When current flows away from arrowheads (axes), downward deflection occurs in EKG
When current flows perpendicular to arrows (axes), no deflection occurs

Figure 5–16.   12-lead EKG leads and waveforms

Table 5–5

Normal 12-lead EKG waveforms	
Lead I	P, Q, R, S, T waveforms are positively deflected (upright)
Lead II	P, Q, R, S, T waveforms are positively deflected (upright)
Lead III	P, Q, R, S, T waveforms are positively deflected (upright)
aVR	P, Q, R, S, T waveforms are negatively deflected
aVL	P and T waves are negative; QRS waveform is biphasic
aVF	P, Q, R, S, T waveforms are positively deflected (upright)
V_1	P and T waves are positively deflected; QRS initiates as negative deflection
V_2	P and T waves are positively deflected; QRS primarily negative deflection with minimal positive deflection
V_3	P and T waves are positively deflected; QRS primarily biphasic with negative deflection being predominant
V_4	P and T waves are positively deflected; QRS primarily biphasic with positive deflection being predominant
V_5	P and T waves are positively deflected; QRS primarily positive with slight negative deflection
V_6	P and T waves are positively deflected; QRS positively deflected

and T wave are negatively deflected but the QRS is biphasic (waveforms are equally positive and negative in deflection). In aVF, all waveforms are positively deflected. In the precordial or chest leads, all P and T waves are positively deflected; however, the QRS waveform initiates as a negative deflection and progresses until it becomes absolutely positive in Lead V_6.

By studying Table 5–5, you will note that the R wave of the QRS complex initially appears as a negative deflection in V_1 and progresses through the V leads to become a totally positive deflection in V_6. This concept is known as normal *R wave progression*.

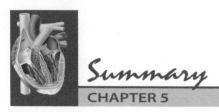

Summary

CHAPTER 5

It is imperative that you remember to always—at ALL times—*observe and treat the patient based on clinical presentation, regardless of the rhythm being observed on the oscilloscope.* Always remember to ask yourself, "How is this rhythm clinically significant to my patient?"

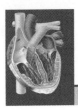

Key Points to Remember

CHAPTER 5

1. An electrode is an adhesive pad that contains conductive gel and is designed to be attached to the patient's skin.

2. Electrodes are connected to the monitor or EKG machine by wires called leads.

3. Leads I, II, and III are known as bipolar leads (standard limb leads), which means that these leads have one positive electrode and one negative electrode.

4. The left arm lead should be placed at a location between the left shoulder and wrist, away from bony prominences.

5. The right lead should be placed between the right shoulder and wrist.

6. The left leg lead should be placed between the left hip and ankle.

7. The right leg lead is placed between the right hip and ankle and is sometimes used as an additional ground lead.

8. In the augmented limb leads, the current flows from the heart outward to the extremities.

9. Augmented leads are referred to as unipolar (having only one true pole) leads and utilize the four limb leads.

10. The chest leads are unipolar and comprise the last six leads on the 12-lead EKG.

11. The chest leads look at the heart via the horizontal (or transverse) plane.

12. The chest leads are also called precordial or V (vector) leads. Proper placement of the V leads is critically important to the correct interpretation of the 12-lead EKG strip.

13. EKG paper is an arrangement of a series of horizontal and vertical lines printed on graph paper and provides a printed record of cardiac electrical activity.

14. EKG paper leaves the machine at a constant speed of 25 mm/sec for a standard 12-lead EKG.

15. Time is measured on the horizontal line of the EKG paper; amplitude, or voltage, is measured on the vertical line.

16. The vertical axis reflects millivolts (two large squares = 1 mV and 1 mV = 10 mm).

17. EKG paper is divided into small squares, each of which is 1 millimeter (mm) in height and width and represents a time interval of 0.04 sec.

18. Darker lines further divide the paper every fifth square, both vertically and horizontally.

19. The squares on the EKG paper represent the measurement of the length of time required for the electrical impulse to traverse a specific part of the heart.

20. A wave or waveform recorded on an EKG strip refers to movement away from the baseline or isoelectric line.

21. Waveforms are represented as a positive deflection (above the isoelectric line) or as a negative deflection (below the isoelectric line).

22. The P wave represents depolarization of both the left and right atria.

23. The PR interval represents the time interval necessary for the impulse to travel from the SA node, through the internodal pathways in the atria, and downward to the ventricles.

24. The QRS complex represents the conduction of the electrical impulse from the bundle of His throughout the ventricular muscle, or ventricular depolarization.

25. The J point is the point at which the QRS complex meets the ST segment.

26. The ST segment is the interval during which the ventricles are depolarized and ventricular repolarization begins.

27. The T wave represents ventricular repolarization.

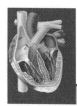

Review Questions
CHAPTER 5

1. Ventricular diastole refers to ventricular:
    a. contraction.
    b. relaxation.
    c. filling time.
    d. pressure ratio.

2. The single-lead electrocardiogram primarily is used to:
    a. determine cardiac output.
    b. detect valvular dysfunction.
    c. evaluate electrical activity in the heart.
    d. detect left-to-right conduction disorders.

3. The PR interval should normally be ___ second or smaller.
    a. 0.10
    b. 0.12
    c. 0.08
    d. 0.20

4. The QRS interval should normally be ___ second or smaller.
    a. 0.20
    b. 0.12
    c. 0.18
    d. 0.36

5. The QRS complex is produced when the:

   a. ventricles repolarize.

   b. ventricles depolarize.

   c. ventricles contract.

   d. both b and c.

6. The normal conduction pattern of the heart follows:

   1. SA node
   2. Purkinje fibers
   3. bundle of His
   4. AV node
   5. bundle branches
   6. internodal pathways

   a. 1, 5, 2, 4, 6, 3

   b. 1, 6, 4, 3, 5, 2

   c. 1, 4, 3, 6, 5, 2

   d. 1, 2, 3, 4, 5, 6

7. The T wave on the EKG strip represents:

   a. rest period.

   b. bundle of His.

   c. atrial contraction.

   d. ventricular contraction.

8. The point at which the QRS complex meets the ST segment is known as the:

   a. delta wave.

   b. end point.

   c. J point.

   d. vector.

9. When interpreting dysrhythmias, the health-care provider should remember that the most important key is the:

   a. PR interval.

   b. rate and rhythm.

   c. presence of dysrhythmias.

   d. patient's clinical appearance.

10. How many cardiac monitor pads are utilized when obtaining a 12-lead EKG?

    a. 10

    b. 12

    c. 3

    d. 6

11. The change of the QRS complex from a negative deflection to a positive deflection in the V leads is called:

   a. the J point.

   b. biphasic.

   c. waveform configuration.

   d. R wave progression.

12. In the aVR lead, the T waveforms are ___ deflected.

   a. positively

   b. biphasic

   c. rarely

   d. negatively

13. In the aVL lead, the T waveforms are ___ deflected.

   a. positively

   b. biphasic

   c. rarely

   d. negatively

14. In the aVF lead, the T waveforms are ___ deflected.

   a. positively

   b. biphasic

   c. rarely

   d. negatively

15. The augmented leads may be referred to as:

   a. unipolar.

   b. bipolar.

   c. multipolar.

   d. vector.

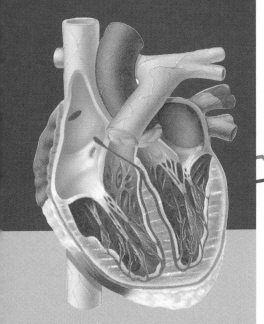

Interpretation of EKG Strips

objectives

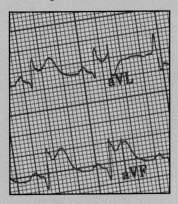

Upon completion of this chapter, the student will be able to:

➤ Recall the general rules to use when correctly identifying heart rhythms

➤ Describe a basic approach for interpretation of EKG strips

➤ Explain the five steps used in interpretation of EKG strips

➤ Explain how to calculate heart rate, given a 6–second strip

➤ Explain the 5 + 3 approach, including

　a. ST elevation

　b. ST depression

　c. Q wave

INTRODUCTION

This is a very significant chapter for you to master in order to fully understand EKG interpretation. The preceding chapters in this text are essential building blocks that lead up to this chapter. The upcoming chapters will focus on application of the rules mastered in this chapter. Therefore, this chapter is critical to your understanding of proper interpretation of an EKG rhythm strip.

For many years now, we have explained to students that the key to learning, interpreting and, most importantly, understanding dysrhythmias is a systematic approach that must be used each and every time a strip is analyzed. Frankly speaking, we do not really expect you to believe that every health-care professional who has been practicing the craft for years *always* applies this five-step systematic approach for every strip they see. However, you are using this book because you wish to learn how to effortlessly interpret dysrhythmias using both 3-lead and 12-lead strips. While you learn this skill, keep in mind that memorization will *not* suffice. You must learn *and* apply the systematic approach to EKG analysis. When you look at a strip, think about and apply the five steps and you should be successful in mastering the art of EKG analysis.

GENERAL RULES

Here are a few basic rules that will assist you in your quest to correctly identify heart rhythms:

➤ *First and most important, look at your patient!* What is the patient's clinical picture, and how is it significant to the rhythm noted on the monitor?
➤ Read EVERY strip from left to right, starting at the beginning of the strip.
➤ Apply the five-step systematic approach that you will learn in this chapter.
➤ Avoid shortcuts and assumptions. A quick glance at a strip will often lead to an incorrect interpretation.
➤ Ask and answer each question in the five-step approach in the order in which it is presented here. This is important for consistency.
➤ You must master the accepted parameters for each dysrhythmia (as described in this book's companion text, *Understanding EKGs: A Practical Approach*) and then apply those parameters to each of the five steps when analyzing the strip.

THE FIVE-STEP APPROACH

There are several appropriate formats for EKG interpretation. The format that we have chosen follows a logical sequence in that we discuss EKG interpretation based first on heart rate and rhythm, followed by analysis of graphic representations of activities as they occur in the electrical conduction system of the heart.

This five-step approach, in order of application, includes analysis of the following:

Step 1:   Heart rate
Step 2:   Heart rhythm
Step 3:   P wave
Step 4:   PR interval
Step 5:   QRS complex

EKG interpretation is more easily accomplished if each step is examined using this approach with each strip. Remember, quick glances can be deceiving.

Step 1: Heart rate

heart rate number of electrical impulses conducted through the myocardium in 60 seconds

Heart rate can be defined as the number of electrical impulses (as represented by PQRST complexes) conducted through the myocardium in 60 seconds (1 min). This analysis should be your first step in the interpretation of an EKG strip. When calculating heart rate, we usually are making reference to the *ventricular* heart rate. However, it is appropriate in certain strips to calculate both the atrial heart rate and the ventricular heart rate.

Simply stated, atrial heart rate can be determined by counting the number of P waves noted, whereas ventricular heart rate is determined by counting the number of QRS complexes. If atrial and ventricular heart rates are dissimilar, it is very important that you calculate both.

Recall now that the sinoatrial (SA) node discharges impulses at a rate of 60 to 100 times per minute. Therefore, a normal heart rate will be noted if the rate is calculated within a range of 60 to 100 beats per minute (BPM). If the rate is less than 60 BPM, it is referred to as **bradycardia.** In contrast, if the heart rate is greater than 100 BPM, the correct term is **tachycardia.** It is important to note that these numbers are simply parameters, or normal ranges, to which you will adhere when analyzing heart rate.

bradycardia heart rate of less than 60 beats per minute

tachycardia heart rate greater than 100 beats per minute

Keep in mind that your patient's clinical picture is critical to proper patient assessment and management. In other words, if your patient's heart rate is 58 BPM, he or she is technically bradycardic, based on normal parameters. The patient's clinical picture, however, may indicate no evidence of hemodynamic compromise. Remember to ask yourself this question: "How is the rhythm significant to the patient's clinical picture?" Often you will find that the patient with a heart rate of 58 BPM is exhibiting no clinical symptomatology at all.

There are two common methods used to determine heart rate by visual examination of an EKG strip. The first and simplest way is called the *6–second method* (Figure 6–1). In order to properly use this method, you must first denote a 6–second interval on an EKG

8 complexes in 6 seconds approximates to 80/min (8 × 10 = 80)

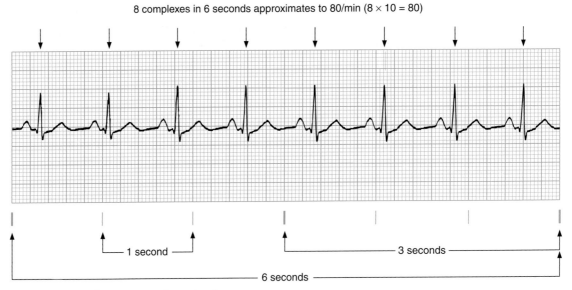

Figure 6–1. The 6–second method

strip. Fortunately, EKG paper is commonly marked in either 3- or 6–second increments. Simply count the number of QRS complexes that occur within the 6–second interval and then multiply that number by 10. If the graph paper does not have 3- or 6–second marks, you can count the number of R waves in 30 large squares and multiply this number by 10. This will yield a close approximation of the patient's heart rate. This method is effective even when the rhythm is noted to be irregular.

The second common method used to determine heart rate by visual examination of an EKG strip is referred to as the *R-R interval method*. This method is most accurate if the heart rhythm is regular; otherwise it is only an estimation of heart rate. Recall from the discussion of EKG graph paper that there are 300 large boxes in a 60-second or 1-minute strip. With this in mind, you should look for a QRS complex (specifically an R wave) that falls on a heavy line on the strip. Then you should count the number of large boxes between the first R wave and the next R wave. After you determine that number, you then divide it into 300. For example, if there are three large boxes between two R waves, you would divide 3 into 300 and realize that the heart rate is 100 BPM (300 divided by 3 = 100). Apply this method to the strip in Figure 6–2.

Remember that the normal heart rate is 60 to 100 BPM. Below 60 BPM is a slow or bradycardic rate, and greater than 100 BPM is considered to be a fast or tachycardic rate. Heart rates can vary depending on many differing factors, including the general health of your patient, stress levels, strenuous exercise, or myocardial compromise. Again, you must constantly assess your patient while assessing his or her EKG strip.

Step 2: Heart rhythm

Step 2 involves evaluating **heart rhythm.** The term *rhythm* can be defined as the sequential beating of the heart as a result of the generation of electrical impulses. Synonyms for the word *rhythm* include: *pattern, guide, model, order,* and *design.* Thus, you can see that calculating the heart rhythm involves establishing a pattern of QRS complex occurrence.

heart rhythm
sequential beating of the heart as a result of the generation of electrical impulses

Heart rhythms are classified as either regular or irregular. Normally, the heart's rhythm is regular. To determine whether the ventricular rhythm is regular, measure the intervals between R waves. To determine whether the atrial rhythm is regular, measure the intervals between P waves. If the intervals vary by less than 0.06 second (or 1.5 small squares), consider the rhythm to be regular. If, however, the intervals are variable by greater than 0.06 second, the rhythm is considered to be irregular.

It may be helpful to use EKG calipers when you initially begin to analyze EKG rhythms. If calipers are not available, you may also measure intervals by making marks

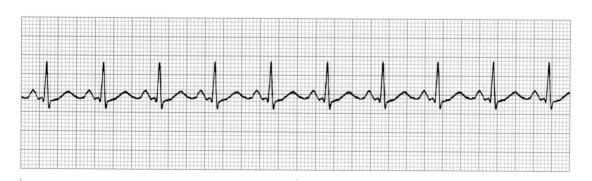

Figure 6–2. Normal sinus rhythm (rate of 100 BPM)

on a piece of paper placed on the EKG strip just below the peak of the R wave. After marking the area where each R wave occurred, look at the marks on your paper to identify a pattern. Then measure the distance between the marks with a ruler. If the marks are relatively equal distances apart, the rhythm is noted to be regular. If the distances between the marks vary noticeably, then the rhythm is probably irregular. Alterations of respiratory rate and depth may produce slight variations in heart rhythms.

Rhythms that are found to be irregular can be further classified as:

➤ **Regularly irregular** — irregular rhythms that occur in a pattern.
➤ **Occasionally irregular** — only one or two R-R intervals are uneven.
➤ **Irregularly irregular** — R-R intervals exhibit no similarity.

Regardless of whether the rhythm is regular or irregular, always remember to ask yourself that all-important question, "How is this rhythm clinically significant to my patient?"

Before moving on to Step 3, take a moment to review Steps 1 and 2. Then look at the strips in Figures 6–3 and 6–4 and calculate the rate and rhythm of each one. After you think you have the answers, ask your instructor or tutor to verify them.

Step 3: P wave

P wave represents depolarization of the left and right atria

First, recall the events that must occur in order to cause the formation of **P waves** on an EKG strip. You learned in Chapter 5 that the P wave is produced when the right and left atria depolarize. Depolarization of the atria is produced when an electrical impulse spreads throughout the atria via the internodal pathways. The P wave is noted as the first deviation from the isoelectric line on the EKG strip and should always be rounded and

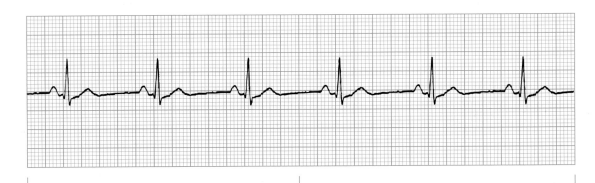

Figure 6–3.   Practice strip for rate and rhythm analysis

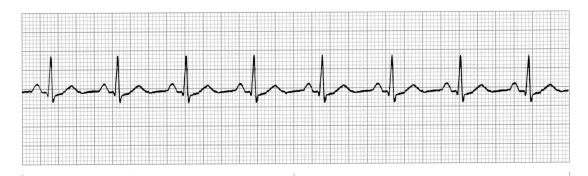

Figure 6–4.   Practice strip for rate and rhythm analysis

upright (positive) in limb Lead II. It will be very helpful in your study of EKG interpretation if you remember the following: *If the P wave is not upright in Lead II, you are not looking at a sinus rhythm (a rhythm that originated in the SA node).*

There are five questions that should be asked when evaluating P waves:

1. Are P waves present?
2. Are the P waves occurring regularly?
3. Is there one P wave present for each QRS complex present?
4. Are the P waves smooth, rounded, and upright in appearance, or are they inverted?
5. Do all the P waves look similar?

Recall now that the SA node is the primary pacemaker of the heart. It is located in the right atrium. If the SA node is pacing or firing at regular intervals, the P waves will also follow at regular intervals. This pattern would then be referred to as a *sinus rhythm.* In this text, the heart rhythms are referenced according to their points of origin.

Step 4: PR interval

The **PR interval** measures the time interval from the onset of atrial contraction to the onset of ventricular contraction, or the time necessary for the electrical impulse to be conducted through the atria and the AV node. Although this component is called the PR interval, it actually includes the entire P wave. The PR interval is measured from the onset (or beginning) of the P wave to the onset of the Q wave of the QRS complex.

The normal length of the PR interval is 0.12 to 0.20 second (three to five small squares). The PR interval should be constant across the EKG strip in order to be considered within normal limits. If the PR interval is shortened (less than 0.12 second), this may be an indication that the usual progression of the impulse was outside the normal route. Prolonged PR intervals (greater than 0.20 second) may indicate a delay in the electrical conduction pathway or an AV block.

There are three questions that should be asked when evaluating PR intervals:

1. Are PR intervals greater than 0.20 second?
2. Are PR intervals less than 0.12 second?
3. Are the PR intervals constant across the EKG strip?

Step 5: QRS Complex

The **QRS complex** represents the depolarization (or contraction) of the ventricles. It is important to note whether all QRS complexes look alike, as this similarity will indicate that the electrical impulses are conducted in a consistent way.

The QRS complex is actually a group of waves, consisting of the following:

➤ **Q wave** — the first negative or downward deflection of this large complex. It is a small wave that precedes the R wave. Often the Q wave is not seen.
➤ **R wave** — the first upward or positive deflection following the P wave. In chest Lead II, the R wave is the tallest waveform noted.
➤ **S wave** — the sharp, negative or downward deflection that follows the R wave.

Refer to Figure 6–5 in order to visualize the appearance of the QRS complex.

The overall appearance of the QRS, as well as its width, can provide important information about the electrical conduction system. When the electrical conduction system is functioning normally, the width of the QRS complex will be 0.12 second (three

PR interval
measures the time interval from the onset of atrial contraction to the onset of ventricular contraction

QRS complex
represents the depolarization (or contraction) of the ventricles

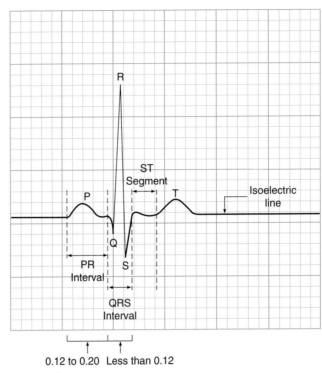

Figure 6–5. EKG waveforms

supraventricular
above the ventricles

small squares) or less (narrow). This normal or narrow QRS complex indicates that the impulse was not formed in the ventricles and is thus referred to as **supraventricular** or above the ventricles. Wide QRS complexes (greater than 0.12 second or three small squares) indicate that the impulse is either of a ventricular origin or a supraventricular origin with aberrant (deviating from the normal course or pattern) conduction.

There are three questions that should be asked when evaluating QRS intervals:

1. Are QRS intervals greater than 0.12 second (wide)? If so, the complex may be ventricular in origin.
2. Are QRS intervals less than 0.12 second (narrow)? If so, the complex is most probably supraventricular in origin.
3. Are the QRS complexes similar in appearance across the EKG strip?

It is important to realize that the shape of QRS complexes will vary slightly in individual patients, depending on factors such as heart shape and size, health of the myocardium, and location and placement of electrodes.

THE 5 + 3 APPROACH

It is imperative that you learn and remember the five basic steps to correctly interpret an EKG, and you must now build on your knowledge in order to incorporate the correct interpretation of the 12-lead EKG strip. We call this approach the **5 + 3 approach.**

5 + 3 approach
a combination of the basic five steps to EKG interpretation plus analysis of the ST segment and Q wave

You will recall that the basic five steps include:

Rate	Rhythm	P wave	PR interval	QRS complex

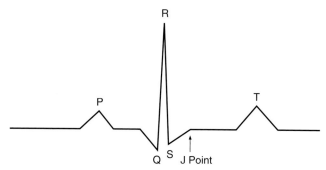

Figure 6–6.   The J point

Now it's time to learn the 5 + 3 approach:

Rate	Rhythm	P wave	PR interval	QRS complex

Plus

ST depression	ST elevation	Q wave

In order to learn each of the three new steps, we will look carefully at the ST segment, as well as the Q wave. The ST segment begins with the end of the QRS complex and ends with the onset of the T wave. The normal ST segment is usually consistent with the isoelectric line of the EKG strip. It is during the period of the ST segment that ventricular repolarization is occurring. The point where the QRS complex meets the ST segment is commonly referred to as the *J point* (Figure 6–6).

In Figure 6–5, notice the location of the ST segment in the EKG. By visualizing the exact location of the ST segment, you will have a reference point as we discuss ST segment depression and elevation.

ST SEGMENT DEPRESSION

ST segment depression occurs due to myocardial ischemia, secondary to myocardial tissue hypoxia (low level of oxygen). Hypoxia results in altered repolarization, which directly contributes to the development of ST segment depression. Significant ST segment depression is characterized by a dip below the isoelectric line of 1 to 2 millimeters or one to two small boxes on the EKG graph paper (Figure 6–7). The effect of hypoxia on repolarization may (or may not) produce an inversion of the T wave. It is important to note and to reiterate that ST segment depression may be seen alone or with accompanying inversion of the T wave. As a rule, the larger the area of ischemic tissue, the more significant the EKG findings will be.

You, as a health-care provider, must realize that appropriate and timely intervention is imperative if your patient is to receive the ultimate in quality patient care. Simply stated, if your index of suspicion is heightened by evidence of clinical and/or EKG findings, you must immediately administer 100% oxygen to the patient. Although there are many sophisticated, state-of-the-art equipment modalities available

ST segment depression characterized by a dip below the isoelectric line of 1 to 2 millimeters or one to two small boxes on the EKG graph paper

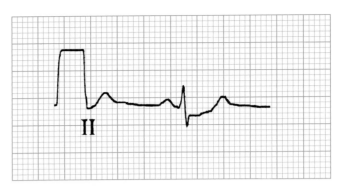

Figure 6–7. ST segment depression

to today's health-care provider, nothing—repeat, nothing—is more important than oxygen administration. This is especially true if your patient is complaining of chest pain and/or has a history of previous cardiac events.

Although the most common cause of ST segment depression is myocardial ischemia, you should understand that there are other causes. These include, but are not limited to:

➤ Ventricular hypertrophy.
➤ Intraventricular conduction defects.
➤ The medication digitalis (also commonly called Lanoxin or Digoxin).

Pathophysiologically, you should realize that the time when the patient's EKG strip demonstrates ST segment depression is one of the more critical times to strive for reversal of the myocardial ischemia. At this point there is no irreversible injury to the myocardium. As you proceed through the subsequent chapters of this textbook, you will often see the phrase "Time is muscle" or "Time is myocardium." The more literal interpretation of this phrase simply says to you, the heath-care provider, that the criticality of immediate oxygen administration cannot be overemphasized. The patient's outcome may quite literally depend on it. The longer the time it takes for intervention to occur, the greater the possibility of irreparable muscle damage.

ST SEGMENT ELEVATION

ST segment elevation
characterized by a rise above the isoelectric line of 1 to 2 millimeters or one to two small boxes on the EKG graph paper

Our reference to **ST segment elevation** will presume that the patient did not receive the necessary oxygen in a timely and appropriate manner. Thus, the succession from hypoxia to ischemia to injury will progress. At this point, the ST segment will become elevated. Significant ST segment elevation is characterized by a rise above the isoelectric line of 1 or 2 millimeters or one or two small boxes on the EKG graph paper (Figure 6–8).

The most common cause of ST segment elevation is myocardial injury, secondary to acute myocardial infarction. Other causes may include:

➤ Coronary artery vasospasm (Prinzmetal's angina).
➤ Pericarditis (EKG evidence is usually present in all leads).
➤ Ventricular aneurysm.
➤ Early repolarization (in young children).

As a general rule, ST segment elevation will occur within the first 1 to 2 hours after the onset of myocardial hypoxia, if the patient is not properly managed. At this point, you must be reminded that IT IS NOT TOO LATE to intercede. Although the myocardial hy-

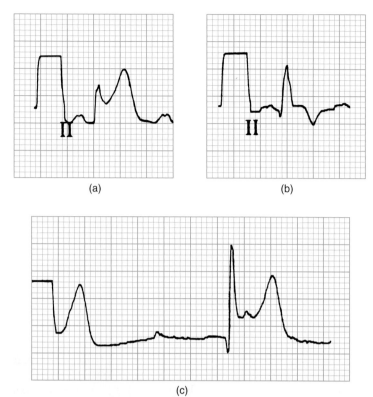

Figure 6–8.   ST segment elevation (a); ST segment elevation with T wave inversion (b); ST segment elevation with tall T wave (c)

Table 6–1

Myocardial tissue hypoxia: early treatment measures

Basic Interventions	Advanced Interventions
Calm and reassure patient.	Administer oxygen.
Administer oxygen.	Initiate cardiac monitoring.
Prehospital—notify ALS backup (as indicated).	Obtain a 12-lead EKG.
	Establish an IV lifeline.

poxia is showing signs of progression, the tissue damage at this point is not irreparable. Thus, early intervention and appropriate management are critical to your patient's outcome. Early intervention includes, but is not limited to, the interventions listed in Table 6–1.

Q WAVE

The development of the **pathologic Q wave** indicates irreversible tissue damage, or death of the myocardial tissue. A pathologic Q wave is defined as a width greater than or equal to one small box (1 millimeter) or depth greater than one-third of the R wave in the same lead. Following myocardial infarction (MI) and inadequate intervention, and as a result of absence of depolarization current from dead myocardial tissue, a deep Q wave may be seen.

pathologic Q wave a Q wave that is equal to or greater than 0.04 second (one small box) in width and has a depth of greater than one-third of the height of the succeeding R wave

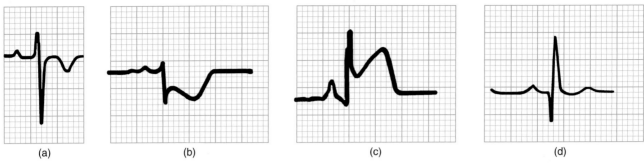

Figure 6–9. The evolution of an MI: EKG changes

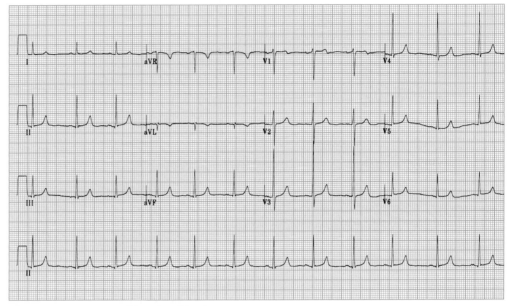

Figure 6–10. Normal 12-lead EKG

The appearance of a pathologic Q wave is an ominous sign and most commonly indicates a more discouraging patient outcome. This is true because at this point, myocardial tissue damage has occurred and may be significant. After several months, fibrous scarring will replace the infarcted tissue. The presence of scar tissue in and around the myocardium may hamper the heart's mechanical and/or electrical activity.

Figure 6–9 shows the EKG changes that occur at each stage of an MI. Figure 6–10 shows a normal 12-lead EKG for comparison.

You must understand that, when considering the 5 + 3 approach, the final three steps must be carefully considered. It is imperative to your understanding of 12-lead EKG interpretation that you note the evidence (or the lack thereof) of each of the steps. In other words, ask yourself the questions:

1. Is there evidence of ST segment depression and, if so, in which leads does it appear?
2. Is there evidence of ST segment elevation and, if so, in which leads does it occur?
3. Is there evidence of Q waves and, if so, in which leads do the Q waves appear, and are the Q waves pathologic or nonpathologic?

You should be aware that evidence in *each* of the + 3 steps may not be present. In other words, an EKG may demonstrate ST segment depression, ST segment elevation, and pathologic Q waves in previously specified leads, allowing you to unequivocally identify a specific type of myocardial infarction. However, a single finding in one step of the + 3 approach may also be indicative of an early myocardial infarction. A clear example could be the presence of ST segment depression in a specific lead group, with no other findings in the + 3 approach.

Assessment of the patient's clinical presentation (signs and symptoms) is critical in determining the presence of an acute myocardial infarction. In addition, you must remember that EKG changes that are the most indicative of the presence of an acute myocardial infarction include ST segment elevation and presence of a pathologic Q wave. Recall the important point that "Time is muscle" and act accordingly.

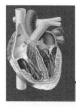

Summary
CHAPTER 6

As this chapter emphasizes, a systematic approach to rhythm interpretation—be it 3-lead EKGs or 12-lead EKGs—is a critical component of proper identification of the various rhythms. You have now been introduced to the concept of 12-lead EKG interpretation by virtue of the simple addition of the + 3 step in the basic five-step approach. In subsequent chapters, you will practice the application of the 5 + 3 approach until you attain mastery-level competency. Again, remember to ask your instructor/tutor to clarify any points that may tend to confuse you. Now is the time to ask questions!

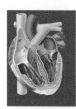

Key Points to Remember
CHAPTER 6

1. Look at your patient's condition.

2. Read every strip from left to right.

3. Apply the 5 + 3 approach.

4. Avoid shortcuts.

5. Ask and answer each step in the 5 + 3 approach.

6. Heart rate is defined as the number of electrical complexes conducted through the myocardium in 60 seconds.

7. Heart rhythm is defined as the sequential beating of the heart as a result of the generation of electrical impulses.

8. The P wave is produced when the right and left atria depolarize.

9. The PR interval measures the time interval from the onset of atrial contraction to the onset of ventricular contraction.

10. The QRS complex represents the depolarization of the ventricles.

11. ST depression occurs due to myocardial ischemia secondary to myocardial tissue hypoxia.

12. ST elevation is a rise above the isoelectric line of 1 mm to 2 mm and indicates injury.

13. Pathologic Q waves are defined as a width greater than or equal to 1 mm or a depth greater than one-third of the R wave in the same lead. Their appearance indicates death of myocardial tissue.

Review Questions
CHAPTER 6

1. The sinoatrial node is located in the:
   a. right atrium.
   b. right ventricle.
   c. Purkinje fiber tract.
   d. atrioventricular septum.

2. The intrinsic firing rate of the AV node is ___ per minute.
   a. 15–25
   b. 25–35
   c. 35–45
   d. 40–60

3. The intrinsic firing rate of the SA node in the adult is ___ per minute.
   a. 20–60
   b. 40–80
   c. 60–100
   d. 80–100

4. The 12-lead EKG is used to evaluate all of the following *except:*
   a. pulse rate.
   b. valvular dysfunction.
   c. electrical activity in the heart.
   d. isolate waveforms indicative of an MI.

5. The PR interval should normally be ___ second or smaller.
   a. 0.10
   b. 0.12
   c. 0.08
   d. 0.20

6. The QRS interval should normally be ___ second or smaller.

    a. 0.20

    b. 0.12

    c. 0.18

    d. 0.36

7. ST segment depression indicates:

    a. myocardial ischemia.

    b. coronary vasospasm.

    c. Prinzmetal's angina.

    d. chronic pericarditis.

8. The QRS complex is produced when the ventricles:

    a. repolarize.

    b. depolarize.

    c. contract.

    d. both b and c

9. The normal conduction pattern of the heart follows:

    1. SA node
    2. Purkinje fibers
    3. bundle of His
    4. AV node
    5. bundle branches
    6. internodal pathways

    a. 1, 5, 2, 4, 6, 3

    b. 1, 6, 4, 3, 5, 2

    c. 1, 4, 3, 6, 5, 2

    d. 1, 2, 3, 4, 5, 6

10. ST segment elevation is a primary indicator of:

    a. ventricular atrophy.

    b. ventricular hypertrophy.

    c. myocardial injury.

    d. atrial aneurysm.

11. The T wave on the EKG strip represents:

    a. rest period.

    b. bundle of His.

    c. atrial contraction.

    d. ventricular contraction.

12. When interpreting dysrhythmias, you should remember that the most important key is the:

a. PR interval.

b. rate and rhythm.

c. presence of dysrhythmias.

d. patient's clinical appearance.

13. The point where the QRS complex meets the ST segment is commonly referred to as the:

a. J point.

b. midpoint.

c. T wave.

d. U wave.

14. The most common cause of ST segment depression is myocardial ischemia. Other causes may include all of the following *except:*

a. interatrial conduction defects.

b. ventricular hypertrophy.

c. digitalis toxicity.

d. interventricular conduction defects.

15. The development of pathologic Q waves indicates:

a. irreversible tissue ischemia.

b. coronary artery vasospasm.

c. third-degree block.

d. irreversible tissue damage.

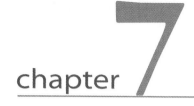

chapter 7

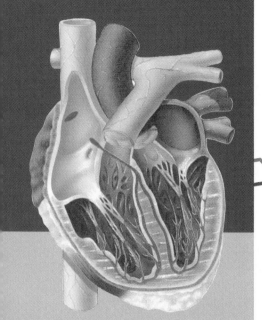

Acute Myocardial Infarction

objectives

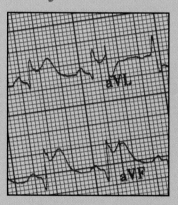

Upon completion of this chapter, the student will be able to:

➤ Discuss the anatomy (structure) and function of the coronary arteries

➤ Discuss the anatomy (structure) and function of the coronary veins

➤ Discuss guidelines for differentiating angina pectoris from acute myocardial infarction based on

   a. Clinical presentation

   b. EKG findings

➤ Discuss chest pain based on signs and symptoms

➤ Describe the standard treatment modalities for cardiac-related chest pain

➤ Describe the noncardiac causes of chest pain

➤ Review the clinical significance of acute myocardial infarction

➤ Relate the critical components of the assessment of a suspected AMI patient

INTRODUCTION

Cardiac emergencies, including acute myocardial infarction (AMI), continue to be one of the nation's leading causes of death. Heart attacks and other cardiac emergencies affect more than 5 million individuals each year. More than 1 million deaths each year are directly attributed to heart disease. Your understanding of 12-lead EKGs will enhance your ability to assess and treat the patient who presents with chest pain in a more time-efficient manner. In this chapter, you will review the coronary artery and vein anatomy. You also will learn the critical aspects of differentiating cardiac versus noncardiac causes for chest pain, as well as its management.

CORONARY ANATOMY

Understanding the structure and functions of the coronary arteries and the coronary sinus is a critical component of 12-lead EKG interpretation. The importance of these structures will be reviewed and further emphasized in this chapter.

   The right and left coronary arteries arise and branch off from the proximal portion of the aorta. They function to transport oxygenated blood throughout the heart muscle (myocardium). The coronary vessels receive their blood supply from the aorta during ventricular diastole (relaxation).

   There are two main branches of the coronary arteries that are located on the surface of the heart. Usually smaller than the left coronary artery, the right coronary artery does not supply as large a portion of the heart muscle with blood as does the left coronary artery. It should be noted that there is a significant degree of individual variance in the normal coronary artery distribution. It is from these important structures that blood is supplied to the myocardial tissues by way of small penetrating arterioles. (See Figure 7–1

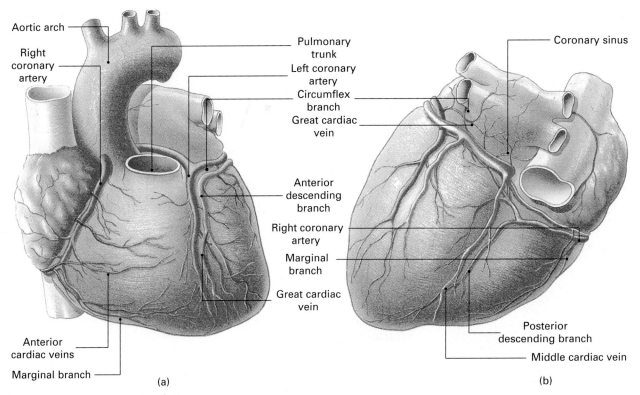

Figure 7–1. Coronary circulation

for an illustration of coronary circulation, Table 7–1 for the divisions or branches of the coronary arteries, and Table 7–2 for the distribution of blood supply to the myocardium.)

Left coronary artery

As the left coronary artery leaves the aorta, it immediately divides into the left anterior descending artery and the circumflex artery. The anterior descending artery is the major branch of the left coronary artery and supplies blood to most of the anterior part of the heart. A marginal branch of the left coronary artery supplies blood to the lateral wall of the left ventricle. The circumflex branch of the left coronary artery extends around to the posterior side of the heart, and its branches supply blood to much of the posterior wall of the heart. Each of these divisions has numerous branches that form a network of blood vessels, which in turn serve to provide oxygenation of designated portions of the myocardium.

Right coronary artery

The right coronary artery extends from the aorta around to the posterior portion of the heart. Branches of the right coronary artery supply blood to the lateral wall of the right ventricle. A branch of the right coronary artery called the *posterior interventricular artery* or *posterior descending artery* lies in the posterior interventricular region and supplies blood to the posterior and inferior part of the heart's left ventricle. The right coronary artery branches also supply oxygen-rich blood to a portion of the electrical conduction system.

Collateral circulation allows for an alternate path of blood flow in the event of vascular occlusion and is a protective mechanism. Numerous **anastomoses** (communication between two or more vessels) between various branches of the coronary arteries allow for collateral circulation. The body's innate ability to develop collateral circulation

collateral circulation a protective mechanism, allows for an alternate path of blood flow in the event of vascular occlusion

anastomoses communications between two or more vessels

Table 7–1

Coronary artery divisions/branches

Left Coronary Arteries	Right Coronary Arteries
Left anterior descending	Posterior descending
Marginal	Marginal
Circumflex	

Table 7–2

Distribution of blood supply to the myocardium

Left Coronary Arteries	Right Coronary Arteries
Anterior left ventricular wall	Lateral wall of the right ventricle
Lateral wall of the left ventricle	A portion of the electrical conduction system
Posterior wall of the left ventricle	Posterior wall of left ventricle
Left interventricular septal wall	Inferior wall of left ventricle

enables select individuals to compensate for atherosclerotic deposits in their coronary arteries, thereby allowing them to remain virtually asymptomatic for extended periods.

Coronary sinus (great cardiac vein)

Draining the myocardial tissue on the left side of the heart is the great cardiac vein. A smaller cardiac vein drains the right margin of the heart. Toward the posterior part of the coronary sulcus (ditch), these veins converge and empty into a large venous cavity called the coronary sinus. The **coronary sinus** is a short trunk that serves to receive deoxygenated blood from the major veins of the myocardium. This trunk empties into the right atrium. The coronary veins roughly correspond positionally with the coronary arteries throughout the myocardium.

coronary sinus
passage that receives deoxygenated blood from the major veins of the myocardium

PATHOLOGY

Now that you have reviewed the anatomy of the coronary circulation, it is time to discuss various pathologies that result from coronary insufficiency.

Angina pectoris

angina pectoris
pain that results from a reduction in blood supply to myocardial tissue

Angina pectoris is described as pain that results from a reduction in blood supply to myocardial tissue. The pain is typically temporary. If blood flow is quickly restored, little or no permanent change or damage may result. Angina is characterized by chest pain or discomfort deep in the sternal area and is often described as heaviness, pressure, or moderately severe pain. It is quite often mistaken for indigestion. This pain can be referred to the neck, lower jaw, or left shoulder, arm, and fingers.

Angina pectoris most often results from narrowed and/or hardened coronary arterial walls. The reduction of blood flow results in a reduced supply of oxygen to cardiac muscle cells. The pain is often predictably associated with exercise, due to the increased pumping activity of the heart, which requires more oxygen that the narrowed blood vessels cannot supply.

Frequently, angina pectoris is relieved by rest and/or medications such as nitroglycerin. **Nitroglycerin** causes blood vessel dilation, which consequently reduces the workload of the heart, thus reducing the need for oxygen because the heart has to pump blood against a lesser pressure. The blood tends to remain in the dilated blood vessels; consequently, a diminished blood supply is returned to the heart for distribution.

nitroglycerin
medication that causes blood vessel dilation, reducing the workload of the heart and the need for oxygen

Acute myocardial infarction

acute myocardial infarction (AMI)
condition that results from a prolonged lack of blood flow to a portion of the myocardial tissue, which leads to a lack of oxygen

An **acute myocardial infarction (AMI)** results from a prolonged lack of blood flow to a portion of the myocardial tissue and results in a lack of oxygen. Eventually, myocardial cellular death will follow unless immediate interventions are initiated. Myocardial infarctions vary with the amount of myocardial tissue and the portion of the heart that is affected. If blood supply to cardiac muscle is reestablished within 10 to 20 minutes, there usually will be no permanent injury. If oxygen deprivation lasts longer, cellular death most likely will result. Within 30 to 60 seconds after blockage of a coronary blood vessel, functional changes will become evident. The electrical properties of the cardiac muscle will be altered and the ability of the cardiac muscle to function properly will be lost.

Table 7–3

Differential symptomology of angina versus AMI	
Signs/Symptoms—Angina Pectoris	**Signs/Symptoms—Acute Myocardial Infarction**
Chest Pain: short duration—usually lasts 3–10 minutes; usually relieved by nitroglycerin	Chest Pain: usually lasts more than 2 hours; not relieved by nitroglycerin
Brought on by stress or exercise and relieved by rest	Usually not precipitated by exercise or stress; not relieved by rest
May be accompanied by dysrhythmias	Usually accompanied by dysrhythmias
Patients usually do not have nausea, vomiting, or diaphoresis	Patients commonly complain of nausea, vomiting and are often profoundly diaphoretic

The most common cause of myocardial infarctions is **thrombus** formation that blocks a coronary artery. Coronary arteries narrowed by atherosclerotic damage provide one of the conditions that increase the likelihood of myocardial infarction. Atherosclerotic lesions partially block blood vessels, resulting in disorderly blood flow due to the rough surfaces of the lesions. These changes increase the probability of thrombus formation.

Signs and symptoms of an acute myocardial infarction may be quite similar to those of angina pectoris (Table 7–3). Clear differences include the facts that the pain caused by an AMI lasts longer and is usually not relieved by rest.

thrombus
stationary blood clots that can lead to vessel occlusion

Cardiac versus noncardiac chest pain

Chest pain of cardiac origin may present in various ways. As discussed previously in this chapter, this type of chest pain may be indicative of serious illness, myocardial ischemia, or myocardial injury, or may simply indicate stress or exercise-related hypoxia.

Chest pain is the most common presenting symptom of cardiac disease, as well as the most common patient complaint. Chest pain of cardiac origin is typically described as "crushing," "squeezing," or "tightness" and is commonly associated with nausea, vomiting, and **diaphoresis** (profuse sweating). The pain is often located substernally and may radiate to the jaw(s), shoulder(s), arm(s), and finger(s).

Chest pain from an acute myocardial infarction may escalate in intensity. Patients may express a feeling of impending doom and may exhibit extreme anxiety.

A common obstacle to timely intervention by the health-care provider when dealing with a patient who complains of chest pain is denial. Patients often deny the possibility that they may indeed be experiencing a heart attack, with thoughts such as "It can't happen to me." Often patients prefer to believe that they are merely experiencing indigestion and that these symptoms will be gone by morning. Unfortunately, it may be the patient, rather than the symptoms, who is gone by morning. With proper public education, many lives have been saved that otherwise would have been lost. This is due in large part to the simple fact that many thousands of laypersons have been certified in the skill of cardiopulmonary resuscitation (CPR).

chest pain the most common presenting symptom of cardiac disease and the most common patient complaint

diaphoresis
profuse sweating

neuropathy the inability to perceive pain due to destruction of nerve endings

It should be noted that in special circumstances, patients may experience no chest pain at all and still have sustained a myocardial infarction. Primarily, this is true in the diabetic patient with advanced **neuropathy,** which is caused by the destruction of nerve endings and results in the inability to perceive pain. The scenario with which diabetic patients may present is often congestive heart failure. Some elderly patients also may experience an AMI without chest pain; most commonly their only presenting symptom will be the complaint of profound weakness.

STANDARD TREATMENT MODALITIES

fibrinolytic therapy the use of agents to activate enzymes that dissolve a thrombus

The primary goal of management of the patient with symptomatic chest pain is to strive to interrupt the infarction process. This can be achieved through interventions such as immediate and effective oxygen administration, pain alleviation, management of dysrhythmias, and the initiation of aspirin therapy. The initiation of thrombolytic or **fibrinolytic therapy** in order to limit the progression of the infarct is based on local and state protocols in conjunction with physician intervention. New research has questioned the efficacy of the immediate initiation of thrombolytic therapy when availability of and access to a cardiac catherization lab is immediate.

Without a doubt, the most important drug any patient with chest pain can receive is oxygen. Time and again, in this and other textbooks, you will see this statement simply because it is true and critically important to the viability of your patient.

Considerations regarding treatment include:

➤ Administer 100% oxygen.
➤ Establish an intravenous (IV) lifeline according to local protocols.
➤ Measure oxygen saturation level (pulse oximetry), if equipment is available.
➤ Perform continuous cardiac monitoring.
➤ Provide pain control and management (i.e., nitroglycerin, morphine sulfate, Demerol, etc.) according to local protocols.
➤ Initiate aspirin therapy.
➤ Initiate fibrinolytic therapy and/or immediate access to cardiac catherization.

Remember that the focus of assessment and treatment of the patient who presents with chest pain centers on the immediate oxygenation of hypoxic tissue. Treatment initiatives will vary depending upon your patient's specific situation. However, you must focus on continual and thorough assessment until such time that the patient is clinically stable.

NONCARDIAC CAUSES OF CHEST PAIN

Causes of noncardiac chest pain are numerous. However, remember that chest pain is cardiac in nature until proven otherwise, especially in the prehospital arena. Some of the causes of noncardiac chest pain include (but are not limited to) the following:

➤ **Pleurisy** — inflammation of the covering of the lungs (pleura).
➤ **Costrochondritis** — inflammation of intercostal muscles (located between ribs).
➤ **Pericarditis** — inflammation of the pericardial sac (surrounding the heart).
➤ **Myocardial contusion** — secondary to chest trauma (high incidence of dysrhythmias).

➤ **Muscle strain** — secondary to overstretching of the chest wall muscles.
➤ **Trauma** — secondary to injury to the chest wall and/or organs contained within the chest.

Examples of chest injuries secondary to trauma include:

➤ **Hemothorax** — the collection of blood within the pleural cavity.
➤ **Pneumothorax** — the collection of air within the pleural cavity.
➤ **Hemopneumothorax** — the collection of blood and air within the pleural cavity.
➤ **Tension pneumothorax** — air trapped in the thoracic cavity without an escape route; pressure builds and affects the lungs, heart, and other vital organs.

Chest trauma can produce severe chest pain and may indicate a serious condition that requires immediate intervention. Any patient who exhibits chest pain, regardless of the clinical presentation, should be monitored for the possible occurrence of dysrhythmias. Remember the old adage about an ounce of prevention? When dealing with chest pain, this adage definitely applies because TIME IS MUSCLE.

CLINICAL SIGNIFICANCE

As mentioned at the beginning of this chapter, cardiac emergencies, including acute myocardial infarctions, continue to be one of the nation's leading causes of death. Thus the significance of the patient's condition, as well as the need for early intervention for patients with suspected AMI, is paramount. An acute myocardial infarction may be a staggering event involving electrical conduction system disturbances, as well as mechanical failure secondary to infarcted tissue.

PATIENT ASSESSMENT

Recall that time is muscle and act accordingly. Thus, timely assessment and management, including immediate oxygen administration, must be rapidly initiated and completed within a 10-minute time interval. Your initial assessment and evaluation should focus on the patient's general appearance. You will probably note that patients who are experiencing an AMI will tend to remain quiet and still. These patients also tend to prefer a sitting position. The Fowler's or semi-Fowler's position tends to allow the patient to breathe more comfortably and may decrease the workload of the myocardium.

A thorough and timely evaluation and management of the patient's ABCs (airway, breathing, circulation) is imperative. Any problem encountered during this evaluation must be managed quickly, followed by a rapid assessment of the vital signs. Because of the wide variations of the presenting vital signs, the clinician should be aware that vital signs are not necessarily reliable in diagnosing an AMI. In spite of this fact, it is important that you monitor and record these signs at frequent intervals.

One of the most important assessment tools that you will utilize when managing the suspected AMI patient is the cardiac monitor. Dysrhythmias that originate from ischemic and injured myocardial tissues are a common complication of acute myocardial infarctions. It is critical for you to understand that in the clinical setting, dysrhythmias may be simply warning signs or they may signal severe, life-threatening events. In either case, you must not ignore the presence of any abnormal heart rhythm when dealing with a patient who exhibits the textbook clinical presentation of an acute myocardial infarction. Although the three-lead EKG strip will adequately depict the heart rate and rhythm, the 12-lead EKG has the ability to afford a comprehensive picture of the myocardial events occurring during an acute myocardial infarction.

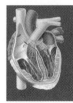

Summary
CHAPTER 7

Your suspicion of an acute myocardial infarction must be based on a combination of a positive 12-lead EKG and the patient's clinical picture (signs and symptoms) in the pre-hospital arena. In the in-hospital setting, these two factors in addition to serum enzyme changes and the development of pathologic Q waves will further assist in your conclusion. Keep in mind, however, that a negative 12-lead EKG does NOT rule out the presence of an AMI. Remember also that any patient who complains of chest pain must be thoroughly evaluated and management continued until the possibility of AMI is ruled out by the physician.

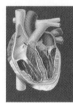

Key Points to Remember
CHAPTER 7

1. The two main branches of the coronary arteries are located on the surface of the heart.
2. The two main branches are the right coronary artery and the left coronary artery.
3. The left coronary artery extends from the aorta and divides into the left anterior descending and the circumflex artery.
4. The right coronary artery extends from the aorta around to the posterior portion of the heart and branches into the posterior descending artery.
5. The coronary sinus is a short trunk that serves to receive deoxygenated blood from the major veins of the myocardium.
6. Angina pectoris is described as the pain that results from a reduction in blood supply to myocardial tissue.
7. Acute myocardial infarction results from the prolonged lack of blood flow to a portion of the myocardial tissue, which results in a lack of oxygen and death of tissue.
8. Chest pain is the most common presenting symptom of cardiac disease.
9. The primary goal of management of the patient with symptomatic chest pain is to strive to interrupt the infarction process.
10. The "time is muscle" adage means that the more time it takes to intervene, the more muscle that may potentially be damaged.

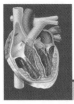

Review Questions
CHAPTER 7

1. The right and left coronary arteries branch off of the:
   a. ventricular artery.
   b. myocardial sulcus.
   c. proximal portion of the aorta.
   d. distal portion of the aorta.

2. Collateral circulation allows for:
   a. alternate path of blood flow in the event of occlusion.
   b. circulation continuum during diastole.
   c. maintaining artery patency during spasms.
   d. the ability of blood flow continuum during systole.

3. The pain of angina pectoris:
   a. is always constant.
   b. is typically temporary.
   c. occurs only during rest.
   d. is never mistaken for indigestion.

4. Myocardial infarction is:
   a. always temporary.
   b. usually diagnosed within 24 hours.
   c. age limited in most patients.
   d. due to myocardial cell death.

5. The most common cause of an AMI is:
   a. coronary vasospasms.
   b. atherosclerotic lesions.
   c. thrombus formation.
   d. arteriosclerotic blebs.

6. In acute myocardial infarctions, chest pain is long in duration and not relieved by nitroglycerin.
   a. True
   b. False

7. Patients experiencing an acute myocardial infarction will always complain of chest pain.

   a. True

   b. False

8. ST segment elevation is a primary indicator of:

   a. ventricular atrophy.

   b. ventricular hypertrophy.

   c. myocardial injury.

   d. atrial aneurysm.

9. The T wave on the EKG strip represents:

   a. rest period.

   b. bundle of His.

   c. atrial contraction.

   d. ventricular contraction.

10. When interpreting dysrhythmias, you should remember that the most important key is the:

    a. PR interval.

    b. rate and rhythm.

    c. presence of dysrhythmias.

    d. patient's clinical appearance.

11. The primary goal of management of the patient with symptomatic chest pain is to:

    a. interrupt the infarction process.

    b. augment the infarction process.

    c. institute thrombolytic therapy.

    d. increase myocardial oxygen consumption.

12. Management of a patient who is suspected of having sustained a myocardial contusion should:

    a. focus primarily on the associated and isolated chest injury.

    b. be similar to the treatment administered to a suspected MI patient.

    c. only be initiated at the definitive care facility following transport.

    d. completed in the prehospital arena, prior to transport to the hospital.

13. The 12-lead EKG is utilized to:

    a. rule out the presence of an acute MI.

    b. confirm the presence of an acute MI.

    c. identify dysrhythmias and contractile force.

    d. identify mechanical causes of dysrhythmias.

14. Timely assessment and management including immediate oxygen administration
must be rapidly completed within a ___ minute time interval.

   a. 5

   b. 10

   c. 12

   d. 15

15. The most important drug any patient experiencing chest pain can receive is:

   a. nitroglycerin.

   b. aspirin.

   c. oxygen.

   d. morphine.

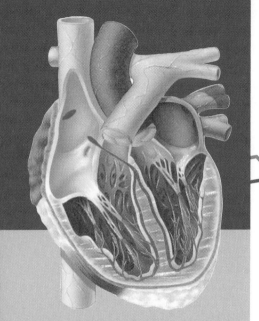

Myocardial Ischemia, Injury, and Necrosis

objectives

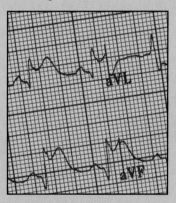

Upon completion of this chapter, the student will be able to:

➤ Describe the importance of timely treatment and transport of a patient with a suspected acute myocardial infarction (AMI)

➤ Define myocardial ischemia

➤ Discuss myocardial ischemia, including

  a. Signs and symptoms

  b. EKG changes

➤ Define myocardial injury

➤ Discuss myocardial injury, including

  a. Signs and symptoms

  b. EKG changes

➤ Define myocardial infarction (necrosis)

➤ Discuss myocardial infarction (necrosis), including

  a. Signs and symptoms

  b. EKG changes

➤ Review the clinical significance of myocardial ischemia, injury, and necrosis

INTRODUCTION

"Time is muscle" is a term that is used worldwide to indicate the importance of timely intervention into a scenario wherein the patient is suspected to be experiencing an acute myocardial infarction. The less time it takes to start definitive treatment, the less muscle that will be lost. Conversely, it can be viewed as follows: the more time it takes to start definitive treatment, the more myocardial muscle is lost. This chapter will focus on the changes that occur at the cellular level as a result of oxygen deprivation. In addition, we will discuss specific EKG changes that can be anticipated as a result of myocardial ischemia, myocardial injury, and necrosis of the myocardial tissues.

TIME IS MUSCLE (MYOCARDIUM)

As stated in Chapter 7, the fundamental goal of management of the patient with symptomatic chest pain is to strive to interrupt the infarction process. It is important to reiterate that this can be achieved through interventions such as appropriate oxygen administration, pain management, and recognition and treatment of dysrhythmias. Based on standard inclusion/exclusion criteria and local protocol, thrombolytic (fibrinolytic) therapy and/or **angioplasty** may be needed to limit the progression of the infarct.

angioplasty procedure used to alter the structure of a vessel either surgically or by dilating it with a balloon inside the lumen

As repeatedly stated, the most important drug that any patient with chest pain can receive is oxygen. Time and again, in this text and other books, you will see that statement—simply because it is true and it is critically important to your patient's outcome.

At the risk of being redundant, we feel it is critical for you to remember that the focus of assessment and treatment of the patient who presents with chest pain centers on the immediate oxygenation of hypoxic tissue. Treatment initiatives will vary depending upon your patient's specific situation. However, you must focus on continual and thorough assessment until such time that the patient is clinically stable.

INFARCT REGIONS AND DEFINITIONS

Typically, the damage caused by an acute myocardial infarction evolves into three distinct sectors (Figure 8–1). From outside to inside, these sectors include the ischemic area, the injured area, and the infarcted area:

➤ **Myocardial ischemia** — deprivation of oxygen and other nutrients to the heart muscle (myocardium); tendency to produce repolarization abnormalities.
➤ **Myocardial injury** — injury (damage) to the heart muscle (myocardium); most commonly results from and follows myocardial ischemia.
➤ **Myocardial necrosis** — death of the myocardial tissue (myocardial infarction).

Myocardial Ischemia

Myocardial ischemia may also be defined as either of the following:

➤ temporary shortage of oxygen at the cellular level, or
➤ transient absence of blood supply to the myocardial tissues.

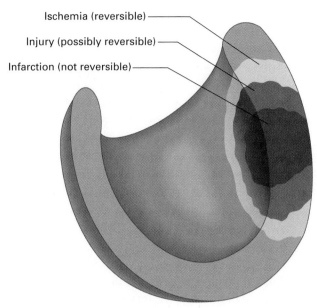

Ischemia (reversible) ——

Injury (possibly reversible) ——

Infarction (not reversible) ——

Figure 8–1. Sectors of damage from myocardial infarction (MI)

Whichever definition you prefer to learn, the most substantive point that you must learn and understand is that the lack or absence of oxygen to the myocardial cells can be a life-altering event if left uncorrected.

Ischemic changes cause a delay in the depolarization and repolarization of the cells around the area of infarct. The human body reacts to this event by eliciting chest pain. In addition, other signs and symptoms indicative of myocardial ischemia may include fatigue, diaphoresis, and varying degrees of anxiety. Once proper intervention has transpired and the return of adequate blood flow and reoxygenation is accomplished, the pain typically subsides and the myocardial cells return to a normal or near-normal state.

EKG changes with myocardial ischemia include ST segment depression, T wave inversion, or peaked T wave (Figure 8–2). The most significant and frequently identifiable of these EKG changes is the **ST segment depression,** which usually occurs in two or more contiguous leads. The ST segment depression is characterized by a dip below the isoelectric line of 1 to 2 millimeters or one to two small boxes on the EKG graph paper. Recall that the **J point** is the point on the EKG strip where the QRS complex meets the ST segment. ST segment depression typically reverts to normal following the administration of oxygen if this intervention corrects the myocardial hypoxia. ST segment depression may be evident on a 12-lead EKG strip following both angina and strenuous exercise.

ST segment depression characterized by a dip below the isoelectric line of 1 to 2 millimeters or one to two small boxes on the EKG graph paper

J point the point on the EKG strip where the QRS complex meets the ST segment

Myocardial injury

Because "time is muscle," the continuum of the hypoxic state of the myocardial cells will cause progression to myocardial injury. At this time in the event, the injured cells are still viable and salvageable. However, the cells will die if the hypoxic state is not quickly alleviated. Myocardial injury can be extensive enough to produce a decrease in electrical conduction and/or pump (mechanical) function.

Without appropriate intervention, at this point in the myocardial event, the patient's signs and symptoms may intensify slightly. In addition to the signs and symptoms

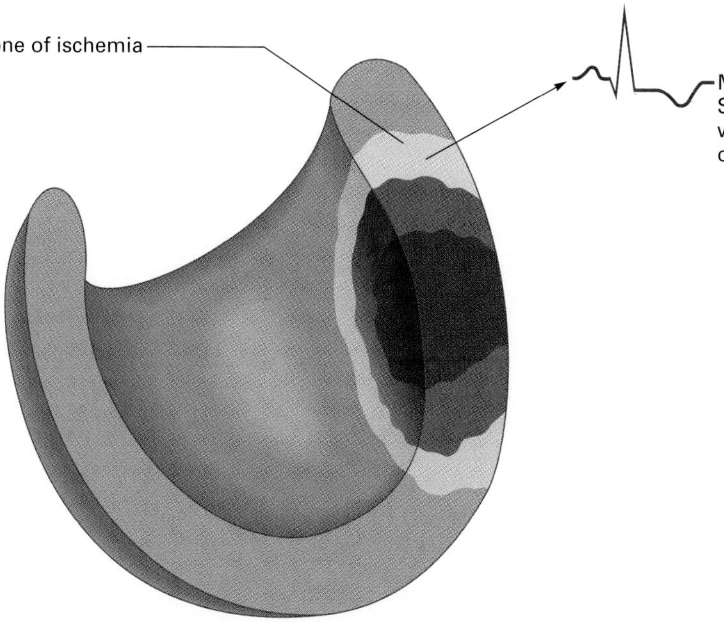

Zone of ischemia —————

Myocardial ischemia causes
ST segment depression with or
without T wave inversion as result
of altered repolarization

Figure 8–2. EKG changes reflecting myocardial ischemia

listed previously, the patient may continue to complain of chest pain of increased magnitude. Clinically, you may note that the patient becomes pale and his or her anxiety level may increase. In addition, it is at the point that some patients may begin to complain of **dyspnea** (difficulty in breathing).

EKG changes with myocardial injury include ST segment elevation and/or T wave inversion (Figure 8–3). The most significant and frequently identifiable of these EKG changes is **ST segment elevation,** which usually occurs in two or more contiguous leads. The ST segment elevation is characterized by a rise above the isoelectric line of 1 to 2 millimeters or one to two small boxes on the EKG graph paper.

ST segment elevation provides the primary indication of myocardial injury in progress. There may also be **T wave inversion** suggestive of the presence of ischemia. ST segments are elevated in the leads that represent the area of injury and may be depressed in the opposite leads.

Myocardial necrosis

As the myocardial ischemia and injury continue uncorrected, some cells will begin to sustain irreversible damage and infarct. At this point, cellular death (necrosis) occurs and the patient will experience a myocardial infarction. It is critical at this point that you, the health-care provider, realize that at the point of myocardial necrosis the myocardial tissue and cells will not—CANNOT—return to normal, even when reoxygenation is initiated. The necrotic cells become scar tissue and do not respond to electrical stimulus or provide any contractile functions. This is the point that we must strive *not* to allow the patient to reach. Now you may better comprehend the concept "time is muscle."

Signs and symptoms of an acute myocardial infarction are numerous. Recall that the precipitating event of an AMI is often a thrombus. As discussed in detail in Chapter 7, the most common presenting sign or symptom of AMI is substernal or epigastric chest pain. Other common signs and symptoms include diaphoresis, anxiety, dyspnea, nausea, vomiting, **pallor,** general weakness, and **malaise.** As a health-care provider, be aware that some patients who are experiencing an AMI will express a feeling of impending

dyspnea difficulty breathing

ST segment elevation characterized by a rise above the isoelectric line of 1 to 2 millimeters or one to two small boxes on the EKG graph paper

T wave inversion negative deflection of the T wave below the isoelectric line

pallor paleness

malaise generalized feeling of discomfort and fatigue

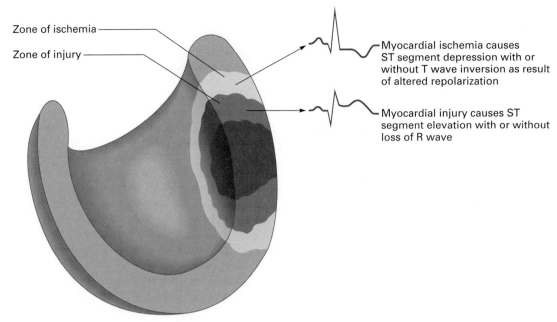

Zone of ischemia
Zone of injury

Myocardial ischemia causes ST segment depression with or without T wave inversion as result of altered repolarization

Myocardial injury causes ST segment elevation with or without loss of R wave

Figure 8–3. EKG changes reflecting myocardial injury

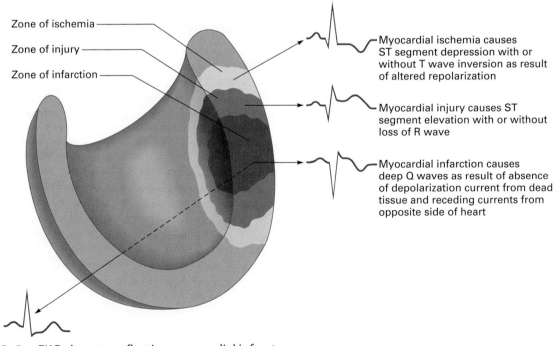

Zone of ischemia
Zone of injury
Zone of infarction

Myocardial ischemia causes ST segment depression with or without T wave inversion as result of altered repolarization

Myocardial injury causes ST segment elevation with or without loss of R wave

Myocardial infarction causes deep Q waves as result of absence of depolarization current from dead tissue and receding currents from opposite side of heart

Figure 8–4. EKG changes reflecting myocardial infarct

pathologic Q wave a Q wave that is equal or greater than 0.04 second (one small box) in width and has a depth of greater than one-third of the height of the succeeding R wave

doom. If a patient tells you that he or she is going to die, you would be well advised to believe the patient. Many times they will do just that.

The development of the **pathologic Q wave** often begins within the first 2 hours after the MI and, in most cases, is complete within 24 hours. Q waves occur because of the absence of a depolarization wave as a result of necrotic tissue. One of the more reliable EKG changes noted when a patient is experiencing an AMI is the presence of pathologic Q waves (Figure 8–4). However, you should realize that the appearance of the pathologic Q wave is a later finding than is the development of ST segment elevation. Pathologic Q waves can be found on a 12-lead tracing as long as 6 to 12 months post-MI. Therefore, the presence of a pathologic Q wave does not indicate (in and of itself) the age of an MI.

A Q wave is considered abnormal if it is equal to or greater than 0.04 second (one small box) in width and has a depth of greater than one-third of the height of the succeeding R wave. It must be emphasized that the size of the pathologic Q wave depends on the degree of infarct that the myocardial muscle has sustained. If damage is very minimal, the pathologic Q wave may not develop. There are also non-Q wave MIs, which we will discuss in a later chapter.

CLINICAL SIGNIFICANCE

As emphasized in Chapter 7, all chest pain is considered clinically significant and thus must be managed in a timely and appropriate manner. Although you are not expected to definitively diagnose an acute myocardial infarction in the prehospital arena, or in the emergency department (ED) or intensive care unit (ICU) for that matter, it is critically important that you learn and commit to memory the various signs and symptoms that will be exhibited as the patient progresses from myocardial ischemia through the myocardial injury event and, finally (without proper intervention), into the myocardial necrotic state.

Thus, timely assessment and management, including immediate oxygen administration, must be rapidly initiated and completed within a 10-minute interval. Your initial assessment and evaluation should focus on the patient's general appearance. *Remember that time is muscle and act accordingly.*

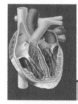

Summary
CHAPTER 8

Now that the phrase "time is muscle" has been explained in detail, you should have gained a new appreciation of its meaning. Understanding the pathophysiology of ischemia, injury, and necrosis will help you to appreciate the significance of prompt and appropriate intervention. When dealing with a patient who is complaining of chest pain, it is your utmost responsibility to act quickly and appropriately to provide optimal-quality patient care.

Key Points to Remember
CHAPTER 8

1. The fundamental goal of the management of the patient who has symptomatic chest pain is to strive to interrupt the infarction process.

2. Myocardial ischemia is the deprivation of oxygen and other nutrients to the heart muscle.

3. Myocardial ischemia EKG changes include ST segment depression, T wave inversion, or peaked T waves.

4. Myocardial injury is damage to the myocardium resulting from, and following, myocardial ischemia.

5. Myocardial injury EKG changes include ST segment elevation and/or T wave inversion.

6. Myocardial necrosis is death of the myocardial tissue.

7. Myocardial necrosis is in most cases indicated on the EKG with a pathologic Q wave.

8. A pathologic Q wave is identified when it is equal or greater than 0.04 second in width and has a depth of greater than one-third of the height of the succeeding R wave.

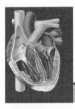

Review Questions
CHAPTER 8

1. The coronary arteries receive oxygenated blood from the:
   a. aorta.
   b. coronary sinus.
   c. pulmonary veins.
   d. pulmonary arteries.

2. Signs and symptoms the health-care provider may expect to observe in a patient with necrotic heart tissue could include:
   a. dysrhythmias.
   b. congestive heart failure.
   c. cardiogenic shock (severe).
   d. All of the above are possible.

3. The function of the chordae tendineae and papillary muscles is to:
   a. prevent backflow of blood into the ventricles.
   b. protect the coronary orifices when the aortic valve opens.
   c. prevent backflow of blood into the atrium.
   d. facilitate backflow of blood from the aorta.

4. The right atrium receives blood from the myocardium via the:
   a. left marginal branch.
   b. inferior vena cava.
   c. great cardiac vein.
   d. internal carotid artery.

5. The coronary sinus returns deoxygenated blood from the:

   a. aorta.

   b. myocardium.

   c. pulmonary veins.

   d. pulmonary arteries.

6. Most cardiac dysrhythmias are caused by ischemia secondary to hypoxia; therefore the most appropriate drug to give a patient with any dysrhythmia is:

   a. oxygen.

   b. D5W.

   c. lidocaine.

   d. morphine.

7. Defined as death of the myocardial tissue, a myocardial infarction commonly results from:

   a. myocardial necrosis.

   b. myocardial injury.

   c. myocardial ischemia.

   d. muscle oxygenation.

8. EKG changes that may be anticipated as a result of myocardial ischemia, injury, and/or necrosis of the myocardial tissues include all of the following *except:*

   a. PR interval prolongation.

   b. ST segment elevation.

   c. ST segment depression.

   d. pathologic Q wave.

9. The development of pathologic Q waves often begins within the first 2 hours after the MI and, in most cases, is complete within ___ hour(s).

   a. 1

   b. 1/2

   c. 24

   d. 48

10. ST segment depression may be evident on a 12-lead EKG strip following both angina and strenuous exercise.

    a. False

    b. True

11. EKG changes of significance with myocardial ischemia include ST segment depression, T wave inversion, or ___ wave.

    a. depressed T

    b. peaked T

    c. peaked P

    d. inverted P

12. Chest pain should be considered to be cardiac in origin and managed accordingly until proven otherwise.

   a. True

   b. False

13. With myocardial injury, the most significant and frequently identifiable change is:

   a. ST depression.

   b. ST elevation.

   c. pathologic Q waves.

   d. peaked T waves.

14. Deprivation of oxygen and other nutrients to the heart muscle may be defined as myocardial:

   a. injury.

   b. ischemia.

   c. necrosis.

   d. infarction.

15. A Q wave is considered abnormal if it is equal to or greater than 0.04 second (one small box) in width and has a depth of ____ of the height of the succeeding R wave.

   a. 30% or less

   b. 15% or less

   c. 45% or more

   d. 25% or more

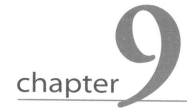

chapter 9

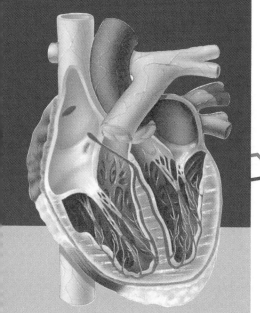

Interpretation of Inferior MIs

objectives

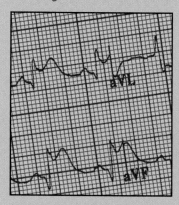

Upon completion of this chapter, the student will be able to:

➤ Review the anatomy and physiology of the heart, with particular emphasis on

   a. Coronary circulation

   b. Degree of myocardial wall involvement (i.e., transmural and subendocardial)

➤ Identify the lead-specific ST elevation parameters

➤ Recognize the EKG changes related to an inferior infarction

➤ Describe the clinical significance of inferior MIs

INTRODUCTION

In this book's earlier chapters and/or in the companion book, *Understanding EKGs: A Practical Approach* 2nd ed., you learned the essential parameters of basic dysrhythmia interpretation. As we move through this textbook, the picture becomes a bit more complex. We recognize now that critical therapeutic management of acute myocardial infarction depends on rapid recognition and correct determination of the **infarct** area. Consequently, the role of the nonphysician intervener as a skilled interpreter of the 12-lead EKG is becoming increasingly significant, because the 12-lead EKG can be used to identify the area of the heart affected by the infarct.

There currently exists an extensive amount of knowledge specific to cardiology, including electrocardiology. We would like you to understand that this text focuses on the recognition and interpretation of 12-lead EKGs; we do not presume to include all aspects of a 12-lead EKG in this approach. Rather, we wish to provide you with a practical and workable knowledge of the parameters of basic 12-lead EKG interpretation.

In this chapter, we begin our discussion of the specific types of myocardial infarctions that your patients may experience. We consciously elected to begin the presentation with the discussion of inferior MIs. In our clinical experience, it appears that inferior MIs are the most common types of infarcts encountered in the emergent setting.

ANATOMY AND PHYSIOLOGY REVIEW

This is a perfect time for you to go back and review Chapters 1 and 2 of this text. You should pay particular attention to the discussion of the coronary circulation (Figure 9–1). A thorough understanding of the anatomy and physiology of the heart is essential to your comprehension of 12-lead EKG interpretation.

Recall now that the heart is perfused with oxygenated blood through a process known as coronary circulation. This process involves the two main coronary arteries that branch off the aorta. Remember also that the two main coronary arteries are called the *left main coronary artery* and the *right main coronary artery* (Table 9–1). These vital structures supply the heart muscle, or myocardium, with freshly oxygenated blood (i.e., blood rich with oxygen). **Inferior wall infarctions** are involved with the right coronary artery. Because of this important association, we will now review the distribution areas of the coronary arteries (Table 9–2).

To review once again, inferior wall infarctions are commonly associated with the *right* coronary artery. The right coronary artery extends from the aorta around to the posterior part of the heart. Branches of the right coronary artery furnish blood to the lateral wall of the right ventricle. A branch of the right coronary artery called the *posterior interventricular artery* or *posterior descending artery* lies in the posterior interventricular region and supplies blood to the posterior and inferior part of the heart's left ventricle. The right coronary artery branches also supply oxygen-rich blood to a portion of the electrical conduction system.

infarct necrosis of tissue following loss of blood supply

inferior wall infarction interruption of the supply of oxygen-rich blood to the inferior myocardial wall involved with the right coronary artery

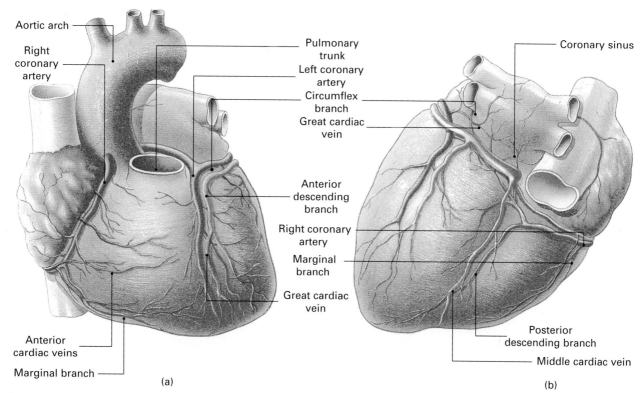

Figure 9–1. Coronary circulation

Table 9–1

Coronary artery divisions/branches	
Left Coronary Arteries	**Right Coronary Arteries**
Left anterior descending	Posterior descending
Marginal	Marginal
Circumflex	

Table 9–2

Distribution of blood supply to the myocardium	
Left Coronary Arteries	**Right Coronary Arteries**
Anterior left ventricular wall	Lateral wall of the right ventricle
Lateral wall of the left ventricle	A portion of the electrical conduction system
Posterior wall of the left ventricle	Posterior wall of left ventricle
Left interventricular septal wall	Inferior wall of left ventricle

TRANSMURAL VERSUS SUBENDOCARDIAL INFARCTIONS

As you may recall from Chapter 7, MIs usually follow the occlusion of a severely narrowed atherosclerotic coronary artery. Many factors may contribute to the occlusion, including atherosclerotic plaques, platelet activation, vasospasms, and formation of thrombi (blood clots). The majority of MIs (90%) are the result of thrombi formation.

Myocardial infarctions may be classified as either transmural or subendocardial. **Subendocardial infarctions** are commonly referred to as *nontransmural.* **Transmural infarctions** (literally translated "across the wall" infarctions) involve the entire full thickness of the ventricular wall, extending from the endocardium to the epicardial surface. It has long been accepted that the area of infarct begins in the subendocardium, possibly because this area has the highest myocardial oxygen demand, yet the least supply of blood at any given time. Once begun, and if not quickly disrupted, the infarction progresses outward in a wavelike motion until full involvement of the entire myocardium has occurred.

Subendocardial or nontransmural infarctions involve only a portion of the ventricular wall, most commonly the subendocardial layer closest to the endocardium. For purposes of this discussion, recall that the coronary arteries lie on the surface of the heart at the endocardium. Thus, interruption of the supply of oxygen-rich blood will adversely affect the subendocardial (deeper) layers of the heart more readily than the superficial layers.

Once again consider the Q wave. It is commonly accepted that if the Q wave pattern exhibits no changes in an EKG strip taken within 24 hours of an infarction, a subendocardial or nontransmural infarction is suggested. However, if the normal appearance of a Q wave has been significantly altered within 24 hours of the onset of the infarction, a transmural infarction has likely occurred. Understand, however, that not all transmural infarctions develop Q waves and that some nontransmural infarctions may cause Q wave abnormalities. Figure 9–2 illustrates both a subendocardial infarction and a transmural infarction along with relevant EKG tracings.

LEAD-SPECIFIC ST ELEVATION

The leads that record electrical impulses generated from the heart's electrical conduction system actually "view" or "look at" specific areas of damaged myocardium. These leads are called **facing leads.** EKG findings of infarction may occur in a single lead or in a combination of leads; however, for these findings to be significant, evidence should be in two or more contiguous leads. Leads II, III, and aVF visualize the inferior (nearest the diaphragm) surface of the heart.

In addition, Leads II, III, and aVF are anatomically adjacent (or bordering); that is, all three leads view adjoining tissues located in the inferior region of the left ventricle. If ST segment elevation is noted in two leads (i.e., Lead II and V_1) that are not adjacent, your index of suspicion for myocardial infarction would be a bit diminished, because these two leads view different areas of the heart. If ST segment elevation is noted in the lower limb leads (Leads II, III, and aVF), this finding is indicative of inferior myocardial infarction involving the inferior wall of the left ventricle. ST segment elevation is an extremely relevant finding in the recognition of an MI in the initial hours of occurrence.

In simpler terms, if your patient is exhibiting clinical signs and symptoms consistent with a myocardial infarction AND you notice that ST segment elevation is present

subendocardial infarction involves only a portion of the ventricular wall, most commonly the subendocardial layer closest to the endocardium. Also called nontransmural infarction

transmural infarction involves the entire full thickness of the ventricular wall, extending from the endocardium to the epicardial surface

facing leads leads that "view" or "look at" specific areas of damaged myocardium

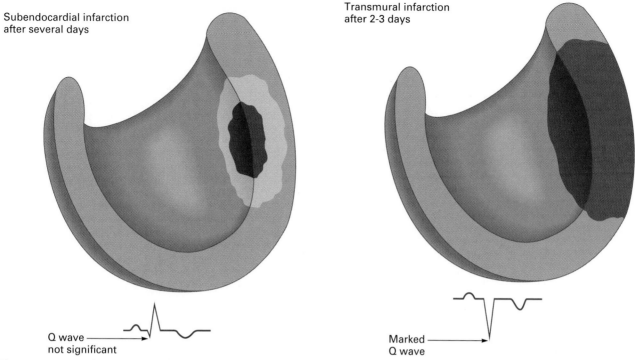

Subendocardial infarction
after several days

Transmural infarction
after 2-3 days

Q wave
not significant

Marked
Q wave

Figure 9–2. Subendocardial and transmural infarctions with relevant EKG tracings

in Leads II, III, and aVF, your index of suspicion regarding the presence of an inferior MI should begin to increase.

You will also notice the presence of ST segment depression in the **reciprocal leads.** Reciprocal leads are those that record the electrical impulse formation in uninvolved myocardium directly opposite the involved myocardium.

Now, it is time for you to look at and study a 12-lead EKG strip that illustrates ST segment elevation (Leads II, III, and aVF) and reciprocal changes (Leads I, aVL, V_2, and V_3). (See Figure 9–3.). Recall that in Chapter 6 we discussed a systematic approach to EKG interpretation. We advised you then and we will repeat this advice now: Always, always follow the logical and workable 5 + 3 approach in order to correctly interpret 12-lead EKG strips. The first five steps include the systematic approach to basic EKG interpretation; for analysis of a 12-lead EKG strip, we have added three additional steps: ST segment depression, ST segment elevation, and pathologic Q wave.

You will recall that the basic five steps are:

reciprocal leads
leads that record electrical impulses in myocardial cells opposite involved myocardium

Rate	Rhythm	P wave	PR interval	QRS complex

The 5 + 3 approach is:

Rate	Rhythm	P wave	PR interval	QRS complex

PLUS

ST segment depression	ST segment elevation	Q wave

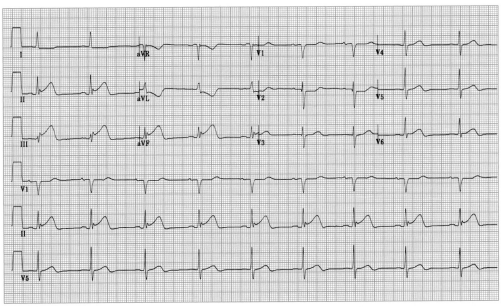

Figure 9–3. Example of 12-lead EKG illustrating changes consistent with inferior MI

Now, apply the steps in the 5 + 3 approach to the strip in Figure 9–3:

Rate: _____

Rhythm: _____

P wave: _____

PR interval: _____

QRS complex: _____

ST segment depression: _____

ST segment elevation: _____

Q wave: _____

We hope you came up with the following answers. If so, you are well on your way!

Rate: 54	*Rhythm:* regular	*P wave:* present; upright	*PR interval:* 0.16 sec (four small boxes)	*QRS complex:* 0.04 sec (one small box)

PLUS

ST segment depression: Leads I, aVL, V₂, V₃	*ST segment elevation:* Leads II, III, aVF	*Q wave:* nonpathologic (within normal limits)

Interpretation: inferior MI, as evidenced by ST segment elevation in Leads II, III, and aVF.

EKG CHANGES RELATED TO AN INFERIOR INFARCTION

EKG changes that occur in reciprocal leads are termed *reciprocal changes.* A potential diagnosis of myocardial infarction may be reinforced by the presence of reciprocal changes. Reciprocal changes in the anterior (V_3 and V_4) and lateral walls, as noted in Leads I and aVL and/or V_5 and V_6, may be noted in the event of an inferior infarction.

In addition to the occurrence of ST segment elevation, T wave inversion and the evolution of significant Q waves in Leads II, III and aVF may also indicate inferior myocardial infarction. As a novice and a student learning the parameters of 12-lead EKG interpretation, it is imperative that you realize the necessity of focusing on lead-specific ST changes.

Although it is important that you look for and recognize pathologic Q waves, you must realize that the appearance of these Q waves indicates that significant muscle damage has already occurred. By the time you see a pathologic Q wave on a 12-lead EKG strip, you should recognize that the MI may have occurred hours previous to this discovery. Nonetheless, in the absence of other findings (i.e., ST segment elevation), the observation of a pathologic Q wave finding must be accompanied by particular attention to the patient's current signs and symptoms, as well as a thorough assessment of the patient's previous medical history.

If the lateral wall is also damaged, EKG changes may be seen in Leads V_5 and V_6. Study Figure 9–4 in order to visualize the appearance of the EKG waveform changes that may be indicative of inferior infarcts.

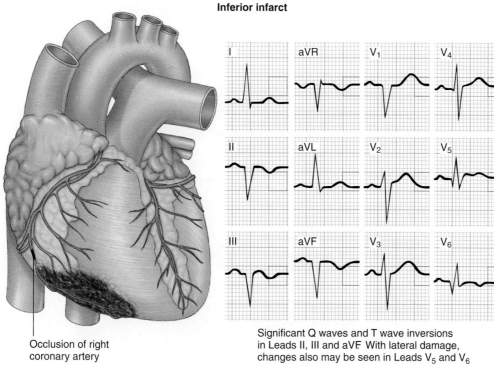

Inferior infarct

Occlusion of right
coronary artery

Significant Q waves and T wave inversions
in Leads II, III and aVF With lateral damage,
changes also may be seen in Leads V_5 and V_6

Figure 9–4. Inferior infarct

CLINICAL SIGNIFICANCE OF INFERIOR MIs

Remember that your main focus in dealing with 12-lead EKGs in the prehospital and emergent settings is *early recognition and early intervention.* Therefore, EKG findings consistent with ST segment elevation, which is indicative of ongoing injury, will serve as the hallmark for you to detect or identify an acute MI in the early hours.

As you have learned, early recognition and prompt treatment may prevent the extension of an MI. Your knowledge of EKG changes will enhance your ability to appropriately manage patients who present with chest pain and aberrant EKG patterns.

Remember always that your patient's clinical picture is the primary focus of your concern. Is your patient clinically stable or unstable? A patient who is clinically stable will generally be alert and oriented and will present vital signs that are within normal limits for that particular patient. He or she may or may not complain of chest pain during your initial encounter. However, the patient who is clinically unstable may present with an altered level of consciousness, moderate to severe chest pain, and blood pressure alterations.

right ventricular infarction (RVI) a complication that occurs in approximately 40% of inferior MIs and indicates a larger infarction that most likely involves both ventricles

If your patient is hypotensive and is exhibiting EKG changes consistent with an inferior myocardial infarction, consider the possibility of **right ventricular infarction (RVI).** RVI is a complication that occurs in approximately 40% of inferior MIs and indicates a larger infarction that most likely involves both ventricles. RVI should be suspected in patients who present with changes in Leads II, III, and aVF because these changes are indicative of an inferior MI. Whenever these EKG changes are noted and are accompanied by the presence of hypotension, distended neck veins, and lung sounds that are relatively clear upon auscultation, you must have a high index of suspicion that RVI is present.

If you suspect that your patient has developed RVI, an EKG with right-sided chest leads should be obtained. Do this by placing the V leads on the right side of the chest (Figures 9–5 and 9–6). However, the V leads most commonly utilized include V$_4$R and V$_5$R. This view allows the EKG leads to look directly at the right ventricle and to show ST segment elevation created by the infarct.

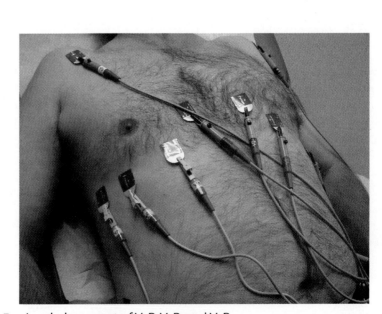

Figure 9–5. Lead placement of V$_3$R, V$_4$R, and V$_5$R

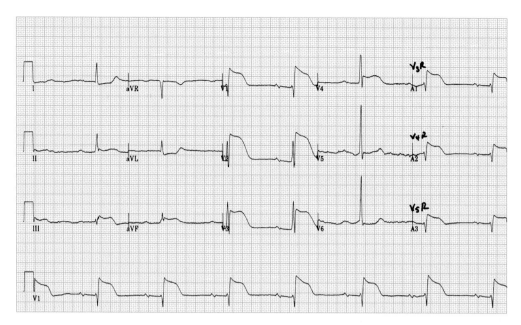

Figure 9–6.   15-lead EKG

If you recall both the structure and function of the heart's lower chambers (the ventricles), you may remember that the ventricles function primarily to propel blood through both the pulmonary and systemic circulation. You will realize that any damage to or weakness of the ventricles will compromise the force with which the ventricles contract. Blood flow may thus be interrupted in the ventricles and ultimately compromise perfusion.

When considering the management of the patient who presents with indications of RVI, the health-care provider should seek physician intervention for guidance. In an effort to increase preload, the administration of a fluid bolus in conjunction with morphine and/or nitroglycerin may be indicated. Be aware that the administration of nitrates will produce vasodilation, which may produce hypotension. Management of patients with RVI will be dependent upon the treatment preferences of the attending physicians.

Be aware also that RVI may exist without being extensive enough to exhibit significant hemodynamic compromise. This is due to the fact that there are various degrees of severity of RVI. Careful attention to the assessment of your patient is imperative.

As mentioned many times in this text, the significance of early intervention for patients with suspected AMI cannot be overemphasized. Recall yet again that time is muscle, and act accordingly. Timely assessment and management, including immediate oxygen administration, must be rapidly initiated and completed within a 10-minute time interval whenever feasible. Your initial assessment and evaluation, whether in the prehospital or in-hospital arena, should focus on the *most* important diagnostic tool—the patient's general appearance.

A thorough and timely evaluation and management of the patient's ABCs is imperative. Any problem encountered during this evaluation must be managed quickly, followed by a rapid assessment of vital signs. Note that vital signs are unreliable as predictors of AMI. They vary greatly and need to be interpreted in correlation with the patient's status. In spite of this fact, it is important that you monitor and record vital signs at frequent intervals.

Another very important assessment tool that you will utilize when managing the suspected AMI patient is the cardiac monitor. You must be particularly alert to the presence of EKG changes, as well as the occurrence of dysrhythmias that originate from ischemic and injured myocardial tissues, as these are common occurrences with acute myocardial infarctions.

Your suspicion of an acute inferior MI must be based on a combination of a definitive 12-lead EKG and the patient's clinical appearance and signs and symptoms. Remember to keep in mind that a negative 12-lead EKG does NOT rule out the presence of an AMI. Remember also that any patients who complain of chest pain must be thoroughly evaluated and their management continued until the possibility of AMI is ruled out by the physician.

Summary
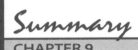
CHAPTER 9

In our collective years of clinical experience, it is clear to us that an inferior MI is the most common type of MI encountered. This particular type of MI can also involve the right ventricle. This event may be evidenced by obtaining a right-sided EKG. The injury pattern will involve Leads II, III, and aVF with reciprocal changes in the lateral and anterior leads. The necessity for and importance of early intervention is paramount when dealing with a patient who is experiencing an inferior MI. This critical intervention may be the key to salvaging myocardial tissue and to ultimately preventing the extension of the infarction damage.

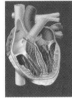
Key Points to Remember
CHAPTER 9

1. The two main coronary arteries are the left main coronary artery and the right main coronary artery.
2. The left coronary artery branches off into the left anterior descending, the marginal, and circumflex arteries.
3. The right coronary artery branches off into the posterior descending and marginal arteries.
4. Transmural infarctions involve the entire full thickness of the ventricular wall.
5. Subendocardial or nontransmural infarctions involve only a portion of the ventricular wall.
6. Leads II, III, and aVF visualize the inferior surface of the heart.
7. ST elevation in Leads II, III, and aVF indicate an inferior infarction.
8. Reciprocal leads are those that record the electrical impulse formation in uninvolved myocardium directly opposite from involved myocardium.
9. Reciprocal changes with inferior MI may include ST depression in V_3, V_4, and/or Leads I, aVL, and/or V_5 and V_6.

10. Right ventricular infarction is a complication that occurs in 40% of inferior MIs and indicates involvement of both ventricles.

11. V leads placed on the right side of the chest allow the EKG leads to "look at" the right ventricle.

Review Questions
CHAPTER 9

1. Two primary structures are responsible for delivering oxygen-rich blood to the myocardium. These structures are the:

   a. coronary sinuses.

   b. cerebral sinuses.

   c. coronary arteries.

   d. cerebral arteries.

2. There are ___ main coronary arteries.

   a. six

   b. three

   c. four

   d. two

3. Inferior wall infarctions are associated with the:

   a. right coronary artery.

   b. left coronary artery.

   c. bundle of His.

   d. coronary sinus.

4. Myocardial infarctions may be classified as either transmural or:

   a. supraendocardial.

   b. subendocardial.

   c. endocardial.

   d. precardial.

5. Subendocardial infarctions are commonly referred to as:

   a. full thickness.

   b. transmural.

   c. nontransmural.

   d. transdermal.

6. Leads that record electrical impulses generated from the heart's electrical conduction system, and that "look at" specific areas of damaged myocardium, are called ___ leads.

   a. reciprocal

   b. facing

   c. viewing

   d. specific

7. EKG findings of infarction may occur in a single lead or in a combination of leads.

   a. True

   b. False

8. The most important diagnostic tool that you can use when assessing and treating a patient with a suspected inferior MI is the:

   a. 12-lead EKG machine.

   b. cardiac enzyme.

   c. patient's clinical appearance.

   d. patient's presenting vital signs.

9. ST segment elevation is noted in the limb leads, Leads II, III, and aVF. This finding is indicative of ___ myocardial infarction.

   a. anterior

   b. lateral

   c. superior

   d. inferior

10. EKG Leads that record the electrical impulse formation in uninvolved myocardium directly opposite from the involved myocardium are called ___ leads.

    a. facing

    b. viewing

    c. reciprocal

    d. endocardial

11. If your patient is hypotensive, and is exhibiting EKG changes consistent with an inferior myocardial infarction, you should consider the possibility of ___ infarction.

    a. right atrial

    b. left atrial

    c. right ventricular

    d. left interatrial

12. Any patient who complains of chest pain must be thoroughly evaluated and management continued until the possibility of AMI is ruled out by the physician.

    a. True

    b. False

13. Reciprocal leads for the inferior MI are Leads:

  a. II and III.

  b. V_1 and V_2.

  c. aVL and aVF.

  d. I and aVL.

14. When obtaining a right-sided EKG, the leads that should be moved are:

  a. V_3, V_4, and V_5.

  b. V_1, V_2, and V_3.

  c. V_5, V_6, and V_7.

  d. I, II, and III.

15. A non-Q wave MI is consistent with:

  a. full thickness.

  b. montransmural.

  c. transmural.

  d. endocardial.

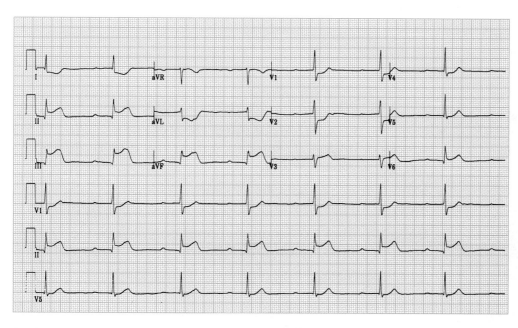

Review strip

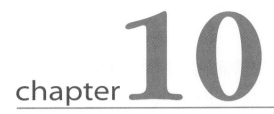

Interpretation of Anterior MIs

objectives

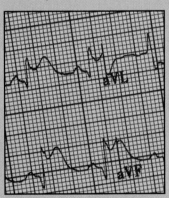

Upon completion of this chapter, the student will be able to:

➤ Describe the anatomy of the coronary arteries, with special emphasis on the description and distribution of the left coronary artery

➤ Identify the lead-specific ST segment elevation relative to anterior MIs, as well as anterolateral and anteroseptal MIs

➤ Describe other EKG changes commonly associated with anterior MIs, as well as anterolateral and anteroseptal MIs

➤ Identify the clinical significance of anterior MIs

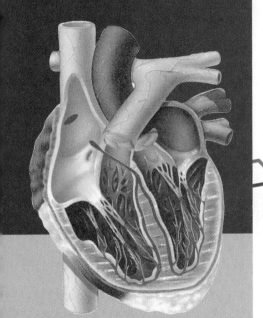

INTRODUCTION

Generally, myocardial infarctions that involve the mass of the left ventricle are considered quite serious. This consideration is based on the fact that the left ventricle of the heart is considered to be the workhorse of the heart—that is, it performs the important function of supplying the entire body with oxygen-rich blood. Consequently, you must be familiar with the indicators that lead you to suspect both inferior and anterior MI events. **Anterior MIs** tend to involve a larger muscle mass than do inferior MIs. Chapter 9 discussed inferior MIs. In this chapter, you will learn about anterior, anteroseptal, and anterolateral MIs.

anterior MIs the interruption of blood supply to the anterior myocardial wall; primarily involves the left anterior descending artery

ANATOMY OF THE CORONARY ARTERIES

The discussion of anterior MIs will primarily involve the *left coronary artery;* therefore, this anatomy review will focus on reviewing the branches and areas of the heart supplied by the left coronary artery (Figure 10–1). As we discussed in Chapter 7, as the left coronary artery leaves the aorta, it immediately divides into the left anterior descending (LAD) artery and the circumflex artery. The anterior descending artery (located immediately to the left of the interventricular septum) is the major branch of the left coronary artery and supplies blood to most of the anterior wall of the left ventricle.

A marginal branch of the left coronary artery supplies blood to the lateral wall of the left ventricle. The circumflex branch of the left coronary artery extends around to

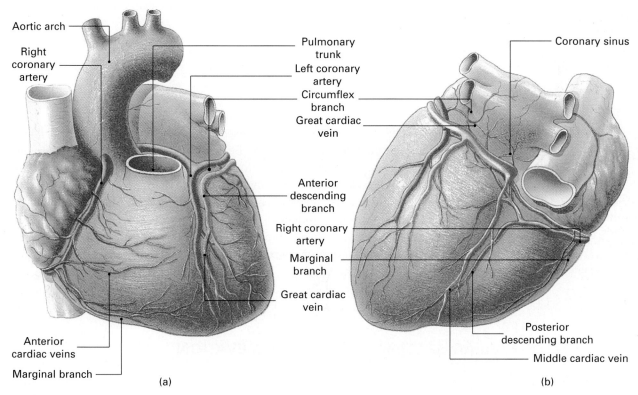

(a)   (b)

Figure 10–1.   Coronary circulation

Table 10–1

Coronary artery divisions/branches

Left Coronary Arteries	Right Coronary Arteries
Left anterior descending	Posterior descending
Marginal	Marginal
Circumflex	

Table 10–2

Distribution of blood supply to the myocardium

Left Coronary Arteries	Right Coronary Arteries
Anterior left ventricular wall	Lateral wall of the right ventricle
Lateral wall of the left ventricle	A portion of the electrical conduction system
Posterior wall of the left ventricle	Posterior wall of left ventricle
Left interventricular septal wall	Inferior wall of left ventricle

the posterior side of the heart and its branches supply blood to much of the posterior wall of the heart. Each of these divisions has numerous branches that form a network of smaller arteries and arterioles.

As a reminder, we would like for you to look once again at Tables 10–1 and 10–2.

"WIDOWMAKER"

You should remember that the left anterior descending (LAD) artery is the largest of the coronary arteries in the majority of patients. Because of its size and the large amount of myocardium that it supplies, massive infarction of cardiac tissue can result if the LAD becomes totally occluded. Because of the potential for massive infarction, the LAD is sometimes called the **widowmaker,** the implications of which are disturbing and obvious.

widowmaker
term used to illustrate the serious result of total occlusion of the left anterior descending artery

A higher incidence of cardiogenic shock and mortality has been associated with anterior and septal infarctions. In addition, LAD occlusion is notably associated with the development of second- and third-degree heart blocks. In certain cases, pacing appears to be clinically indicated; however, due to the significant degree of muscle damage, electrical activity may be affected, but mechanical function will most likely not respond.

LEAD-SPECIFIC ST SEGMENT ELEVATION

As a brief review, the EKG leads that record electrical impulses generated from the heart's electrical conduction system actually "view" or "look at" specific areas of damaged myocardium. These leads are called *indicative* or *facing leads.*

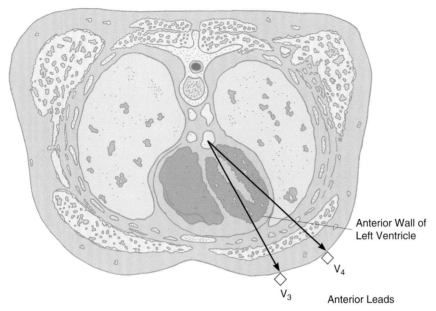

Figure 10–2.   Cross-section of the heart with chest leads and associated myocardial wall areas

Again, as a reminder, EKG findings of infarction may occur in a single lead or in a combination of leads; however for these findings to be significant, evidence should be in two or more contiguous leads. Leads V_3 and V_4 are the indicative (facing) leads that visualize the anterior wall of the heart's left ventricle (Figure 10–2). The reciprocal leads for an anterior MI are Leads II, III, and aVF; however, most often there are usually no significant reciprocal lead EKG changes with anterior MI.

Remember that only rarely do MIs involve the anterior wall exclusively. Most often, either the septal or lateral walls of the ventricles are involved in an acute anterior MI. Leads V_1, V_2, V_3, and V_4 will illustrate ST segment elevation in the face of an **anteroseptal MI.** (Septal MIs will be discussed in Chapter 11.) This finding often indicates a larger mass of myocardial muscle involvement than does an isolated finding in V_3 and V_4. Leads V_3, V_4, V_5, V_6, I, and aVL will illustrate ST segment elevation in the event of an **anterolateral MI.** (Lateral MIs will be discussed in Chapter 12.) This finding also indicates a larger degree of ventricular wall involvement than does the isolated finding in V_3 and V_4. Both anteroseptal and anterolateral MIs will be discussed in more detail in subsequent chapters.

ST segment elevation is an extremely relevant finding in the recognition of an MI in the initial hours of occurrence. In simpler terms, if your patient is exhibiting clinical signs and symptoms consistent with a myocardial infarction AND you notice that ST segment elevation is present in Leads V_3 and V_4, your index of suspicion regarding the presence of an anterior MI should begin to increase.

Now look at and study a 12-lead EKG strip that illustrates ST segment elevation (Lead V_3 and V_4). Note that there are no reciprocal changes in Leads II, III, and aVF. Again, recall the Chapter 6 discussion about the systematic approach to EKG interpretation. Remember that you should always follow the logical and workable 5 + 3 approach in order to correctly interpret 12-lead EKG strips. The first five steps include the systematic approach to basic EKG interpretation; for analysis of a 12-lead EKG strip, we have added three additional steps: ST segment depression, ST segment elevation, and pathologic Q wave.

anteroseptal MI
involves decreased blood supply to the interventricular septum and the anterior wall of the left ventricle; illustrated by ST segment elevation in Leads V_1, V_2, V_3, and V_4

anterolateral MI
involves decreased blood supply to the lateral wall of the left ventricle in conjunction with proximal occlusion of the left anterior descending artery; illustrated by ST segment elevation in Leads V_3, V_4, V_5, V_6, I, and aVL

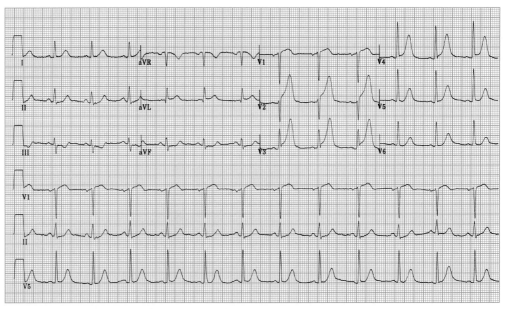

Figure 10–3. Example of 12-lead EKG illustrating changes consistent with anterior MI

You will recall that the basic five steps are:

Rate	Rhythm	P wave	PR interval	QRS complex

The 5 + 3 approach is:

Rate	Rhythm	P wave	PR interval	QRS complex

PLUS

ST segment depression	ST segment elevation	Q wave

Now, apply each of the steps in the 5 + 3 approach to the strip in Figure 10–3:

Rate: _____

Rhythm: _____

P wave: _____

PR interval: _____

QRS complex: _____

ST segment depression: _____

ST segment elevation: _____

Q wave: _____

We hope you came up with the following answers. If so, you are well on your way!

Rate: 74	Rhythm: regular	P wave: present; upright	PR interval: 0.16 sec (four small boxes)	QRS complex: 0.04 sec (one small box)

PLUS

ST segment depression: none	ST segment elevation: Leads V_2, V_3, V_4	Q wave: nonpathologic (within normal limits)

Interpretation: anterior MI, as evidenced by ST segment elevation in Leads V_2, V_3, and V_4

EKG CHANGES COMMONLY ASSOCIATED WITH ANTERIOR MIs

In addition to the occurrence of ST segment elevation, T wave inversion and the evolution of significant Q waves in Leads V_3 and V_4 may indicate anterior myocardial infarction. As a reminder, pathologic Q waves are not an early indicator or EKG finding, but occur as later evidence of myocardial tissue damage.

Another EKG finding indicative of an anterior MI may be absent or poor R wave progression in the V leads. You may recall from the discussion of R wave progression in Chapter 5 that the R wave deflection goes from a negative in V_1 to positive in V_6, with V_3 and V_4 leads being mostly biphasic (the R wave is half negative and half positive or in transitions). As the myocardial muscle cells of the anterior wall begin to die, depolarization gradually decreases until the R wave becomes smaller and smaller and the deflection can ultimately be seen as a Q wave. This occurrence is called *loss of R wave progression.*

CLINICAL SIGNIFICANCE OF ANTERIOR MIs

Infarctions involving the left ventricle are, as stated earlier, primarily categorized based upon whether the inferior or anterior wall of the heart is predominately affected (Figure 10–4). This is an important clinical distinction because the therapeutic and prognostic implications of these two types of infarctions will vary. Because of coronary artery distribution variances, it is a commonly held belief that anterior infarctions tend to be larger than inferior infarctions. Due to this larger degree of myocardial muscle involvement, anterior MIs have a greater predisposition for the development of complications such as lethal ventricular dysrhythmias and **cardiogenic shock.**

In addition, conduction system defects are more common with anterior infarctions. Generally, first-degree AV block and Mobitz Type I second-degree AV block (or Wenckebach) are more common with inferior infarctions, whereas Mobitz Type II second-degree AV block, third-degree AV block, and bundle branch blocks are more common with anterior infarctions.

As you may recall from the discussions of basic dysrhythmias, both first-degree AV block and Mobitz Type I second-degree AV block (or Wenckebach) tend to be transient

cardiogenic shock condition caused by inadequate cardiac output (pump failure)

Anterior infarct

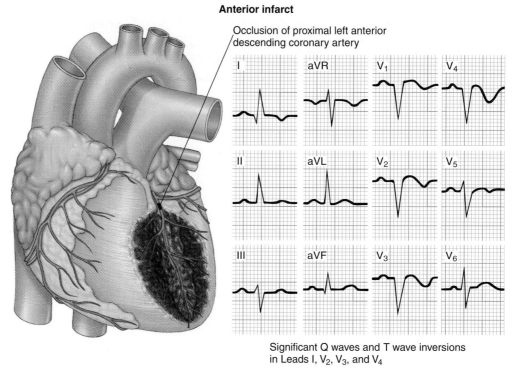

Occlusion of proximal left anterior descending coronary artery

Significant Q waves and T wave inversions in Leads I, V₂, V₃, and V₄

Figure 10–4. Anterior infarct

in nature, whereas Mobitz Type II second-degree AV block, third-degree AV block may need more aggressive treatment, such as artificial pacemaker implantation. Sequential EKGs should be obtained and carefully scrutinized in order to identify indications of a damaged conduction system.

Again, it is important to remind you that early death can occur in patients with acute anterior MIs. This fact is primarily due to congestive heart failure (CHF) within a few days of the initial infarct. Also, there is an increased incidence of the development of sustained ventricular tachycardia (V-tach) or ventricular fibrillation (V-fib) up to 1 to 2 weeks post MI. This is an important fact for the health-care provider to keep in mind, particularly when dealing with a patient who has experienced recurring chest pain and has returned to the hospital after having been discharged with the diagnosis of anterior MI. Your index of suspicion regarding the possible development of CHF or **lethal dysrhythmias** should be increased whenever a patient presents with a medical history of cardiac disease, particularly status post (recent past history of) MI.

You should be aware that the type of autonomic nervous system dysfunction that typically presents clinically in an anterior wall MI results from stimulation of the sympathetic nervous system. Recall that this is the division of the autonomic nervous system that controls the "fight or flight" processes. Thus, anterior infarctions tend to result in hyperactivity of the sympathetic nervous system, resulting in various signs and symptoms including sinus tachycardia and hypertension. Treatment may include medications such as vasodilators or beta blockers.

At this point, you should question yourself as to the significance of sinus tachycardia in the patient who is exhibiting signs and symptoms of an acute MI. Your answer

lethal dysrhythmias
abnormalities in heart rhythms that, if left untreated, result in death

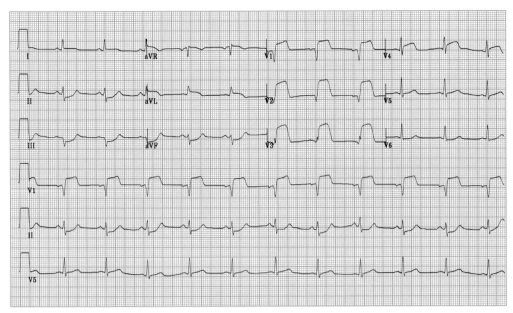

Figure 10–5. Example of 12-lead EKG illustrating changes consistent with anteroseptal MI

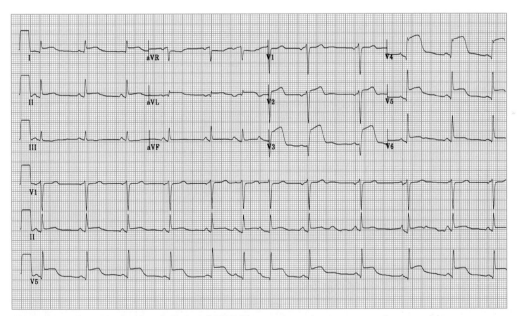

Figure 10–6. Example of 12-lead EKG illustrating changes consistent with anterolateral MI

should center around the issue of myocardial oxygen supply and demand. This simple self-test will reemphasize to you the ultimate importance of early intervention and early oxygenation.

You should now utilize the 5 + 3 approach to evaluate Figures 10–5 and 10–6. Do not hesitate to ask for assistance if you feel unsure about your answer.

EKG Changes in Anterior MIs

ST segment elevation in Leads V_3 and V_4	T wave inversion; pathologic Q waves may be present

EKG changes in anterolateral MIs

ST segment elevation in Leads V_3, V_4, V_5, V_6, I, and aVL	T wave inversion; pathologic Q waves may be present

EKG changes in anteroseptal MIs

ST segment elevation in Leads V_1, V_2, V_3, and V_4	T wave inversion; pathologic Q waves may be present

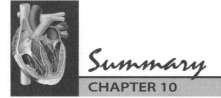

Summary
CHAPTER 10

Anterior MIs occur when the left coronary artery becomes occluded. Anterior MIs are most commonly associated with injury to the septal and lateral wall(s) of the myocardium. This type of infarction is associated with major muscle damage and has an incidence of high morbidity. The anterior MI is evidenced by ST elevation and/or T wave inversion or Q waves in V_3 and V_4. This type of MI often is a precursor to the development of second- and third-degree heart blocks as well as bundle branch blocks.

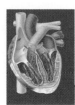

Key Points to Remember
CHAPTER 10

1. An anterior MI will primarily involve the left coronary artery.

2. The left coronary artery divides into the left anterior descending and the circumflex arteries.

3. A marginal branch of the left coronary artery supplies blood to the lateral wall of the left ventricle.

4. The left anterior descending artery is sometimes called the widowmaker because of its size and the large amount of myocardium that it supplies.

5. EKG findings in anterior MI are ST elevation in Leads V_3 and V_4 of 1 mm or more of elevation.

6. EKG findings in anteroseptal MI are ST elevation in Leads V_1, V_2, V_3, and V_4 of 1 mm or more of elevation.

7. EKG findings in anterolateral MI are ST elevation in Leads V_3, V_4, V_5, V_6, and/or Leads I and aVL of 1 mm or more of elevation.

8. Poor R wave progression in the V leads occurs when depolarization gradually decreases until the R wave is ultimately seen as a Q wave.

9. There is an increased incidence of development of sustained ventricular tachycardia or ventricular fibrillation with anterior MIs.

Review Questions
CHAPTER 10

1. The ___ of the heart is considered to be the "workhorse" of the heart.
   a. right ventricle
   b. left ventricle
   c. left atrium
   d. right atrium

2. Generally, anterior MIs tend to involve a larger muscle mass than do inferior MIs.
   a. True
   b. False

3. A ___ branch of the left coronary artery supplies blood to the lateral wall of the left ventricle.
   a. central
   b. peripheral
   c. marginal
   d. secondary

4. The ___ branch of the left coronary artery extends around to the posterior side of the heart and its branches supply blood to much of the posterior wall of the heart.
   a. marginal
   b. descending
   c. ascending
   d. circumflex

5. Because of its size and the large amount of myocardium that it supplies, massive infarction may result if the ___ becomes totally occluded.

   a. LAD

   b. CAD

   c. RAD

   d. MBD

6. Because of the potential for massive infarction, the LAD is sometimes called the *widowmaker.*

   a. True

   b. False

7. Leads V_3 and V_4 visualize the ___ wall of the heart's left ventricle.

   a. medial

   b. lateral

   c. anterior

   d. posterior

8. If your patient is exhibiting clinical signs and symptoms consistent with a myocardial infarction AND you notice that ST segment elevation is present in Leads ___, your index of suspicion regarding the presence of an anterior MI should begin to increase.

   a. V_2 and aVL

   b. V_1 and aVF

   c. V_3 and V_4

   d. V_5 and V_6

9. Regarding the systematic approach to EKG interpretation, you should always follow the logical and workable ___ in order to correctly interpret 12-lead EKG strips.

   a. six-step approach

   b. 5 + 3 approach

   c. 5 + 2 approach

   d. four-step approach

10. In addition to the occurrence of ST segment elevation, ___ and the evolution of significant Q waves in Leads V_3 and V_4 may indicate anterior myocardial infarction.

    a. T wave elevation

    b. loss of T wave

    c. prolonged PR interval

    d. T wave inversion

11. Due to the large degree of myocardial muscle involvement, ___ MIs have a greater predisposition for the development of complications such as lethal ventricular dysrhythmias and cardiogenic shock.

    a. posterior   c. lateral

    b. anterior   d. inferior

12. Anterior infarctions tend to result in hyperactivity of the sympathetic nervous system.
   a. True
   b. False

13. Anterior MIs are associated with the development of:
   a. sinus dysrhythmias.
   b. first-degree heart blocks.
   c. wandering atrial pacemakers.
   d. third-degree heart blocks.

14. Loss of R wave progression rarely occurs with anterior MIs.
   a. True
   b. False

15. The reciprocal Lead changes in the anterior MI, though uncommon, are:
   a. I, II, and aVR.
   b. II, III, and aVF.
   c. II, III, and aVL.
   d. I, aVR, and aVL.

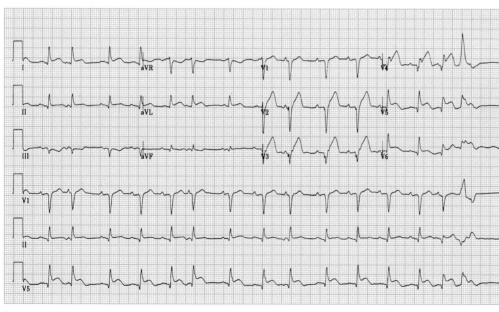

Review strip

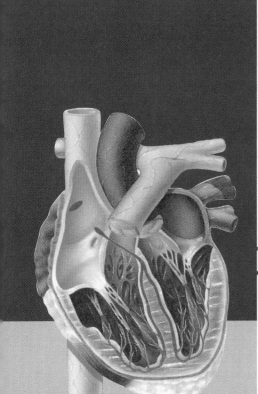

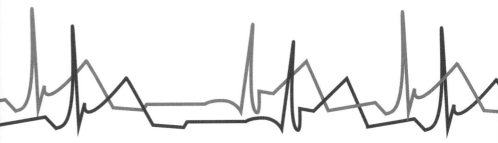

Interpretation of Septal MIs

objectives

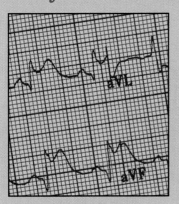

Upon completion of this chapter, the student will be able to:

➤ Describe the anatomy of the interventricular septum

➤ Discuss the anatomy and distribution of the left coronary artery

➤ Identify the lead-specific ST segment elevation relative to septal MIs

➤ Identify the lead-specific ST segment elevation relative to anteroseptal MIs

➤ Describe other EKG changes commonly associated with septal MIs, as well as anteroseptal MIs

➤ Identify the clinical significance of septal MIs

INTRODUCTION

Pure (or isolated) septal MIs are a less common occurrence than the other types of MIs we discuss in this text. Generally, an MI that involves the interventricular septum will also involve the left ventricle of the heart. Because there can be 12-lead EKG evidence of a septal infarct, we feel that you should be familiar with the indicators that lead to suspicion of both septal and anteroseptal MI events. Thus, we will briefly discuss septal MIs.

ANATOMY OF THE INTERVENTRICULAR SEPTUM AND THE CORONARY ARTERIES

Our discussion of **septal MIs** will primarily involve the *left coronary artery* as described in previous chapters. As the left coronary artery leaves the aorta, it immediately divides into the left anterior descending (LAD) artery and the circumflex artery. The anterior descending artery is the major branch of the left coronary artery and supplies blood to most of the left side of the interventricular septum. The LAD also has six branches called **septal perforating arteries.** These perforating arteries supply the anterior two-thirds of the interventricular septum. Still other branches of the LAD are called **diagonal arteries.** These arteries supply blood to the anterolateral wall of the left ventricle. If occlusion of the LAD occurs high enough in the septum to inhibit circulation to the septal wall, you may note interventricular conduction disturbances. This is true because the main trunk of the right bundle branch and both major fascicles of the left bundle branch lie within the interventricular septum.

As mentioned in earlier chapters, the anatomy of some individuals varies slightly, especially with respect to the distribution areas of the coronary arteries. With this in mind, you should realize that the posterior descending artery, which may be derived from the right coronary artery but is sometimes derived from the left circumflex artery, supplies the superior posterior portion of the interventricular septum.

The heart is generally thought of as a single organ with two halves. The left and right halves of the heart each contain one atrium and one ventricle and are divided by a wall called the *septum.* Technically the heart contains two septa (plural of *septum*): the interatrial septum, which is located between and divides the two atria, and the interventricular septum, which is located between and divides the two ventricles. The interventricular septum is larger than the interatrial septum, just as the ventricles are larger than the atria. The interventricular septum has a thicker muscle mass toward the apex (bottom) of the heart and a thin membranous part toward the atria. Figure 11–1 provides a view of the anatomy of the heart. Refer to this figure to visualize the location of the septum.

septal MIs interruption of oxygen-rich blood supply to the interventricular septum

septal perforating arteries supply the anterior two-thirds of the interventricular septum

diagonal arteries supply blood to the anterolateral wall of the left ventricle

LEAD-SPECIFIC ST SEGMENT ELEVATION

Recall the EKG leads that record electrical impulses generated from the heart's electrical conduction system actually view precise areas of damaged myocardium. Remember also that these leads are called *indicative* or *facing leads.*

Also recall that EKG findings of infarction may occur in a single lead or in a combination of leads; however for these findings to be significant, evidence should be in two or more contiguous leads. Leads V_1 and V_2 visualize the interventricular septum of the heart (Figure 11–2). Most often there is no significant reciprocal lead EKG changes with septal MIs.

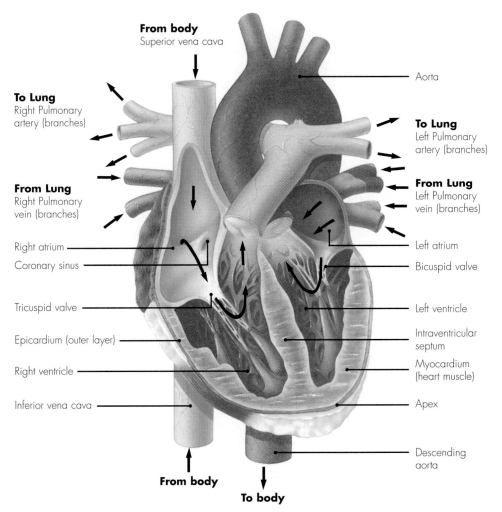

Figure 11–1. Anatomical structures of the heart

You should remember that only rarely do MIs involve *only* the septum. Most often, either the anterior or lateral wall of the ventricles are also involved in an acute septal MI. Leads V_1, V_2, V_3, and V_4 will illustrate ST segment elevation in the face of an anteroseptal MI. This finding often indicates a larger mass of myocardial muscle involvement than does an isolated finding in V_1 and V_2.

Now look at and study a 12-lead EKG strip that illustrates ST segment elevation (Leads V_1 and V_2). Note that there are no reciprocal changes in Leads II, III, and aVF. As you may recall from Chapter 6, you must always follow the logical and workable 5 + 3 approach in order to correctly interpret 12-lead EKG strips. The first five steps include the systematic approach to basic EKG interpretation. For analysis of a 12-lead EKG strip, we have suggested the addition of the following three steps: ST segment depression, ST segment elevation, and pathologic Q wave.

You should recall that the basic five steps are:

Rate	Rhythm	P wave	PR interval	QRS complex

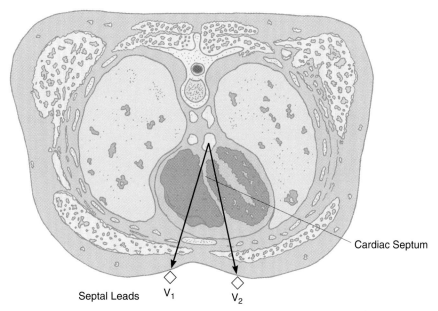

Figure 11–2.   Cross-section of the heart with chest leads and associated myocardial wall areas

The 5 + 3 approach is:

Rate	Rhythm	P wave	PR interval	QRS complex

PLUS

ST segment depression	ST segment elevation	Q wave

Now, systematically apply each of the steps in the 5 + 3 approach to the strip in Figure 11–3:

Rate: _____

Rhythm: _____

P wave: _____

PR interval: _____

QRS complex: _____

ST segment depression: _____

ST segment elevation: _____

Q wave: _____

Are you comfortable with your answers? We hope you came up with the following ones. If so, you are definitely getting there!

Rate: 61	**Rhythm:** regular	**P wave:** present; negative deflection	**PR interval:** 0.12 sec (three small boxes)	**QRS complex:** 0.08 sec (two small boxes)

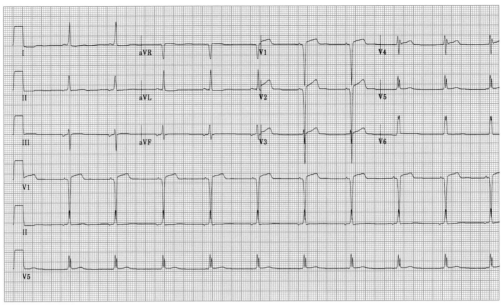

Figure 11–3. Example of 12-lead EKG illustrating changes consistent with septal MI

PLUS

ST segment depression: none	ST segment elevation: Leads V_1 and V_2	Q wave: pathologic in V_1 and V_2

Interpretation: septal MI, as evidenced by ST segment elevation and pathologic Q waves in Leads V_1 and V_2.

EKG CHANGES COMMONLY ASSOCIATED WITH SEPTAL MIs

pure septal MIs recognized by the development of QS complexes in Leads V_1 and V_2

Although rare, **pure septal MIs** are recognized by the development of QS complexes in Leads V_1 and V_2. Normally, the R wave in V_1 is small yet significant, as it represents the depolarization of the ventricular septum. Another important point to realize is that while the septum is a thick muscular wall, it is actually a part of the left ventricle. In Lead V_2, the R wave is expected to increase and become more positive (above the iso-electric line). This change or progression demonstrates that the septum is functioning sufficiently well to allow for electrical conduction. This R wave progression is important in your analysis of the V leads. The absence of an R wave in V_2 should increase your index of suspicion for a septal infarction. This concept is referred to as *poor R wave progression*. The EKG shown in Figure 11–3 illustrates this concept.

In addition to the occurrence of ST segment depression or elevation, T wave inversion and the evolution of significant Q waves in Leads V_1 and V_2 may indicate septal MI. As a reminder, pathologic Q waves are not an early indicator (EKG finding), but occur as later evidence of myocardial tissue damage.

As the myocardial muscle cells of the septum wall begin to die, depolarization gradually decreases until the R wave becomes smaller and smaller and the deflection can ultimately be seen as a Q wave. Again, this occurrence is known as *loss of R wave progression*.

CLINICAL SIGNIFICANCE OF SEPTAL MIs

Therapeutic and prognostic implications of septal MIs will be primarily based on the clinical picture of your patient. Due to the location of significant conduction components in the interventricular septum, the predisposition for the development of complications such as conduction system dysrhythmias is relatively common with septal infarctions. Generally, Mobitz Type II second-degree AV block, third-degree AV block, and bundle branch blocks are the conduction dysrhythmias associated with septal infarctions. As you will recall from the discussions of basic dysrhythmias, Mobitz Type II second-degree AV block and third-degree AV block may need more aggressive treatment, such as artificial pacemaker implantation. Again, your consideration of intervention modalities must be based on your patient's clinical picture.

Recall that pure septal MIs are infrequent; rather, EKG changes will most commonly indicate the involvement of either the anterior or lateral wall in conjunction with septal wall infarctions.

The 12-lead EKG in Figure 11–4 is an example of anteroseptal injury as indicated by ST segment elevation with T wave inversion in Leads V_1, V_2, V_3, and V_4.

EKG changes in septal MIs

ST segment elevation in Leads V_1 and V_2	Poor R wave progression in the V leads

EKG changes in anteroseptal MIs

ST segment elevation in Leads V_1, V_2, V_3, and V_4	Poor R wave progression in the V leads

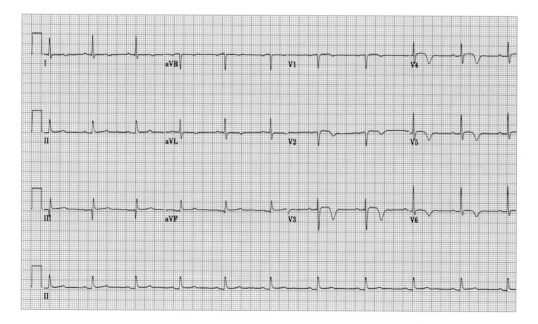

Figure 11–4.   Example of 12-lead EKG illustrating changes consistent with anteroseptal MI

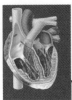

Summary
CHAPTER 11

This chapter has focused on the understanding of septal MIs and the interpretation of specific EKG indicators. You now should understand that septal MIs are less common than other types of MIs. You also should understand that septal MIs most often occur due to occlusion in the left coronary artery.

Key Points to Remember
CHAPTER 11

1. Septal MIs will primarily involve the left coronary artery.

2. The left coronary artery divides into the left anterior descending and the circumflex arteries.

3. The left anterior descending artery has branches of its own. They are the septal perforating arteries and the diagonal arteries.

4. The leads on the EKG specific for septal MI are Leads V_1 and V_2.

5. The leads on the EKG for the anterioseptal MI are Leads V_1, V_2, V_3, and V_4.

6. Pathologic Q waves are not an early indicator but occur as later evidence of myocardial tissue damage.

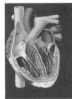

Review Questions
CHAPTER 11

1. Pure (or isolated) septal MIs are a more common occurrence than other types of MI.
   a. True
   b. False

2. Generally, an MI that involves the interventricular septum will also involve the ___ of the heart.
   a. left ventricle   c. left atrium
   b. right ventricle   d. right atrium

3. The left anterior descending artery has six branches called septal ___ arteries.

   a. penetrating

   b. protruding

   c. perforating

   d. piercing

4. Other branches of the LAD are called ___ arteries and supply blood to the anterolateral wall of the left ventricle.

   a. perforating

   b. marginal

   c. dissecting

   d. diagonal

5. The left and right halves of the heart are divided by a wall called the:

   a. schism.

   b. bridge.

   c. septum.

   d. ridge.

6. The ___ septum is located between and divides the two atria.

   a. interatrial

   b. interarterial

   c. intratrial

   d. intraarterial

7. The ___ septum is located between and divides the two ventricles.

   a. interatrial

   b. interventricular

   c. intraventricular

   d. interarterial

8. Leads ___ visualize the interventricular septum of the heart.

   a. V_4 and V_6

   b. V_2 and V_3

   c. V_5 and aVF

   d. V_1 and V_2

9. Pathologic Q waves are not an early indicator or EKG finding, but occur as later evidence of myocardial tissue damage.

   a. True

   b. False

10. To diagnose an acute septal MI, evidence of ___ must be present in Leads V_1 and V_2.

a. ST segment depression

b. ST segment elevation

c. pathologic Q waves

d. Any of the above.

11. Pathologic Q waves are indicative of early onset of acute MI.

a. True

b. False

12. Electrical conduction system dysrhythmias are a common occurrence in patients with septal MIs.

a. True

b. False

13. The left coronary artery leaves the aorta and immediately divides into the left anterior descending artery and the ___ artery.

a. diagonal

b. perforating

c. circumflex

d. marginal

14. The reciprocal leads for the septal MI are Leads I, II, and III.

a. True

b. False

15. ST elevation in Leads V_1, V_2, V_3, and V_4 are indicative of ___ MI.

a. pure septal

b. anteroposterior

c. anterolateral

d. anteroseptal

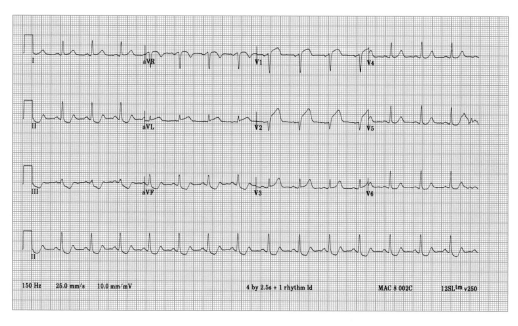

150 Hz   25.0 mm/s   10.0 mm/mV   4 by 2.5s + 1 rhythm ld   MAC 8 002C   12SL^{tm} v250

Review strip

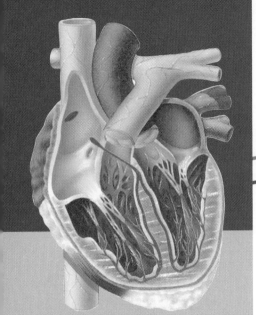

Interpretation of Lateral MIs

objectives

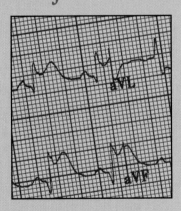

Upon completion of this chapter, the student will be able to:

➤ Describe the anatomy of the left ventricle

➤ Discuss the anatomy and distribution of the left coronary artery

➤ Identify the lead-specific ST segment elevation relative to lateral MIs

➤ Identify the lead-specific ST segment elevation relative to anterolateral MIs

➤ Identify the lead-specific ST segment elevation relative to inferolateral MIs

➤ Describe other EKG changes commonly associated with lateral MIs, as well as anterolateral and inferolateral MIs

➤ Identify the clinical significance of lateral MIs

INTRODUCTION

Pure (or isolated) lateral MIs are *not* common; rather, infarction of the lateral wall of the left ventricle usually involves the anterior, inferior, or posterior wall of the left ventricle. Because there can be 12-Lead EKG evidence of a lateral wall infarct, we want you to be familiar with the indicators that lead to suspicion of both lateral and anterolateral MI events. Thus, we will briefly discuss lateral MIs.

ANATOMY OF THE LEFT VENTRICLE AND THE CIRCUMFLEX BRANCH OF THE LEFT CORONARY ARTERY

Our discussion of lateral MIs primarily involves the circumflex branch of the left coronary artery. By way of review, as the left coronary artery leaves the aorta, it immediately divides into the left anterior descending (LAD) artery and the circumflex artery. If occlusion of the circumflex artery occurs, lateral wall infarction will result. The anterior descending artery is the major branch of the left coronary artery and supplies blood to most of the left side of the interventricular septum. Other branches of the LAD are called *diagonal arteries;* these arteries supply blood to the anterolateral wall of the left ventricle.

The anatomy of some individuals varies slightly, especially with respect to the distribution areas of the coronary arteries. With this in mind, you should realize that the posterior descending artery, which may be derived from the right coronary artery but is sometimes derived from the left circumflex artery, supplies the superior posterior portion of the interventricular septum.

In approximately 10% of the general population, the circumflex artery, rather than the right coronary artery, runs along the underside of the heart to form the posterior descending artery. Thus, the lateral wall of the left ventricle is variably supplied by the circumflex artery, the LAD, or a branch of the right coronary artery.

When the lateral wall is involved with proximal occlusion of the LAD, this is termed an *anterolateral MI.* When the lateral wall is involved with a branch of the right coronary artery, this is termed an *inferolateral* (diaphragmatic surface of the heart) *MI* or *posterolateral* (superior posterior surface of the heart) *MI.* Myocardial infarctions of the lateral wall of the heart most commonly occur as a result of an extension of anterior and/or inferior wall MIs.

Recall that of the two ventricles, the left is thicker and more muscular. This anatomical variance between the left and right ventricles is appropriate, based on the function of each. The left ventricle of the heart is the workhorse, because it has the responsibility for supplying sufficient blood to perfuse the body. Thus, when the myocardium of the left ventricle is severely compromised, the patient's clinical condition may deteriorate. Note the location of the lateral wall of the heart in Figure 12–1.

LEAD-SPECIFIC ST SEGMENT CHANGES

Leads V_5, V_6, I, and aVL visualize the lateral wall of the heart. Although occasionally reciprocal changes may be present in V_1, most often there is no significant reciprocal lead EKG changes with lateral MIs.

Leads V_3, V_4, V_5, and V_6 will illustrate ST segment elevation in the face of an anterolateral MI. This finding often indicates a larger mass of myocardial muscle involvement than does an isolated finding in Leads V_5, V_6, I, and aVL. Leads II, III, aVF, V_5, and V_6 will illustrate ST segment elevation in the face of an inferolateral MI.

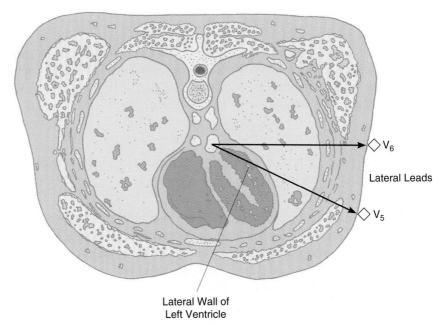

Figure 12–1.   Cross-section of the heart with chest leads and associated myocardial wall areas

Look at and study the 12-Lead EKG strip that illustrates ST segment elevation (Lead V$_5$, V$_6$, I, and aVL) in Figure 12–2. Note that there are no reciprocal changes in Leads II, III, and aVF. Remember that you should always follow the logical and workable 5 + 3 approach in order to correctly interpret 12-Lead EKG strips.

The basic five steps are:

Rate	Rhythm	P wave	PR interval	QRS complex

The 5 + 3 approach is:

Rate	Rhythm	P wave	PR interval	QRS complex

PLUS

ST segment depression	ST segment elevation	Q wave

Now, systematically apply each of the steps in the 5 + 3 approach to the strip in Figure 12–2:

Rate: _____

Rhythm: _____

P wave: _____

PR interval: _____

QRS complex: _____

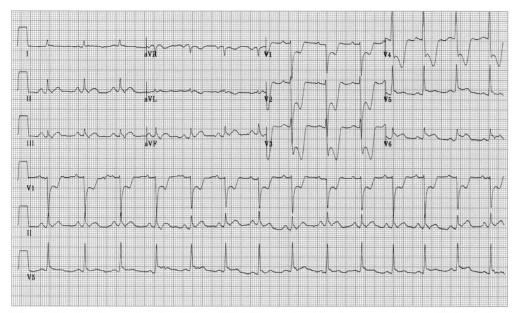

Figure 12–2. Example of a 12-Lead EKG illustrating changes consistent with lateral MI

ST segment depression: _____

ST segment elevation: _____

Q wave: _____

Do your answers match the ones listed below? If not, go back to recalculate your findings, remembering to follow the 5 + 3 approach.

Rate: 83	Rhythm: regular	P wave: present; upright	PR interval: 0.16 sec (four small boxes)	QRS complex: 0.08 sec (two small boxes)

PLUS

ST segment depression: Leads V_1, V_2, V_3, V_4	ST segment elevation: Leads V_5, V_6, I, and aVL	Q wave: nonpathologic (within normal limits)

Interpretation: lateral MI, as evidenced by ST segment elevation in Leads V_5, V_6, and aVL.

EKG CHANGES COMMONLY ASSOCIATED WITH LATERAL MIs

Pure lateral MIs, although rare, are recognized by the development of ST elevation in Leads V_5, V_6, I, and aVL. In Lead V_2, the R wave is expected to increase and become more positive (above the isoelectric line). This change or progression demonstrates that the septum is functioning sufficiently well to allow for electrical conduction. R wave progression is important in your analysis of the V leads. The absence of an R wave in

V_2 should increase your index of suspicion for a lateral infarction. This concept is referred to as *poor R wave progression.*

In addition to the occurrence of ST segment elevation, T wave inversion and the evolution of significant Q waves in Leads V_5, V_6, I, and aVL may indicate lateral MI. As a reminder, pathologic Q waves are not an early indicator or EKG finding, but occur as later evidence of myocardial tissue damage.

CLINICAL SIGNIFICANCE OF LATERAL MIs

Again, remember that the process of myocardial injury in an acute MI is time dependent. Salvage of myocardial muscle tissue is likely possible if blood flow is restored, but intervention must occur early. Therapeutic and prognostic implications of lateral MIs will be primarily based on the clinical picture of your patient.

Due to the location of significant conduction components in the interventricular septum, the predisposition for the development of complications such as conduction system dysrhythmias is relatively common with lateral infarctions. Generally, Mobitz Type II second-degree AV block, third-degree AV block, and bundle branch blocks are the conduction dysrhythmias associated with lateral infarctions. As you will recall from the discussions of basic dysrhythmias, Mobitz Type II second-degree AV block and third-degree AV block may need more aggressive treatment, such as artificial pacemaker implantation. Again, your consideration of intervention modalities must be based on your patient's clinical picture.

Recall that pure lateral MIs are infrequent; rather, EKG changes will most commonly indicate the involvement of either the anterior or posterior wall, in conjunction with lateral wall infarctions.

The EKG in Figure 12–3 depicts an anterolateral MI. Note the ST segment elevation in Leads V_3, V_4, V_5, V_6, I, and aVL.

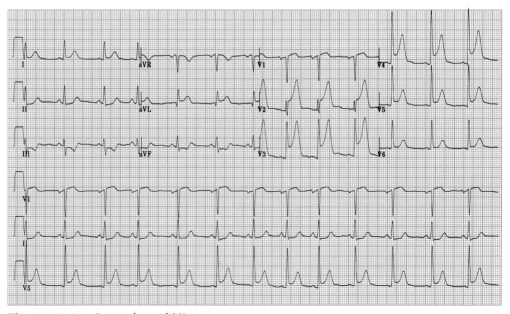

Figure 12–3.   Anterolateral MI

The EKG in Figure 12–4 is included in this chapter to point out the significant ST segment elevation that is present, as well as the accompanying ST segment depression. Collectively, these findings manifest the presence of EKG changes indicative of an anterior, inferior, and lateral MI. Note also the "tombstone" appearance of the ST segment elevation in V$_3$ and V$_4$. ST segment elevation that resembles the appearance of a tombstone signifies that the occurring ischemia and injury is massive in nature and is a very serious and acute finding.

Another example of a lateral MI, in this case accompanied by EKG changes indicative of inferior and posterior MI, is illustrated in Figure 12–5.

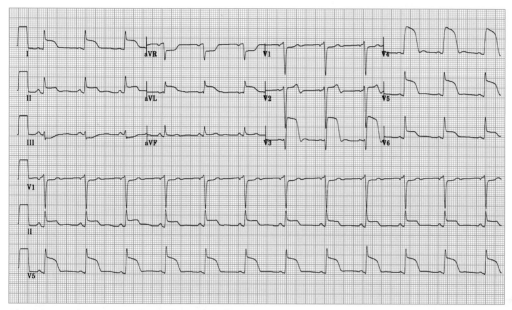

Figure 12–4. Anterior inferior lateral MI

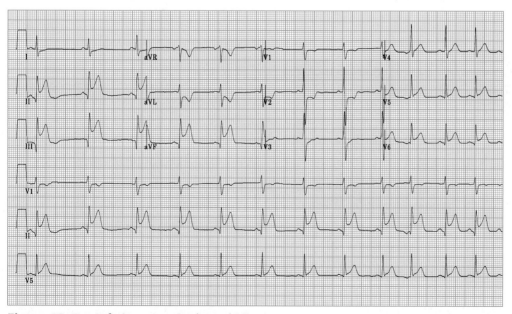

Figure 12–5. Inferior posterior lateral MI

EKG changes in lateral MIs

ST segment elevation in Leads V_5, V_6, I, and aVL	T wave inversion; development of pathologic Q waves

EKG changes in anteroseptal MIs

ST segment elevation in Leads V_3, V_4, V_5, V_6, I, and aVL	T wave inversion; development of pathologic Q waves; poor R wave progression

Summary
CHAPTER 12

You now understand that pure lateral MIs are uncommon and are most often associated with anterior, posterior, or septal MIs. The changes that are seen in pure lateral MIs include ST elevation in Leads V_5, V_6, I, and aVL. You also now have a better understanding of how the progression of the R wave is affected during a lateral infarction.

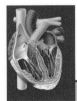

Key Points to Remember
CHAPTER 12

1. Lateral MIs primarily involve the circumflex branch of the left coronary artery.

2. If occlusion of the circumflex artery occurs, a lateral wall infarction will result.

3. Leads V_5, V_6, Lead I, and aVL visualize the lateral wall of the heart, may illustrate ST segment elevation of 1 mm or more, and indicate a lateral MI.

4. Leads V_3, V_4, V_5, and V_6 illustrate ST segment elevation of 1 mm or more and indicate an anterolateral MI.

5. Leads II, III, aVF, V_5, and V_6 illustrate ST segment elevation of 1 mm or more and indicate an inferolateral MI.

6. Poor R wave progression should increase the index of suspicion for a lateral infarction.

7. Lateral MIs predispose for the development of conduction system dysrhythmias.

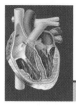

Review Questions

CHAPTER 12

1. Pure lateral MIs are uncommon; infarction of the lateral wall of the left ventricle usually involves the:

   a. anterior or inferior wall of the right atrium.

   b. inferior and posterior wall of the left atrium.

   c. posterior and superior wall of the left ventricle.

   d. anterior, inferior, and posterior wall of left ventricle.

2. The anatomy of some individuals varies slightly, especially with respect to the distribution areas of the coronary arteries.

   a. True

   b. False

3. Myocardial infarction or myocardial ischemia may be produced by:

   a. sudden increase in myocardial workload.

   b. spasms of the coronary arteries.

   c. coronary artery occlusion.

   d. All of the above.

4. Therapeutic and prognostic implications of lateral MIs will be primarily based on the:

   a. clinical picture of your patient.

   b. serum cardiac enzyme levels.

   c. 3-lead EKG tracing.

   d. patient's vital signs.

5. Due to the location of significant conduction components in the interventricular septum, the predisposition for the development of complications such as conduction system dysrhythmias is relatively common with lateral infarctions.

   a. True

   b. False

6. ST segment elevation that resembles the appearance of a tombstone signifies that the occurring ischemia and injury is massive in nature and is a very serious and acute finding.

   a. True

   b. False

7. When the lateral wall is involved with proximal occlusion of the LAD, this is termed a(n) ___ MI.

   a. posterolateral   c. anterolateral

   b. anteroseptal   d. posteroseptal

8. Myocardial infarctions of the lateral wall of the heart most commonly occur as a result of an extension of anterior and/or inferior wall MIs.

   a. True

   b. False

9. Leads ___ visualize the lateral wall of the heart.

   a. V_1, V_2, II, and V_3

   b. V_3, V_4, I, and aVF

   c. V_2, V_4, II, and aVR

   d. V_5, V_6, I, and aVL

10. The interatrial septum is a thick muscular wall that is actually a part of the left ventricle.

    a. True

    b. False

11. Pure lateral MIs are infrequent; thus, EKG changes will commonly indicate the involvement of either the anterior or lateral wall in conjunction with lateral wall infarctions.

    a. True

    b. False

12. ST segment depression may be indicative of:

    a. cerebral hypoxia.

    b. myocardial ischemia.

    c. unstable angina.

    d. ventricular atrophy.

13. Pathologic Q waves indicate:

    a. ischemia.

    b. necrosis.

    c. atrophy.

    d. hypoxia.

14. The concept of poor R wave progression refers to the absence of R waves in Lead:

    a. V1.

    b. V_2.

    c. aVF.

    d. aVR.

15. When the lateral wall is involved with proximal occlusion of the LAD, this is termed a(n) ___ MI.

   a. anterolateral

   b. posterolateral

   c. anteroseptal

   d. right-sided

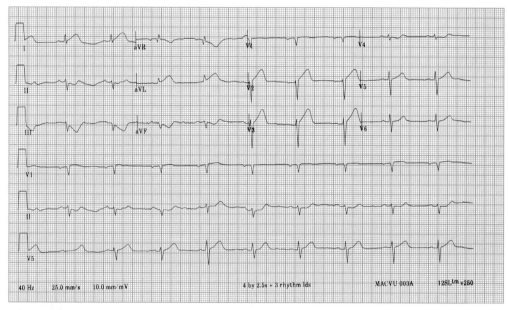

Review strip

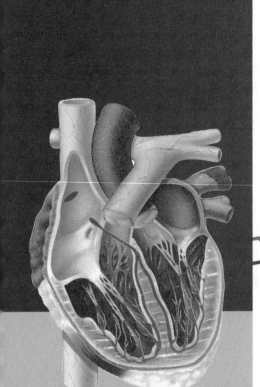

chapter 13

Interpretation of Posterior MIs

objectives

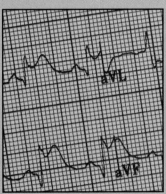

Upon completion of this chapter, the student will be able to:

➤ Describe the anatomy of the left ventricle

➤ Discuss the anatomy and distribution of the right coronary artery

➤ Identify the lead-specific ST segment elevation relative to posterior MIs

➤ Describe other EKG changes commonly associated with posterior MIs

➤ Discuss the significance and use of the 15-lead EKG

➤ Identify the clinical significance of posterior MIs

INTRODUCTION

In the previous chapters we discussed the 12-lead EKG indications that will manifest each specific type of MI; however, in the posterior MI there are no facing or indicative leads that are monitored in the standard 12-lead EKG. In other words, there are no leads that view or "look at" the posterior wall. Therefore, when considering the possibility of posterior wall MIs, expect to assess reciprocal leads rather than indicative leads. It is wise to remember that most often posterior MIs do not occur as isolated incidents, but more commonly occur in conjunction with infarction of the lateral and/or inferior wall of the left ventricle. Posterior wall MIs are most commonly associated with inferior wall MIs.

CORONARY ARTERY ANATOMY REVIEW

Remember that the two main coronary arteries are called the *left main coronary artery* and the *right main coronary artery.* Recall also that these vital structures supply the myocardium with freshly oxygenated blood.

    Posterior MIs, or posterior wall infarctions, may involve the right coronary artery, which extends from the aorta around to the posterior part of the heart. Branches of the right coronary artery furnish blood to the lateral wall of the right ventricle. In the vast majority of patients, a branch of the right coronary artery called the *posterior interventricular artery* or *posterior descending artery* lies in the posterior interventricular region and supplies blood to the posterior and inferior part of the heart's left ventricle. In a small percentage of patients (approximately 10%), the posterior descending artery arises from the circumflex branch of the posterior descending artery.

    The right coronary artery branches also supply oxygen-rich blood to a portion of the electrical conduction system. If occlusion of the right coronary artery occurs, the result may be either a posterior wall MI, an inferior wall MI, or a posteroinferior MI.

posterior MI
involves a decrease in oxygen-rich blood supply from the right coronary artery to the posterior wall of the left ventricle

LEAD-SPECIFIC ST SEGMENT CHANGES

There are no indicative or facing leads that view the posterior wall of the left ventricle; therefore detection of a posterior wall MI may tend to be a bit confusing to the student. We want to be sure that you understand the parameters to evaluate in order to correctly interpret EKG changes that occur in the 12-lead EKG of a patient who is indeed experiencing a posterior wall MI (Figure 13–1).

    Based on your knowledge of cardiac anatomy, recall that the anterior portion of the heart muscle lies directly opposite the posterior portion of the muscle mass. Now recall that we referred to reciprocal leads as those that "mirror" the facing or indicative leads. Quite literally, what this statement means to you is that because there are no facing leads on the standard 12-lead EKG to detect ST segment elevation and/or Q waves, you must look at the posterior wall's reciprocal leads (V_1, V_2, V_3, and V_4) or modify the 12-lead EKG.

    Again, remember that the reciprocal leads are the mirror image of the facing or indicative leads. Therefore, if the posterior portion of the heart is injured and ST elevation is present, then one could surmise that in the reciprocal leads, the ST segments would appear depressed or directly opposite of their appearance in the facing leads.

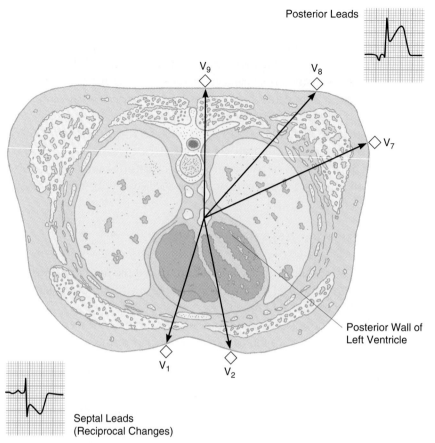

Figure 13–1. Cross-section of the heart with associated chest leads and myocardial wall

THE MIRROR TEST

Although it may not be frequently used in the clinical area, one of the oldest and more proven methods of viewing posterior MI EKG changes would involve the use of an actual mirror. In order to conduct the **mirror test,** place the mirror above the V leads of the 12-lead EKG tracing and observe the image in the mirror for the presence of ST segment elevation (the opposite finding suspected with a posterior MI). By employing the mirror test, you should be able to recognize a posterior infarction by the changes it produces in the anterior leads.

mirror test
method used to view posterior myocardial infarction EKG changes

ANOTHER TRICK FOR IDENTIFYING POSTERIOR MIs

Another method of identifying ST segment elevation is to simply hold the 12-lead EKG up to the light, upside down and backwards. In other words, hold the EKG in both hands with the tracing facing you. Then flip the paper over, being sure that the tracing is facing the light. Now look for ST segment elevation in V_1, V_2, V_3, and V_4.

POSTERIOR V LEADS

Another method for interpreting posterior MIs is to actually utilize posterior leads. This method is quite often used after the standard 12-lead EKG has been obtained, especially if a posterior MI is suspected. Most commonly, posterior Leads V_7, V_8, and V_9 are employed to obtain a posterior view. This is done by taking Leads V_4, V_5, and V_6 and moving them around toward the back or posterior side of the patient's body. This is sometimes referred to as a **15-lead EKG.**

Simply place the patient in the right lateral recumbent position for a brief time in order to apply the posterior leads. To properly place the V_7 lead, you should move the V_4 lead to the posterior axillary position, which is located directly posterior to V_6. For proper placement of V_8, move the V_5 lead and place it at the midscapular line. To place V_9 in its proper position, move the V_6 lead to the left at the midline of the back, approximately two centimeters to the left of the spine (Figure 13–2).

After the posterior leads are applied, the patient may again be placed in the supine and resting position. Clinical experience has proven that the patient will rest more quietly and comfortably in the supine position. This position will also tend to maximize the patient's feeling of security and minimize the possibility of muscle tremors, which often lead to artifact.

15-lead EKG
method used to interpret posterior MIs using posterior Leads V_7, V_8, and V_9

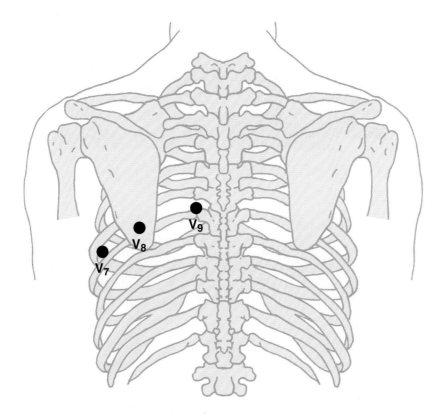

V_7—5th intercostal space, posterior axillary line
V_8—5th intercostal space, midscapular line
V_9—5th intercostal space, 2 cm left of spinal column

Figure 13–2. Posterior V lead placement

Newer EKG machines on the current market (such as the Marquette 5000) allow the operator to key in the 15-lead EKG option (Figure 13–3). The operator then adds three leads to the acquisition module and connects those to V_7, V_8, and V_9. The EKG machine will then print a 15-lead EKG.

Figure 13–4 shows an illustration of a 15-lead EKG. You will note that after careful evaluation of this EKG, there are 15 rather than 12 leads on this strip.

As with most other procedures in the medical profession, documentation is critically important when utilizing posterior lead placement. The 12-lead EKG machine will not recognize the absence of Leads V_4, V_5, and V_6; nor will the machine recognize the

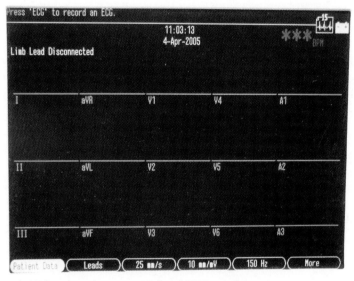

Figure 13–3. A 15-lead option to a 12-lead EKG machine

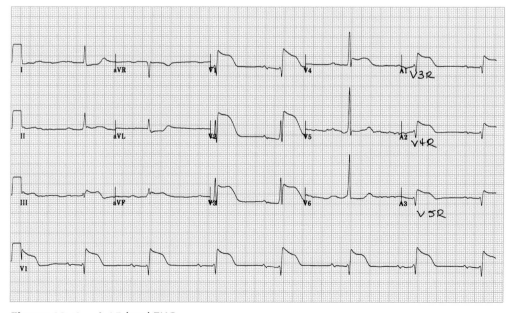

Figure 13–4. A 15-lead EKG

presence of Leads V_7, V_8, and V_9. Therefore, you must mark directly on the 12-lead tracing to indicate that a posterior lead EKG was obtained. V_4 is marked out and V_7 is written in its place. The same holds true with V_5, which becomes V_8, and with V_6, which becomes V_9.

It is imperative for you to understand that utilization of the newer 15-lead EKG machine dictates that you still must document the posterior leads on the tracing. The tracing will print and label the first 12 leads, followed by the posterior leads, labeled as A_1, A_2, and A_3. These represent and must be documented as V_7, V_8, and V_9. Also understand that the machine's internal computer will not recognize the posterior leads; thus, the EKG must always be carefully studied and interpreted by the evaluator.

You must understand that a misdiagnosis can occur if a posterior lead EKG is not properly marked (Figure 13–5). As you have undoubtedly heard numerous times, *documentation is critical.*

Now it is time to apply the knowledge you have gained in this chapter to the interpretation of an EKG strip that illustrates evidence of both inferior and posterior wall changes. Always follow the logical and workable 5 + 3 approach in order to correctly interpret 12-lead EKG strips. Here it is again as a reminder:

The 5 + 3 approach is:

Rate	Rhythm	P wave	PR interval	QRS complex

PLUS

ST segment depression	ST segment elevation	Q wave

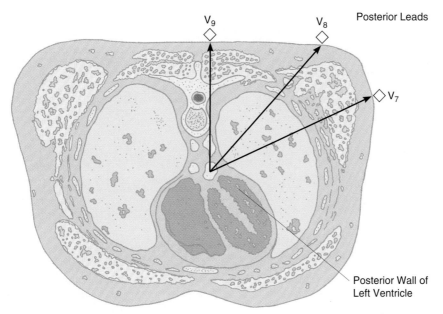

Figure 13–5.   Cross-section of heart with posterior leads and myocardial wall

Now, systematically apply each of the steps in the 5 + 3 approach to the strip in Figure 13–6:

Rate: _____

Rhythm: _____

P wave: _____

PR interval: _____

QRS complex: _____

ST segment depression: _____

ST segment elevation: _____

Q wave: _____

See if your answers match the ones listed as follows:

Rate: 77	**Rhythm:** irregular	**P wave:** present; negative deflection	**PR interval:** 0.16 sec (four small boxes)	**QRS complex:** 0.04 sec (one small box)

PLUS

ST segment depression: Leads V₁, V₂, V₃, V₄	**ST segment elevation:** none present	**Q wave:** nonpathologic (within normal limits)

Interpretation: pure posterior MI, as evidenced by ST segment depression.

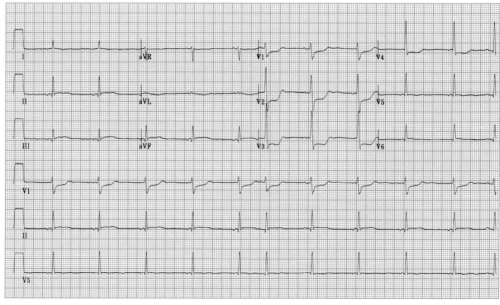

Figure 13–6. A 12-lead EKG tracing illustrating changes consistent with posterior MI

EKG CHANGES RELATED TO POSTERIOR MIs

In the early stages of a suspected posterior MI, you would observe for ST segment depression in Leads V_1, V_2, and V_3 (reciprocal leads; Figure 13–7). Other findings could include the development of tall R waves in the reciprocal leads. When tall R waves are noted in Lead V_1, this finding should prompt you to think of posterior infarction. In the earlier stages of a posterior MI, the presence of tall R waves should be evidenced in conjunction with the presence of ST segment depression. In the latter stages, the tall R wave may be present, but the ST segment depression may have diminished and returned to the baseline.

CLINICAL SIGNIFICANCE OF POSTERIOR MIs

Interpretation of a standard 12-lead EKG obtained from a patient who is suspected of having experienced a posterior MI depends on evidence of ST segment depression in the reciprocal leads (V_1, V_2 V_3, and/or V_4). Various studies have suggested that the placement of posterior chest leads is superior to the standard 12-lead EKG in the recognition of posterior MIs.

The efficacy of prehospital posterior 12-lead EKGs has not been proven. This is true in part because of the difficulty encountered in properly positioning the patient for placement of the posterior leads. However, applying posterior leads in a controlled environment such as an emergency department may be done with relative ease, as described earlier in this chapter.

Again, it is important to remind you that pure posterior MIs are rarely encountered. Rather, in most circumstances EKG evidence will include the presence of either a lateral

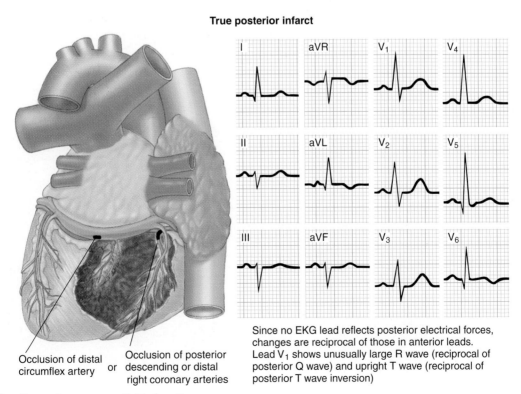

True posterior infarct

Occlusion of distal circumflex artery   or   Occlusion of posterior descending or distal right coronary arteries

Since no EKG lead reflects posterior electrical forces, changes are reciprocal of those in anterior leads. Lead V_1 shows unusually large R wave (reciprocal of posterior Q wave) and upright T wave (reciprocal of posterior T wave inversion)

Figure 13–7.   Posterior myocardial infarction

or inferior MI. You must understand that the clinical significance of posterior wall injury, in combination with evidence of inferior infarction, lies in the fact that this association indicates a more extensive infarction. Consequently, a greater risk of complications should be anticipated.

When considering the clinical symptomology of posterior wall infarction, recall that the major area involved in this event is the left ventricle. Based on your knowledge of the anatomy and physiology of the left ventricle, you may reason that necrosis of portions of the left ventricular wall may lead to the development of serious rhythm disturbances that are indicative of ventricular irritability (e.g., ventricular tachycardia, ventricular fibrillation, premature ventricular contractions) as well as left ventricular heart failure.

If the inferior surface of the myocardium has become involved, the patient may complain of "indigestion." This occurs due to the proximity of the inferior aspect of the myocardium to the diaphragm. It is because of the sensation of indigestion that many patients tend to deny the possibility that they are truly experiencing an MI. Rather, they will often self-medicate with antacids. There is clearly no way to know how many patients have succumbed to acute MIs by virtue of this denial. Ongoing efforts toward public education may tend to negate this behavior. However, this may be a rather optimistic point of view.

It is wise to keep in mind that when dealing with inferior, posterior, and infero-posterior MIs, the presence of high-degree AV blocks (third-degree and second-degree Type II) may be present on admission to the hospital or a short time after admission. This is true because the atrioventricular (AV) node receives its blood supply from the right coronary artery. Consequently, if the right coronary artery becomes occluded, blood flow to the AV node may be impeded.

In Figure 13–8, you should note the presence of ST segment depression V_1, V_2, V_3, and V_4. Also note the ST segment elevation in Leads I, II, and aVF. Then flip the EKG over, hold it up to the light, and note the ST segment elevation in V_1, V_2, V_3, and V_4. It may be more comfortable (or easier) for you to simply copy the page containing Figure 13–8 and then hold the copied page up to the light.

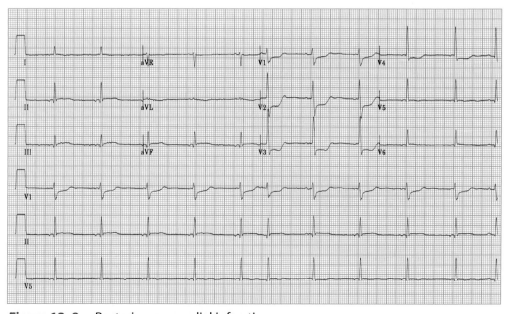

Figure 13–8. Posterior myocardial infarction

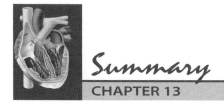

Summary
CHAPTER 13

As the discussion of the specific types of MIs ends with this chapter, there are two more items that we want to share with you. First, look now at Figure 13–9 and note the correlation of the chest leads, right-sided leads, and posterior leads with the anatomy of the heart. This figure illustrates the comprehensive views that are possible with 12- or 15-lead EKG tracings. You may recall that much earlier in this book we used the analogy of taking photographs of the heart while walking around a pedestal. Think of that action as you view Figure 13–9. We believe that by doing this mental exercise you will be able to recognize the various views that can be obtained by a 12-lead EKG tracing.

Another mnemonic or memory aid was formulated by one of our former EMT-Intermediate graduates, Melissa Patterson. Melissa was struggling to recall the acute lead specific injury pattern, so she came up with this: I SAW A LION'S PAW. The first letter of each word stands for:

I	Inferior	Leads II, III, and aVF
SAW	Septal	Leads V_1 and V_2
A	Anterior	Leads V_3 and V_4
LION'S	Lateral	Leads V_5 and V_6
PAW	Posterior	Leads V_1, V_2, V_3, and/or V_4 (ST depression)

Melissa's classmates (and instructor) immediately picked up on this memory aid, and we decided to include it here for your reference.

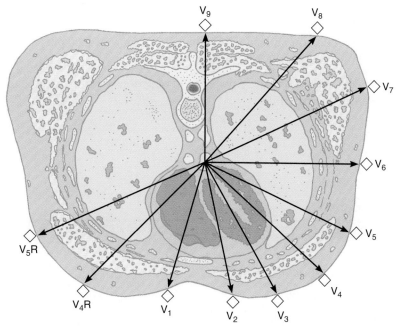

Figure 13–9. Cross-section of heart with associated chest leads, right-sided leads, posterior leads, and myocardial wall

EKG CHANGES IN POSTERIOR MIs

ST segment depression in Leads V_1, V_2, V_3, and/or V_4	Tall R waves

EKG CHANGES IN INFEROPOSTERIOR MIs

ST segment elevation in Leads II, III, and aVF; ST segment depression in Leads V_1, V_2, V_3, and/or V_4	T wave inversion; tall R waves; pathologic Q waves

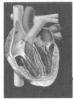

Key Points to Remember
CHAPTER 13

1. Posterior wall infarctions may involve the right coronary artery.

2. Lead-specific ST segment changes for posterior MI will be ST segment depression in Leads V_1, V_2, V_3, and V_4.

3. The anterior portion of the myocardium lies opposite the posterior portion of the muscle mass.

4. Look at the posterior walls. Reciprocal leads will show depression.

5. Posterior V leads will show ST elevation and most commonly are V_7, V_8, and V_9, which are placed on the posterior chest.

6. The 15-lead option on 12-lead EKG units allows for a 12-lead plus three to be performed, showing the posterior leads.

7. Posterior MIs may lead to the development of serious rhythm disturbances indicative of ventricular irritability.

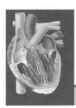

Review Questions
CHAPTER 13

1. ST segment elevation may indicate:

    a. ventricular atrophy.

    b. ventricular hypertrophy.

    c. myocardial injury.

    d. atrial aneurysm.

2. The T wave on the EKG strip represents:

   a. rest period.

   b. bundle of His.

   c. atrial contraction.

   d. ventricular contraction.

3. When interpreting dysrhythmias, remember that the most important key is the:

   a. PR interval.

   b. rate and rhythm.

   c. presence of dysrhythmias.

   d. patient's clinical appearance.

4. If ST segment elevation is noted in the lower limb leads (II, III, and aVF), this finding is indicative of ___ MI.

   a. anterior

   b. lateral

   c. superior

   d. inferior

5. EKG leads that record the electrical impulse formation in uninvolved myocardium directly opposite from the involved myocardium are called ___ leads.

   a. facing

   b. viewing

   c. reciprocal

   d. endocardial

6. If your patient is hypotensive and is exhibiting EKG changes consistent with an inferior MI, consider the possibility of ___ infarction.

   a. right atrial

   b. left atrial

   c. right ventricular

   d. left ventricular

7. The combination of posterior wall injury evidence, in addition to evidence of ___, indicates a more extensive infarction and a greater risk of complications.

   a. anterior wall ischemia

   b. inferior infarction

   c. T wave inversion

   d. prolonged PR interval

8. When dealing with inferior and inferoposterior MIs, the appearance of high-degree AV blocks may be present upon admission to the hospital. Examples of high-degree blocks include ___ blocks.

   a. first-degree   c. third-degree

   b. second-degree Type I   d. Wenckebach (Mobitz I)

9. The 12-lead EKG machine is capable of recognizing the posterior V leads (V_7, V_8, and V_9).
   a. True
   b. False

10. Placement of posterior Lead V_7 is at the level of the:
    a. 7th intercostal space, anterior axilla.
    b. 5th intercostal space, mid-scapula.
    c. 5th intercostal space, posterior axilla.
    d. 3rd intercostal space, mid-axilla.

11. Placement of posterior Lead V_8 is at the level of the:
    a. 7th intercostal space, anterior axilla.
    b. 5th intercostal space, mid-scapula.
    c. 5th intercostal space, posterior axilla.
    d. 3rd intercostal space, mid-axilla.

12. Placement of posterior Lead V_9 is at the level of the:
    a. 7th intercostal space, anterior axilla.
    b. 5th intercostal space, 2 cm left of the spine.
    c. 5th intercostal space, posterior axilla.
    d. 3rd intercostal space, 4 cm lateral to the spine.

13. When considering the possibility of posterior wall MIs, expect to assess reciprocal leads rather than indicative leads.
    a. True
    b. False

14. When tall R waves are noted in Lead V_1, this finding should prompt you to think of inferior infarctions.
    a. True
    b. False

15. When conducting the mirror test, the mirror should be placed ___ the V leads of the 12-lead EKG.
    a. below
    b. beside
    c. above
    d. to the left of

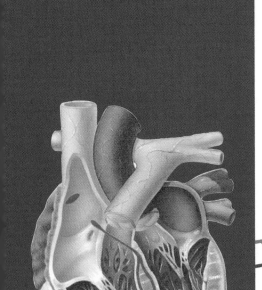

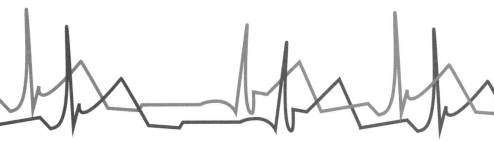

Axis Deviation and Bundle Branch Blocks

objectives

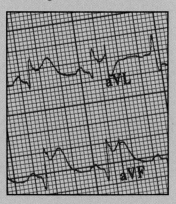

Upon completion of this chapter, the student will be able to:

➤ Define the following terms
  a. Vector
  b. Normal axis
  c. Right axis deviation
  d. Left axis deviation

➤ Identify the causes of right axis deviation

➤ Determine the causes of left axis deviation

➤ Explain the methodology utilized to determine axis deviation

➤ Recall and describe the components of the electrical conduction system of the heart

➤ Identify the characteristics of a right bundle branch block (RBBB)

➤ Identify the characteristics of a left bundle branch block (LBBB)

➤ List causes of bundle branch blocks

➤ Identify the location of MIs that may result in new onset right and left bundle branch blocks

➤ Discuss the clinical significance of bundle branch blocks

INTRODUCTION

A brief discussion of axis deviation is included in this text because this determinant is specific to the 12-lead EKG. Axis deviation cannot be determined with a standard 3-lead EKG. The concept of axis deviation can be very complex. In this text, however, we have elected to employ a simple approach to the basics of axis determination.

EKG LEADS

An EKG machine records the electrical activity of the heart as this activity is detected by various leads attached to the body. In order to detect this electrical activity, a minimum of two electrodes must be utilized. Thus, each lead is made up of a pair of electrodes. Most commonly, one electrode is positive and the other is negative. When an electrical current moves toward the positive electrode, a positive deflection will appear on the recorder. This positive deflection will cause the stylus to move in an upward direction. Conversely, if the electrical current moves away from the positive electrode, this will cause a negative deflection on the EKG machine and the stylus will move downward. You should realize that electrical activity of the heart is a complex combination of both positive and negative current flows. These current flows are depicted graphically on EKG paper as it moves through the EKG machine.

As you will recall, it takes both a negative and a positive lead to be able to create waveforms on an EKG tracing. Recall also that there are three types of EKG leads: bipolar, augmented, and precordial (Table 14–1).

You should remember that the bipolar limb leads and the augmented limb leads (Leads I, II, III, aVR, aVL, and aVF) together comprise the **frontal plane leads.** These leads are placed on the patient's extremities. Frontal plane leads, as their name suggests, record the electrical activity of the heart in the frontal plane of the body. This means that the electrical currents are measured from the top of the heart to the bottom of the heart, or from right to left.

The **precordial leads** (also referred to as chest leads) are V_1, V_2, V_3, V_4, V_5, and V_6. They view the heart in the horizontal plane. In order to envision the horizontal plane, imagine that a cross-section of the body is taken from the front to the back. Now envision the heart as the central point of the cross-section. The electrical current flows from that central point out to each of the V leads. A ground lead is used as a reference point or negative pole. Figure 14–1 provides a view of 12-lead EKG perspectives.

frontal plane leads bipolar limb leads and augmented limb leads (Leads I, II, III, aVR, aVL, and aVF)

precordial leads chest leads (V_1, V_2, V_3, V_4, V_5, and V_6)

Table 14–1

EKG leads

Bipolar limb leads	I, II, and III
Augmented limb leads	aVR, aVL, and aVF
Precordial leads	V_1, V_2, V_3, V_4, V_5, and V_6

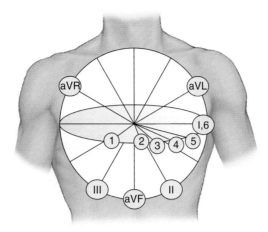

Figure 14–1.   12-lead EKG perspectives

THE HEXAXIAL REFERENCE SYSTEM

The limb leads view the frontal plane. The hexaxial reference system takes Leads I, II, III, aVR, aVL, and aVF and superimposes them over each other to form a 360-degree circle. It is divided into positive and negative sides with the direction of the left arm beginning at zero (0) degrees. It measures clockwise in 30-degree increments until it reaches 180 degrees, and then it begins to measure in the negative range until it returns to zero (0) degrees.

At this time, you should examine the hexaxial reference system as depicted in Figure 14–2 and begin to become acquainted with the leads and their corresponding degree representations.

These degree representations are used to calculate the exact axis of the heart. However, in the emergent situation, finding the exact degree of axis is less important than determining the presence of any deviation in the axis. Therefore, we will now discuss axis deviation.

AXIS DEVIATION

Some of the critical elements involved in axis determination are:
- ➤ **Vector** — a mark (or symbol) that can be used to describe any force having both magnitude and direction; the direction of electrical currents in cardiac cells that are generated by depolarization and repolarization of the atria and ventricles as it spreads from the endocardium outward to the epicardium. Most frequently, arrows are used for this purpose (Figure 14–3). The mean QRS vector is typically represented by a single large arrow.
- ➤ **Lead axis** — the axis of a given lead.
- ➤ **Axis** — the direction of the heart's electrical current from negative to positive.
- ➤ **Mean QRS axis** — the mean (average) of all ventricular vectors is a single large vector with a mean QRS axis, usually pointing to the left and downward. As you

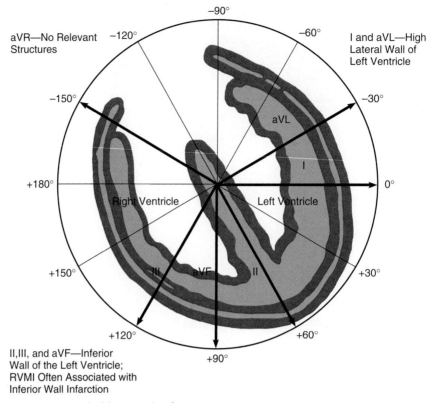

Figure 14–2. Detailed hexaxial reference system

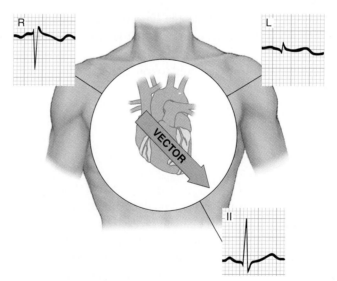

Figure 14–3. Cardiac vector (QRS axis)

look at Figure 14–4, you will see a graphic depiction of the normal or mean QRS axis, which falls between 0 degrees and +90 degrees.

➤ **Axis deviation** — an alteration in the normal flow of current, which represents an abnormal ventricular depolarization pathway and may signify death or disease of the myocardium.

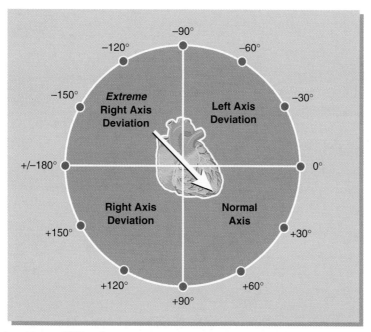

Figure 14–4.   Mean QRS axis

All waveforms have their own axis (i.e., P axis, QRS axis, and T axis). Because the **QRS axis** is usually the largest of the axes (and most commonly measured), and because of the amount of myocardial muscle, it is called the *QRS mean axis* (which is the sum direction of electrical flow through the heart as a whole).

There exists a correlation between axis (vector) and the anatomy of the myocardium. Recall that during normal conduction the impulse travels from top to bottom (or from right to left). In the hexaxial reference chart, the mean axis most commonly flows to a point of +30 degrees, which is located between Lead I and Lead II. When the heart is enlarged (ventricular hypertrophy), or due to disease or death of the muscle, the conduction pattern is altered or deviated, hence the term **axis deviation.**

Remember that the normal QRS axis falls between 0 degrees and +90 degrees. When a change (or shift) occurs, the flow of the electrical current is changed or deviated. When the deviation is between +90 degrees and + or −180 degrees, it is considered a **right axis deviation.** Right axis deviation is caused by several cardiac and/or pulmonary disorders. When the axis is deviated between −90 and + or −180 degrees, it is considered **extreme right axis deviation** (or *indeterminate axis deviation*). This degree of deviation, however, is very rare. When the deviation is between 0 and −90 degrees, this is considered a **left axis deviation.** Left axis deviation is caused by several cardiac disorders. Table 14–2 represents a list of pathophysiological disorders that can cause axis deviation.

There are several methods commonly utilized in the determination of the presence of axis deviation. One method uses only two leads, whereas the other methods may use more than two leads. We feel that in the emergent setting, the two-lead method is more efficient. In the two-lead method, look at Leads I and aVF, as recorded on the 12-lead EKG machine. Table 14–3 and Figure 14–5 illustrate the findings that may be used to quickly calculate the QRS axis.

QRS axis the largest of the axes and the most commonly measured

axis deviation occurs when the conduction pattern is altered due to disease or death of the muscle

right axis deviation an axis deviation between +90 and + or −180 degrees

extreme right axis deviation an axis deviation between −90 and + or −180 degrees. Also called indeterminate axis deviation

left axis deviation an axis deviation between 0 and −90 degrees

Table 14–2

Causes of axis deviation

Right axis deviation may be caused by:	Left axis deviation may be caused by:
COPD	Ischemic heart disease
Pulmonary embolism	Systemic hypertension
Congenital heart disease	Aortic stenosis
Pulmonary hypertension	Disorders of the left ventricle
Cor pulmonale	Aortic valvular disease
	Wolfe-Parkinson-White syndrome

Table 14–3

Two-lead method for determining axis deviation

Axis	Lead I	Lead aVF
Normal	Positive QRS deflection	Positive QRS deflection
Left axis	Positive QRS deflection	Negative deflection
Right axis	Negative QRS deflection	Positive QRS deflection
Extreme right axis	Negative QRS deflection	Negative QRS deflection

Determination of axis is useful in 12-lead EKG interpretation because bundle branch blocks, chamber enlargement, and various other factors can affect the QRS axis.

BUNDLE BRANCH BLOCKS

Review of the electrical conduction system

The electrical conduction system of the heart includes the following components: the SA node, internodal pathways, AV node, AV junction, bundle of His, right and left bundle branches, and the Purkinje's network. Take a moment to refer to Table 14–4 and Figure 14–6 for a brief review of the electrical conduction system, including the inherent firing rates of each of the three pacemakers.

Bundle branches

The right bundle branch runs down the right side of the interventricular septum and terminates at the papillary muscles in the right ventricle. This bundle branch functions to carry electrical impulses to the right ventricle.

Shorter than the right bundle branch, the left bundle branch divides into pathways that spread from the left side of the interventricular septum and throughout the left ventricle. The two main divisions of the left bundle branch are called **fascicles.** The *anterior*

fascicles the two main divisions of the left bundle branch

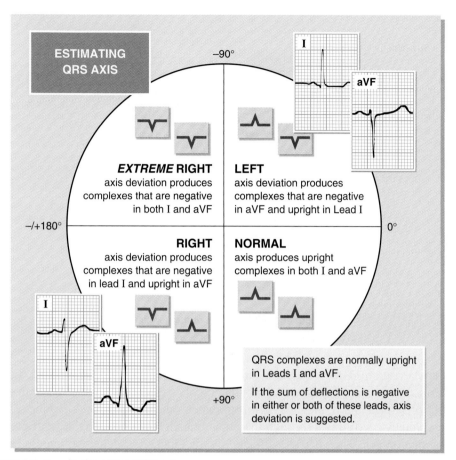

Figure 14–5.   Estimating QRS axis

Table 14–4

		Review of the electrical conduction system of the heart		
SA Node	**Internodal Pathways**	**AV Junction (AV Node and Bundle)**	**Bundle Branches**	**Purkinje's Network**
Firing rate: 60–100 BPM	Transfer impulse from the SA node throughout the atria to the AV junction	Slows impulse; intrinsic firing rate of 40–60 BPM	Two main branches (left and right) transmit impulse to ventricles	Spreads impulses throughout the ventricles; intrinsic firing rate of 20–40 BPM

fascicle carries electrical impulses to the anterior wall of the left ventricle. The *posterior fascicle* spreads the impulses to the posterior ventricular wall.

Normally, the impulse travels simultaneously through the right bundle branch and the left bundle branch, causing depolarization of the interventricular septum and

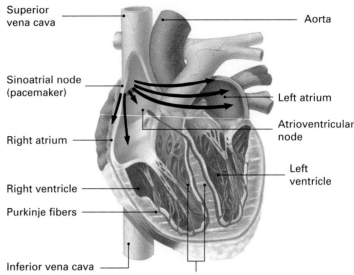

Superior vena cava

Aorta

Sinoatrial node (pacemaker)

Left atrium

Atrioventricular node

Right atrium

Left ventricle

Right ventricle

Purkinje fibers

Inferior vena cava

Right and left branches of the bundle of His

Figure 14–6. Cardiac conduction system

then depolarization of the right and left ventricular muscles. Simply stated, bundle branch blocks represent the abnormal conduction of an electrical impulse through either the right or left bundle branches. Therefore, when one bundle branch is blocked, the electrical impulse will travel through the intact branch and stimulate the ventricle supplied by that branch. The ventricle affected by the blocked or defective bundle branch is activated indirectly by impulses that cross through the interventricular septum from the unaffected branch. There is a delay caused by this alternate route; thus the QRS complex will represent widening beyond the usual time interval of 0.12 second.

Bundle branch blocks may be classified as either complete or incomplete blocks. Though you will not be asked to differentiate between complete and incomplete bundle branch blocks, it is wise for you to know that an **incomplete bundle branch block** is one in which the width of the QRS complex will measure between 0.10 and 0.11 second, whereas a **complete bundle branch block** is one in which the width of the QRS complex will measure 0.12 second or greater.

Right bundle branch block

The occurrence of right bundle branch blocks is a relatively common development. As stated earlier, the right bundle branch leaves the bundle of His and runs down the right side of the interventricular septum to conduct the electrical impulses to the right ventricle. Anatomically, the right bundle branch is relatively thin and more vulnerable to disruption. A relatively small lesion can disrupt the right bundle branch. This disruption primarily occurs secondary to an anteroseptal MI. More rarely, RBBBs can resemble anteroseptal, inferior, or posterior wall MIs, but generally do not block the EKG changes of MIs. When a RBBB occurs, the electrical impulses are prevented from entering the right ventricle directly, causing a delay in depolarization of the right ventricle.

The right ventricle is a low-pressure chamber that pumps deoxygenated blood to the lungs. The muscle mass of the right ventricle is smaller than the left ventricular muscle mass. In the normal EKG, the electrical forces of the right ventricle are overshadowed by the more massive forces of the larger left ventricle. In the case of a right bundle

incomplete bundle branch block one in which the width of the QRS complex measures between 0.10 and 0.11 second

complete bundle branch block one in which the width of the QRS complex will measure 0.12 second or greater

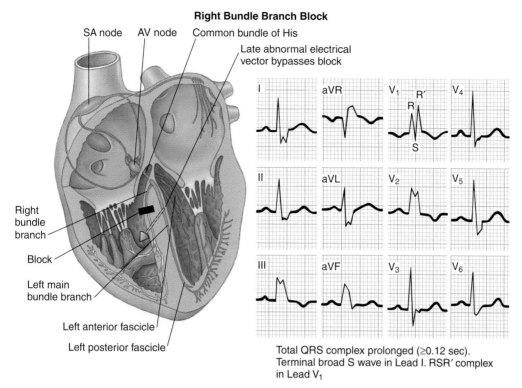

Right Bundle Branch Block

Total QRS complex prolonged (≥0.12 sec).
Terminal broad S wave in Lead I. RSR′ complex
in Lead V$_1$.

Figure 14–7. Right bundle branch block

branch block, right ventricular depolarization occurs after left ventricular depolarization. In this scenario, the impulse is spread from the left ventricle to the right ventricle rather than being stimulated by the right bundle branch.

EKG changes will occur secondary to the disruption of conduction of the electrical impulses through the right bundle branch.

You may expect to see the following EKG changes in conjunction with right bundle branch blocks:

- ➤ Duration of QRS complex 0.12 second or greater (complete block).
- ➤ Duration of QRS complex 0.10 or 0.11 second (incomplete block).
- ➤ QRS axis may be normal or deviated to the right.
- ➤ Small Q waves with normal configuration may be seen in Leads I, aVL, V$_5$, and V$_6$.
- ➤ Small R waves may be present in V$_1$ and V$_2$.
- ➤ Classic RSR pattern (Figure 14–7) or the "M" or "rabbit ears" in Leads V$_1$ and V$_2$.
- ➤ Slurred S waves in Leads I, aVL, V$_5$, and V$_6$ producing qRS pattern in V$_5$ and V$_6$.

Left bundle branch block

The presence of a left bundle branch block may indicate significant myocardial disease. As stated earlier, the left bundle branch is a short, thick, flat left common bundle branch and has two main divisions. The divisions of the left bundle branch are referred to as the *left anterior and posterior fascicles*. The left bundle branch conducts electrical impulses to the left ventricle and the interventricular septum. A widespread lesion is necessary to block the less vulnerable main stem of the left bundle branch. When a left bundle branch block occurs, the left ventricle cannot be depolarized normally.

The electrical impulses are prevented from entering the left ventricle directly because of the disruption of conduction of the electrical impulses through the left bundle branch. Therefore, depolarization must proceed down the right bundle branch and across the interventricular septum from the right to the left ventricle. This abnormal depolarization process via myocardial rather than specialized conduction fibers takes longer, so that QRS complexes are widened and the duration is prolonged.

It will be helpful for you to realize that left bundle branch blocks have the same general orientation as in normal depolarization, traveling from right to left, which is the same direction as most forces in normal depolarization. Left bundle branch blocks may occur secondary to anteroseptal or inferior MIs.

You may expect to see the following EKG changes in conjunction with left bundle branch blocks:

➤ Duration of QRS complex 0.12 second or greater (complete block).
➤ Duration of QRS complex 0.10 or 0.11 second (incomplete block).
➤ QRS axis may be normal or deviated to the left.
➤ Q waves are absent in Leads I, V_5, and V_6.
➤ R waves small to relatively tall; narrow R waves may be present in V_1, V_2, and V_3; tall, wide, slurred R waves present in Leads I, aVL, V_5, and V_6; R waves may be notched.
➤ Classic rSR pattern (Figure 14–8) or the "M" or "rabbit ears" in Leads V_5 and V_6.
➤ Deep, wide S waves in Leads V_1, V_2, and V_3.

The underlying heart disease that produces the block, rather than the conduction abnormality itself, usually determines the patient's progress. As a word of caution, you should be aware that the presence of a left bundle branch block will tend to obscure ischemic changes associated with MI. The possibility of localizing an MI with a 12-lead EKG may be greatly hampered if a left bundle branch block is present.

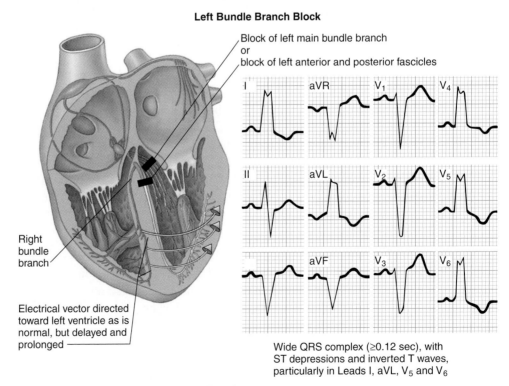

Left Bundle Branch Block

Block of left main bundle branch or block of left anterior and posterior fascicles

Right bundle branch

Electrical vector directed toward left ventricle as is normal, but delayed and prolonged

Wide QRS complex (≥0.12 sec), with ST depressions and inverted T waves, particularly in Leads I, aVL, V_5 and V_6

Figure 14–8. Left bundle branch block

Specifically, LBBBs characteristically mask the Q wave of lateral, inferior, and anteroseptal MIs.

CLINICAL SIGNIFICANCE OF BUNDLE BRANCH BLOCKS

In the prehospital or emergent setting, realize that the presence of EKG evidence indicating bundle branch blocks may not be clinically significant. It is very difficult, if not impossible, to definitively recognize a preexisting bundle branch block merely by obtaining a 12-lead EKG.

However, if you encounter a patient who presents with signs and symptoms of coronary ischemia and, after obtaining a 12-lead EKG tracing on the patient, you note evidence of bundle branch block, your index of suspicion for the possibility that this is a new onset bundle branch block should be heightened.

Therefore, as a health-care provider, you should realize that a new onset of bundle branch block in the face of an acute MI is an important finding.

Research indicates that approximately 15% to 30% of patients experiencing MIs in conjunction with new onset bundle branch blocks may develop complete heart block and an estimated 30% to 70% of these individuals may develop cardiogenic shock. It is also estimated that cardiogenic shock carries an 85% mortality rate. Consequently, you must recognize the clinical significance of new onset bundle branch blocks, particularly when dealing with patients who exhibit symptomology consistent with acute MI.

In order to determine the presence of a new onset bundle branch block, it is necessary for the physician to have access to previous 12-lead EKGs. By viewing a previous 12-lead EKG tracing, the health-care provider can determine the existence (or nonexistence) of a previous bundle branch block. Although this is quite important for the purpose of comparative analysis, it may not always be feasible. For instance, the patient may have never had a 12-lead EKG, may be from another state, or the previous 12-lead may be located in his or her physician's office.

The 12-lead EKGs in Figures 14–9 through 14–12 are graphic representations of right and left bundle branch blocks.

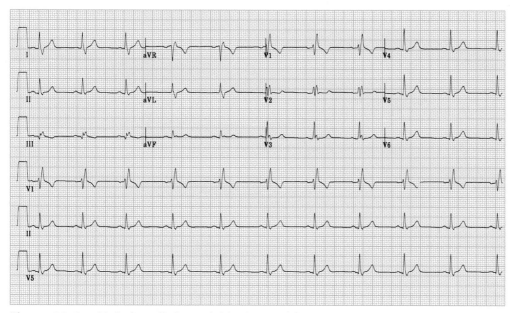

Figure 14–9.   Right bundle branch block, normal axis

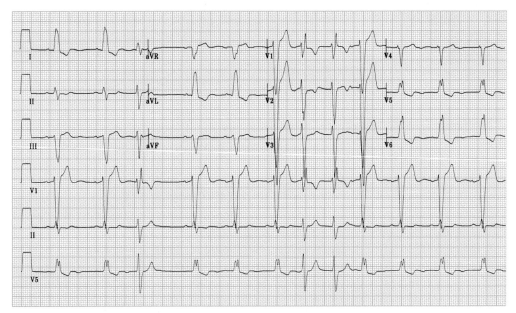

Figure 14–10.   Left bundle branch block, left axis deviation

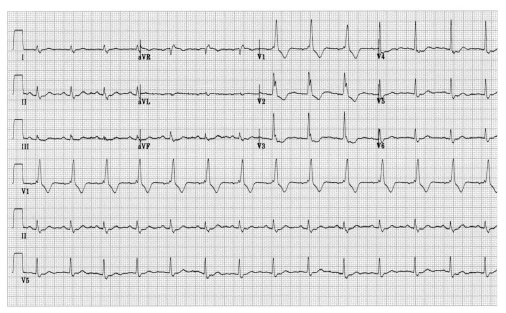

Figure 14–11.   Right bundle branch block, normal axis

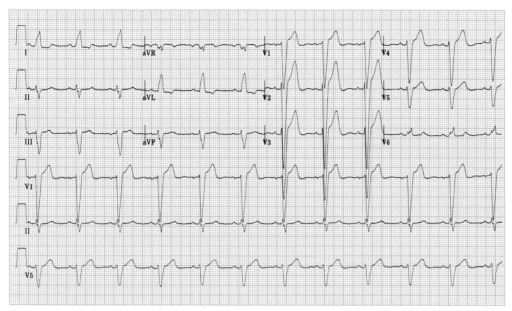

Figure 14–12. Left bundle branch block, left axis deviation

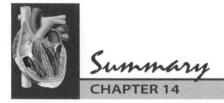

Summary
CHAPTER 14

As you have learned, axis deviation is specific to the 12-lead EKG. Axis deviation is useful in 12-lead interpretation in that bundle branch blocks, chamber enlargement, and various other factors can affect the QRS axis and assist in diagnosing other conditions that effect the heart. You have also learned that bundle branch blocks can effect the ability to interpret an acute MI when these are present as well as the importance if the bundle branch block is a new onset.

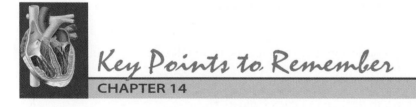

Key Points to Remember
CHAPTER 14

1. The hexaxial reference system takes Leads I, II, III and Leads aVR, aVL, and aVF and superimposes them over each other to form a 360-degree circle.

2. The circle is divided into positive and negative sides with the direction of the left arm beginning at zero (0) degrees.

3. Vector is a mark that can be used to describe any force having both magnitude and direction.

4. Lead axis is the axis of a given lead.

5. A mean QRS axis falls between 0 and +90 degrees.

6. Axis deviation is an alteration in the normal flow of current.

7. Right axis deviation is a deviation between +90 degrees and + or −180 degrees.

8. Extreme right or indeterminate axis deviation is a deviation between −90 and + or −180 degrees.

9. Left axis deviation is a deviation between 0 and −90 degrees.

10. Right axis deviation may be caused by COPD, pulmonary embolism, cor pulmonale, pulmonary hypertension, or congenital heart disease.

11. Left axis deviation may be caused by ischemic heart disease, systemic hypertension, aortic valvular disease, or Wolfe-Parkinson-White syndrome.

12. Normal axis is indicated by a positive QRS deflection in Leads I and aVF.

13. Left axis deviation is indicated by a positive QRS deflection in Lead I and a negative deflection in Lead aVF.

14. Right axis deviation is indicated by a negative QRS deflection in Lead I and a positive QRS deflection in aVF.

15. Extreme right axis deviation is indicated by a negative QRS deflection in Lead I and a negative QRS deflection in aVF.

16. Bundle branch blocks may be classified as either complete or incomplete.

17. Bundle branch blocks can be either a right or left bundle branch block.

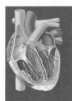

Review Questions
CHAPTER 14

1. In the two-lead method of axis determination, a normal axis is determined by:
   a. negative QRS deflection in Leads I and aVF.
   b. positive QRS deflection in Leads I and aVF.
   c. negative QRS deflection in Lead I and positive QRS deflection in aVF.
   d. negative QRS deflection in Lead I and positive QRS deflection in aVL.

2. In the two-lead method of axis determination, a left axis deviation is determined by:
   a. negative QRS deflection in Leads I and aVF.
   b. positive QRS deflection in Leads I and aVF.
   c. negative QRS deflection in Lead I and positive QRS deflection in aVF.
   d. positive QRS deflection in Lead I and negative QRS deflection in aVF.

3. In the two-lead method of axis determination, a right axis deviation is determined by:

    a. negative QRS deflection in Leads I and aVF.

    b. positive QRS deflection in Leads I and aVF.

    c. negative QRS deflection in Lead I and positive QRS deflection in aVF.

    d. positive QRS deflection in Lead I and negative QRS deflection in aVF.

4. In the two-lead method of axis determination, an indeterminate right axis deviation is determined by:

    a. negative QRS deflection in Leads I and aVF.

    b. positive QRS deflection in Leads I and aVF.

    c. negative QRS deflection in Lead I and positive QRS deflection in aVF.

    d. positive QRS deflection in Lead I and negative QRS deflection in aVF.

5. Which one of the following disease processes can be expected in left axis deviation?

    a. left bundle branch block

    b. pulmonary hypertension

    c. Wolfe-Parkinson-White syndrome

    d. pulmonary embolism

6. Which one of the following disease processes can be expected in right axis deviation?

    a. ischemic heart disease

    b. chronic obstructive pulmonary disease

    c. right bundle branch block

    d. systemic hypertension

7. The right bundle branch runs down the right side of the interventricular septum and terminates at the ___ in the right ventricle.

    a. Purkinje's network

    b. papillary muscles

    c. anterior fascicle

    d. posterior fascicle

8. In the prehospital or emergent setting, you should realize that the presence of EKG evidence indicating bundle branch blocks is always clinically significant.

    a. True

    b. False

9. An incomplete bundle branch block is one in which the width of the QRS complex will measure between 0.10 and 0.11 second.

    a. True

    b. False

10. A complete block is one in which the width of the QRS complex will measure 0.12 second or greater.

   a. True

   b. False

11. In the presence of an acute MI, a right bundle branch block will obscure EKG evidence.

   a. True

   b. False

12. To determine right bundle branch block, the primary EKG leads to observe are:

   a. V_1 and V_2.

   b. V_5 and V_6.

   c. V_2 and V_3.

   d. V_2 and V_4.

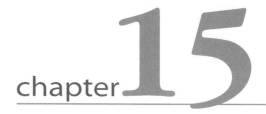

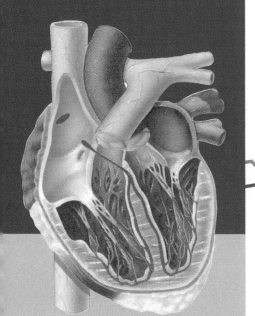

Therapeutic Modalities

objectives

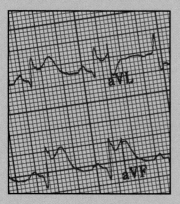

Upon completion of this chapter, the student will be able to:

➤ Discuss the purpose of fibrinolytics in the treatment of myocardial infarction

➤ Describe and list the indications for fibrinolytic therapy

➤ Describe and list the contraindications for fibrinolytic therapy

➤ Review the various fibrinolytic agents and the correct dosage of each agent

➤ Describe the indications for pacing in the emergency situation

➤ Discuss the purpose of transcutaneous pacing

➤ Define cardioversion and defibrillation

➤ Describe the indications for cardioversion

➤ Describe the indications for defibrillation

➤ Review the techniques for cardioversion and defibrillation

INTRODUCTION

Recall that the goal of management of the patient with symptomatic chest pain is to attempt to stop the infarction process. This goal can often be accomplished through interventions such as oxygen administration, pain alleviation, and possibly initiation of *fibrinolytic therapy* (also known as *thrombolytic therapy*) in order to limit the progression of the infarct. Although fibrinolytics were first used in the late 1950s, it was not until the 1980s that they began to be considered the standard in treating acute MIs. Ever-evolving medical research, including recent clinical trials, now strongly suggests that *early percutaneous coronary intervention (PCI)* may indeed be the most comprehensive and effective treatment for the patient who is suspected to have experienced an MI. An obstacle in the use of PCI presents when there is no hospital readily available and equipped for cardiac catherizations. In this chapter, we will discuss the five agents most commonly used today.

We continue to stress that the core component of assessment and treatment of the patient who presents with chest pain centers on the prompt oxygenation of hypoxic tissue. Treatment initiatives will vary depending upon your patient's specific situation; however, you must focus on continual and thorough assessment until such time that the patient is clinically stable.

You will learn in this chapter that one of the more serious side effects of fibrinolytic therapy involves reperfusion dysrhythmias, which may require various interventions such as pharmacologic agents, pacing, cardioversion, and/or defibrillation. Thus, this chapter also will discuss these various modalities.

FIBRINOLYTICS

Fibrinolytics have changed the focus of the initial management of acute MIs in this decade. Stated simply, fibrinolytics dissolve blood clots, which continue to be the leading cause of MIs. This process of "clot busting" allows for the occluded artery to be reopened. As a result, reoxygenation of the ischemic or infarcted tissue will likely occur. You have learned in previous chapters of the critical importance of the *time is muscle* concept. The maximum benefit of fibrinolytic therapy is best achieved when the agent is administered within 6 to 12 hours after the onset of symptoms. Administration of fibrinolytic therapy more than 12 hours after the onset of symptoms is of little benefit.

Several of the fibrinolytic agents that you will likely be encountering when dealing with the emergent treatment of acute MI are described on the following pages.

Indications

Based on specific screening criteria, the administration of fibrinolytics may be indicated for the patient who presents with clinical and EKG evidence of an acute MI. Clinical presentations in patients with suspected acute MIs were discussed in detail in Chapter 8. Based again on the *time is muscle* concept, you will recognize that late EKG changes (i.e., the development of pathologic Q waves) occur hours after the initial insult. To wait for this type of definitive EKG change would therefore be detrimental to

Table 15–1

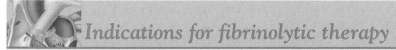

Indications for fibrinolytic therapy

ST segment elevation (1 mm or greater in two contiguous leads).	Clinical presentation: chest pain unrelieved by rest (may radiate), diaphoresis, pallor.

the very purpose of fibrinolytic therapy (early interruption of the MI process). Thus, the most common tool used to indicate the presence of myocardial damage that may lead to infarction is ST segment elevation (Table 15–1).

Screening criteria

Screening criteria for the use of fibrinolytic therapy are very important and essential components of the selection of potential candidates. The major side effect of fibrinolytics therapy is bleeding. These agents not only dissolve the clots located in the coronary arteries, but also the clots in any circulatory system vessel. Consequently, the screening is done to identify those patients who may be susceptible to catastrophic hemorrhage.

Fibrinolytic check sheets are composed of generic lists of patient data, as well as lists of absolute and relative contraindications. The format of the check sheet may vary across the nation. The information inquiry, based on the particular check sheet, is typically completed in the prehospital setting or immediately upon arrival in the critical care areas of the hospital (ED, ICU, CCU).

Contraindications

Although contraindications are numerous and very notable, it is vital to stress the importance of the proven beneficial role of fibrinolytic therapy in the treatment of the acute MI. The major complication of fibrinolytic therapy is hemorrhage, usually a direct result of the mechanism of action of the agent.

Contraindications in the use of fibrinolytic therapy are classified as absolute and relative. *Relative contraindications* are those that the physician must consider in the decision to institute or withhold fibrinolytic therapy. With the existence of as few as one of the *absolute contraindications,* fibrinolytic therapy usually is not initiated. As with any type of therapy, however, the physician must ultimately decide whether the benefits of fibrinolytic therapy outweigh the risks. If the physician decides that fibrinolytic therapy is the treatment modality of choice, he or she must consult the patient regarding this decision and seek to gain permission. Refer to Tables 15–2 and 15–3 for the most commonly used relative and absolute contraindications.

Fibrinolytic agents

Acetylsalicylic Acid (ASA, Aspirin)   Aspirin is one of the most commonly used anti-inflammatory agents. One of the primary mechanisms of action of acetylsalicylic acid is its ability to inhibit the function of platelets. Thus, ASA has gained prominence as a beneficial agent in the treatment of thromboembolic diseases such as acute MI. It has

Table 15–2

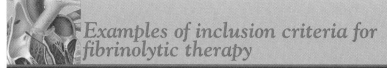

Examples of inclusion criteria for fibrinolytic therapy

Inclusion Criteria

• Age of less than 75 years. (There is diminished benefit in ages greater than 75.)
• Clinical complaints consistent with ischemic-type chest pain.
  • Onset of chest pain occurring within 12 hours.
  • Most benefit from fibrinolysis if given within 6 hours.
  • Little benefit from fibrinolysis if given after 12 hours, unless symptomatic.
• EKG changes
  • ST-segment elevation ≥ or = 1 mm in two or more contiguous limb leads.
  • ST-segment elevation ≥ or = 2 mm in two or more contiguous precordial leads.
  • New or presumably new bundle branch block (BBB).

Table 15–3

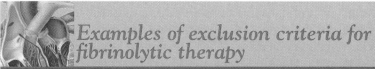

Examples of exclusion criteria for fibrinolytic therapy

Relative Contraindications	Absolute Contraindications
• Severe uncontrolled hypertension at presentation (BP > 180/110). • Other intracerebral pathology. • Current use of anticoagulants. • Recent trauma (previous 8 weeks), including head trauma. • Prolonged and traumatic CPR. • Major surgery (less than 3 weeks prior). • Noncompressible vascular punctures. • Pregnancy. • Active peptic ulcer.	• Unwilling or unable to give informed consent. • Previous hemorrhagic stroke at any time; other strokes or cerebrovascular events within 1 year. • Known intracranial neoplasm. • Active internal bleeding within past 3-week period. • Suspected aortic dissection. • Surgery within previous 2 weeks.

proven highly effective in reducing mortality associated with MI. Aspirin also appears to reduce the rate of nonfatal stroke.

TRADE NAME:	Aspirin.
GENERIC NAME:	Acetylsalicylic acid.
ONSET:	5 to 30 minutes after ingestion.
HALF-LIFE:	2 to 3 hours for low dosages.
DOSAGE:	160 to 325 milligrams (chewable).
SIDE EFFECTS:	**Tinnitus,** dizziness, gastrointestinal (GI) disorders.
PRECAUTIONS:	History of GI disease, renal disease, hepatic disease, chronic alcohol use and abuse.

tinnitus the sound of "ringing in the ears"

Streptokinase (SK)   Streptokinase (SK) was the first fibrinolytic agent on the market and available for use. This agent has a bacterial origin. Anisoylated plasminogen SK activator complex (APSAC) was developed after SK as a hybrid.

TRADE NAME: Streptase.
GENERIC NAME: Streptokinase.
ONSET: Immediate.
PEAK: 20 minutes to 2 hours.
DURATION: 4 hours.
DOSAGE: 1.5 million units in 1-hour infusion.
SIDE EFFECTS: Bleeding, allergic reaction, anaphylaxis, fever, nausea, vomiting.
PRECAUTIONS: Streptase therapy within past 12 months; anaphylaxis may occur; reperfusion dysrhythmias are common.

Tissue Plasminogen Activator (tPA, Alteplase)   tPA/Alteplase has the distinction of being considered a clot-specific agent at low doses. This means that tPA will work on those clots in the coronary arteries that were recently formed and leave other clots in the systemic circulation alone. However, at **therapeutic levels,** tPA does not noticeably decrease the incidence of bleeding when compared to SK or urokinase (UK).

therapeutic level refers to an optimum level of a medication in the blood

TRADE NAME: Activase.
GENERIC NAME: Alteplase, tissue plasminogen activator.
ONSET: Immediate.
PEAK: 45 minutes.
DURATION: 4 hours.
DOSAGE: 15–mg IV bolus over 1 to 2 minutes; then 0.75 mg/kg over 30 minutes (not to exceed 50 mg); then 0.5 mg/kg over 60 minutes (not to exceed 35 mg).
SIDE EFFECTS: Bleeding, allergic reaction (infrequent), fever, nausea, vomiting, hypotension.
PRECAUTIONS: Although very uncommon, anaphylaxis may occur; **reperfusion dysrhythmias** are common.

reperfusion dysrhythmias dysrhythmias that occur after a vessel is reopened and blood flow returned

Retavase   Retavase was approved by the Food and Drug Administration in the latter part of 1996. This fibrinolytic agent is given as a double bolus of 10 units each with the second bolus given 30 minutes after the first.

TRADE NAME: Retavase.
GENERIC NAME: Reteplase, Recombinant.
ONSET: Immediate.
PEAK: 80 minutes.
DURATION: Half-life is 13 to 16 minutes in length.
DOSAGE: 10-unit IV bolus over 1 to 2 minutes; wait 30 minutes then repeat dosage (10-unit IV bolus over 1 to 2 minutes).
SIDE EFFECTS: Bleeding, allergic reactions.
PRECAUTIONS: Heparin and Retavase are incompatible when combined in solution and should not be administered simultaneously in the same IV line. Reperfusion dysrhythmias are common.

TNK (TNKase) TNK-t-PA   TNK-t-PA is the newest fibrinolytic agent on the market, released for use in early 2000. The agent is currently being tested widely in controlled localities.

half-life the time required for the total amount of a drug in the body to diminish by one-half

TRADE NAME:	TNKase (TNK-t-PA).
GENERIC NAME:	Tenecteptase.
ONSET:	16 minutes.
DURATION:	**Half-life** is 13 to 16 minutes in length.
DOSAGE:	0.50- to 0.55-mgm/kg (body weight adjusted) single dose over 10 seconds.
SIDE EFFECTS:	Bleeding, allergic reaction (infrequent), fever, nausea, vomiting, hypotension.
PRECAUTIONS:	Reperfusion dysrhythmias.

Urokinase (UK)   Although urokinase (UK) has been available for a longer period of time than either tPA or APSAC, this agent has been involved in the least amount of trial testing.

EMERGENCY EXTERNAL CARDIAC PACING

One of the most common precautions that you must be aware of is the prevalence of reperfusion dysrhythmias, particularly the bradydysrhythmias. Consequently, a discussion of external cardiac pacing is a necessary component of this chapter.

Although the concept of emergency cardiac pacing has been around for more than a century, the use of this therapy has become much more standard in the past decade. Although there are several different types of cardiac pacing, the type used most often in the emergent setting is called **transcutaneous cardiac pacing (TCP).** Among the more advantageous features of TCP are the minimal occurrence of complications, documented effectiveness, and the small amount of time needed to initiate the therapy.

transcutaneous cardiac pacing (TCP) therapy performed via two large electrode pads placed in an anterior-posterior position on a patient's chest to conduct electrical impulses through the skin to the heart

TCP consists of two large electrode pads that are most commonly placed in an anterior-posterior position on the patient's chest in order to conduct electrical impulses through the skin to the heart. When this method is used, cardiac cells depolarize in a normal fashion. Prior to implementation of TCP, the patient should be placed in a supine position and IV, oxygen, and EKG monitoring must be established. It is essential for the health-care provider to have received either Medical Control orders or orders from the attending physician prior to initiating TCP.

Indications for external cardiac pacing

External cardiac pacing is sometimes indicated for the treatment of certain reperfusion dysrhythmias, such as symptomatic bradycardia and/or heart block associated with reduced cardiac output. Examples of bradydysrhythmias frequently seen following the administration of fibrinolytics include (but are not limited to):

➤ Third-degree (complete) heart block.
➤ Second-degree Mobitz Type II heart block.
➤ Idioventricular rhythm (IVR).
➤ Accelerated idioventricular rhythm (AIVR).
➤ Profound bradycardia (clinically symptomatic).

Table 15–4

Procedure for transcutaneous pacing

Step 1: Ensure monitoring electrodes are in place.

Step 2: Attach pacing electrodes. (Preferred placement is anterior-posterior.)*

Step 3: Turn on the pacing unit. (Method will vary based on type of monitor.)

Step 4: Adjust QRS size to allow monitor to sense the present QRS complex.

Step 5: Set the desired rate (usually 70 to 80 BPM).

Step 6: Set the milliamps (mA) at 70 to 80 mA (usual setting).

Step 7: Increase the mA by increments of 5 to 10 mA (unit dependent) until capture occurs.

Step 8: Assess for capture by observing the characteristically widened QRS complex (Figure 15–1) and assess for presence of carotid pulse.

Step 9: Keep mA at a minimum (5 to 10 mA above level needed for capture).

Step 10: Consider sedation, as per medical direction or local protocol.

* Anterior electrode is placed left of the sternum at the fifth intercostal space, midclavicular. The posterior electrode is placed on the back, to the left of the spine, below the clavicle and in line with anterior electrode (Figure 15–2).

It is important to note that you must carefully observe your patient throughout the initiation of fibrinolytic therapy. In the event that reperfusion dysrhythmias occur following the administration of a fibrinolytic agent, it is imperative that you immediately identify the rhythm. If the rhythm is a bradydysrhythmia and the patient is exhibiting signs and symptoms of hypoperfusion (alterations in mental status, chest pain, decreasing blood pressure), you must consider treating the patient with TCP either in conjunction with or following drug therapy. As always, follow your local protocols and/or medical direction. It is also critical that you make sure your patient is receiving proper and adequate oxygenation.

Table 15–4 lists the steps to perform for transcutaneous cardiac pacing (TCP).

Complications of transcutaneous pacing

One of the more common complications of transcutaneous pacing is pain. With the delivery of electrical current through the skin into the heart, the patient will experience discomfort secondary to both the electrical stimulus and to muscle contractions. It is for this reason that **analgesics** and/or sedatives are often administered prior to and during TCP. Another potential complication that sometimes occurs is failure to capture (when the pacemaker fails to successfully depolarize the myocardium). The major causes of failure to capture in TCP therapy are poor or incorrect pad placement and patient movement.

analgesics agents used to relieve or reduce pain

DEFIBRILLATION

Defibrillation, also known as *asynchronous cardioversion,* is therapeutic by virtue of its ability to terminate fibrillation by passing a current of electricity through the heart's critical mass. Recall that ventricular fibrillation is a life-threatening dysrhythmia. When the heart's critical mass (multiple cells) is discharging independently of other cardiac cells, ventricular fibrillation ensues. Because there is no organization of depolarization or repolarization leading to myocardial contraction, there can be no significant cardiac

defibrillation therapeutic modality by virtue of its ability to terminate fibrillation by passing a current of electricity through the heart's critical mass

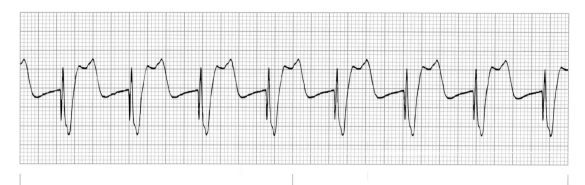

Figure 15–1. Normal capturing pacer rhythm

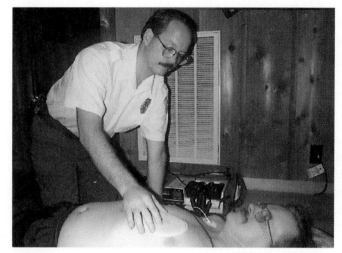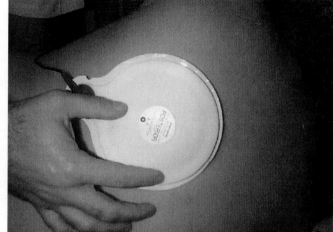

Figure 15–2. Anterior-posterior electrode placement

output. Subsequently, if your patient's heart is unable to produce any output, your patient's viability will soon diminish and perfusion will cease. Without appropriate treatment (airway, oxygen, defibrillation), asystole will soon follow ventricular fibrillation.

It is widely agreed that the most frequent rhythm associated with sudden cardiac death is ventricular fibrillation. Currently, electrical defibrillation is the most effective method of terminating ventricular fibrillation. Because pulseless ventricular tachycardia (VT, V-tach) rapidly deteriorates into ventricular fibrillation (VF, V-fib), if either of these rhythms is left untreated, asystole will rapidly develop. Therefore, both pulseless VT as well as VF must be rapidly controlled with defibrillation.

The success of defibrillation is extremely time dependent. Numerous studies have documented the fact that defibrillation is most successful if delivered within the first minute after cardiac arrest has occurred. Unfortunately, after only 8 to 9 minutes of cardiac arrest, a successful resuscitation occurs in less than 1 out of every 10 attempts. Though CPR is critically important and necessary in a cardiac arrest situation, you should realize that CPR is most effective in maintaining coronary and cerebral blood flow rather than in actually converting ventricular fibrillation. It is important to stress, therefore, that effective CPR must be implemented and maintained until a defibrillator is available. Early defibrillation is essential.

A variety of defibrillators are available for purchase and use in today's market. These various defibrillators have several energy-level settings that the health-care

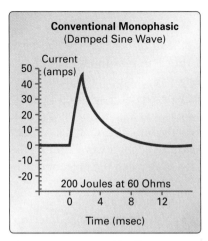
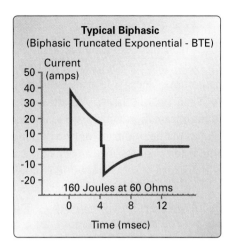

Figure 15–3. Defibrillation waveforms

provider selects before charging the capacitor and delivering the energy. The specific amount of energy is selected based upon patient needs and is measured in **joules,** or watt-seconds. The common maximum energy level used for defibrillation is 360 watt-seconds when using a **monophasic defibrillator.** When utilizing a monophasic defibrillator, the energy is delivered to the heart via the current traveling in one direction, from one paddle to the other in one phase. The monophasic defibrillator was previously utilized in the traditional defibrillator.

The newest defibrillators on the market have a new type of waveform called **biphasic defibrillators** (Figure 15–3). With a biphasic waveform, the current initially travels in one direction during the first phase of the shock and then reverses and travels in the opposite direction for the second phase. Although the monophasic waveform is considered the traditional waveform, market research strongly indicates that biphasic waveforms may be more successful in conversion of ventricular fibrillation. In addition, less energy is delivered by the biphasic current. The exact level of energy for successful conversion of lethal dysrhythmias is yet undetermined.

As you might imagine, the higher the amount of energy selected, the more energy that will be delivered to the heart. You must keep in mind that the more electrical energy delivered to the myocardium, the greater the risk of myocardial damage. It is for this reason that you should elect to begin with an energy level that is likely to convert the rhythm from fibrillation but is not so high that it will cause unnecessary myocardial tissue damage.

When using the monophasic defibrillator for the initial defibrillation attempt in a patient with pulseless VT or VF, the energy used is 200 joules. The second defibrillation attempt should be 200 to 300 joules, and the third and highest energy level is 360 joules. After these three *stacked shocks* have been delivered, successive defibrillations are delivered at 360 joules. (The term **stacked shocks** refers to three consecutive shocks that are delivered without pausing between each defibrillation.) If VF or pulseless VT recur following successful conversion, you should select the energy level that was previously successful.

When using the biphasic defibrillator, the current recommendation is that the provider should use the equivalent biphasic energy dose. You, the care provider, will want to remain attentive to the ever-evolving technology in this field.

joules watt-seconds

monophasic defibrillator a device with which energy is delivered to the heart via current traveling in one direction

biphasic defibrillator a device with which energy is delivered to the heart via current traveling in one direction in the first phase of a shock and then reversing and traveling in the opposite direction

stacked shocks three consecutive shocks that are delivered without pausing between each defibrillation

Transthoracic resistance

As you know, electricity will travel along the pathway of least resistance. The chest can offer a high resistance to electrical flow (called **transthoracic resistance**) during defibrillation attempts. Energy delivered during defibrillation must pass through the chest wall before it reaches the heart. A portion of the energy delivered is used up in overcoming the high transthoracic resistance of the chest. Thus, the amount of current that actually reaches the heart during defibrillation is less than the initial current that was delivered through the paddles. If this resistance to current flow is not lowered during the defibrillation process, a subtherapeutic amount of energy may reach the heart and may thus be unable to defibrillate the critical mass of myocardial tissue.

There are many factors that may determine the amount of transthoracic resistance to current flow. Some of these factors are electrode position, electrode size, interface material between the electrode and the skin, size of the patient, contact pressure, successive defibrillations, and energy-level selection.

Simply making sure that the size of the electrode applied to the patient's chest is the proper size can decrease resistance. Electrode paddles for the adult patient should be 8.5 to 12 cm in diameter. Infant paddles, which clip onto the adult paddle and have a smaller surface area, are typically 4.5 cm. A child-size electrode would be about 8 cm. Whatever size electrode is used, it is essential that there should be no large voids between the chest wall and the paddles.

Two positions are recommended for the placement of defibrillation electrodes. The specific placement recommendations will ensure that the maximum amount of electricity will flow through the myocardium. These positions include the anterior apex placement and the anterior-posterior placement. The **anterior apex placement** is more commonly used simply because it the easier of the two placements to use, especially during a cardiac arrest event. With the anterior-apex placement, the negative electrode is placed to the right of the sternum, just beneath the clavicle and the positive electrode is placed to the left of the nipple of the left thorax in the midaxillary position (Figure 15–4). The **anterior-posterior placement** positions the anterior or negative electrode over the left precordium, with the posterior or positive electrode in the infrascapular space of the left scapula. Both placement positions have proven equally effective in enhancing the amount of energy that reaches the heart muscle.

It is necessary to use some type of commercially available gel pad or electrode gel to eliminate the resistance between the bare chest and the dry metal electrode. Arcing

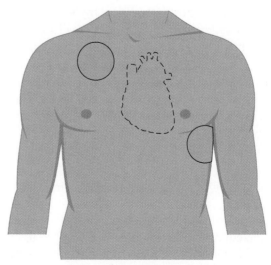

Figure 15–4.   Anterior-apex position of placement of defibrillation electrodes

between paddles (caused by contact between the mediums of each paddle) is a potentially dangerous complication of improperly performed defibrillation. Therefore, only the necessary amount of gel should be used with each paddle.

Another important aspect of successful defibrillation is contact pressure. Attempt to apply approximately 25 pounds of muscle pressure to ensure good contact of the paddle to the conductive medium against the chest. This amount of pressure will also help to eliminate the chance for arcing of the electrical current. (To give yourself some idea of how much pressure is needed, press on a standard bathroom scale, using the muscular strength of your arms only, until you see 25 pounds on the display.) Table 15–5 lists the steps for correctly performing defibrillation.

If the defibrillation attempts were accomplished in the prehospital field, immediately transfer your patient to the definitive care facility, maintaining constant contact with your Medical Control physician. Be very careful and specific with your documentation of the event.

CARDIOVERSION

Remember at all times that your patient's clinical condition will dictate the care you render as an emergency health-care provider. Keeping that important fact in mind, you should maintain constant vigilance on the patient's appearance, as well as his or her vital signs (level of consciousness, pulse rate, respiratory rate, blood pressure). In the emergent setting, you must determine whether your patient is perfusing, as evidenced by the presence of a pulse. It is also imperative that you diligently monitor the patient's EKG pattern.

Indications for emergency synchronized cardioversion are patient dependent and include perfusing ventricular tachycardia that is unstable or unresponsive to drug therapy, paroxysmal supraventricular tachycardia that is unstable or unresponsive to drug therapy, and in some cases, rapid atrial fibrillation. If your patient's condition is hemodynamically unstable, as evidenced by an altered level of consciousness or a decreasing blood pressure, and the cardiac monitor is showing evidence of ventricular tachycardia (with a palpable pulse) or paroxysmal supraventricular tachycardia, then cardioversion should be initiated. Cardioversion should be accomplished following the placement of an IV lifeline and oxygen administration. If time allows, and with permission from Medical Control or the attending physician, the patient should be sedated.

Table 15–5

Procedure for defibrillation

Step 1: Be sure to confirm VF or pulseless VT on the cardiac monitor.

Step 2: Make sure the patient is in a safe location (not surrounded by metal or water).

Step 3: Apply electrode gel to paddles or defibrillator pads to patient's exposed chest.

Step 4: Turn on and charge the defibrillator to 200 joules for the initial shock or clinically equivalent biphasic energy dose.

Step 5: Ensure that electrodes are in the proper position and that proper pressure is applied.

Step 6: Call "clear." LOOK, SAY, SEE CLEAR. Make sure no one is in contact with the patient.

Step 7: Deliver shock by depressing both red buttons simultaneously. (Button color and placement may vary depending on manufacturer.)

Step 8: Reconfirm rhythm on monitor. If VF/VT persists, recharge and repeat steps 5–7, using higher energy levels when using monophasic defibrillators.

synchronized cardioversion
the delivery of an electrical shock to the heart, synchronized so as to coincide with the R wave of the cardiac cycle

Emergency **synchronized cardioversion** is the delivery of an electrical shock to the heart, synchronized so as to coincide with the R wave of the cardiac cycle, thus avoiding the vulnerable relative refractory period. You will recall that during the relative refractory period, the myocardial muscle cells may be capable of accepting a stimulus; whereas in the absolute refractory period, no stimulus can be accepted. Synchronized cardioversion is designed to deliver the shock approximately 10 milliseconds after the peak of the R wave of the cardiac cycle.

With defibrillation, the operator determines when the energy will be delivered. However, with synchronized cardioversion, the exact time of the delivery of electrical current is very specific. The process of synchronization reduces the energy required to terminate dysrhythmias.

Energy requirements for synchronized cardioversion are based on the type of dysrhythmia being treated. Certain dysrhythmias—notably those of atrial origin—can be treated with as little as 10 joules. Most often, if the dysrhythmia is atrial in origin, you should elect to set an initial energy setting of 50 joules equivalent biphasic energy level. If the dysrhythmia appears to be ventricular in origin, it is recommended that the initial energy setting be 100 joules or equivalent biphasic energy level. Always follow your local protocol and allow Medical Control to guide your treatment regime.

Procedure for cardioversion

You will note that when the defibrillator is placed in the synchronized mode, the EKG displayed on the oscilloscope shows a marker denoting where in the cardiac cycle the energy will be discharged. The marker should appear on the R wave of the QRS complex. If the marker does not appear, you must adjust the EKG size until the marker appears atop the R wave or switch to a different lead that depicts a positively deflected R wave. Table 15–6 lists the steps to be followed during synchronized cardioversion.

If the cardioversion was performed in the prehospital field, you should immediately transfer your patient to the definitive care facility, maintaining constant contact with your Medical Control physician. Again, it is important that you carefully and precisely document the event.

Table 15–6

Procedure for synchronized cardioversion

Step 1: Be sure to confirm the presence of appropriate rhythm on the cardiac monitor.

Step 2: Make sure the patient is in a safe location (not surrounded by metal or water).

Step 3: Apply electrode gel to paddles or defibrillator pads to patient's exposed chest.

Step 4: Turn on defibrillator, select the synchronization mode, and set the proper energy level.

Step 5: Ensure that electrodes are in the proper position and that proper pressure is applied.

Step 6: Call "clear." LOOK, SAY, SEE CLEAR. Make sure no one is in contact with the patient.

Step 7: Deliver shock by depressing both red buttons simultaneously and holding until unit discharges. (Button color and placement may vary depending on manufacturer.)

Step 8: Reconfirm rhythm on monitor. If rhythm persists, recharge and repeat steps 5–7, using higher energy levels or equivalent biphasic energy level.

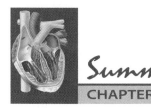

Summary
CHAPTER 15

In this chapter, we have continued to stress that the core component of assessment and treatment of the patient who presents with chest pain centers on the prompt oxygenation of hypoxic tissue. Treatment initiatives will vary depending upon your patient's specific situation. However, you must focus on continual and thorough assessment until the patient is clinically stable. Building on that, we have discussed therapeutic modalities as dictated by the most up-to-date literature.

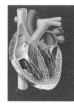

Key Points to Remember
CHAPTER 15

1. Fibrinolytics dissolve blood clots, which are the leading cause of myocardial infarctions.

2. Fibrinolytics are indicated for patients who present with clinical and EKG evidence of an acute myocardial infarction.

3. Fibrinolytics are contraindicated in patients who have had surgery within the last 2 weeks, have known intracranial neoplasm, and have a history of previous CVAs and suspected aortic dissection.

4. Transcutaneous pacing is indicated for patients with symptomatic bradycardia and/or heart blocks associated with reduced cardiac output.

5. Defibrillation or asynchronous cardioversion is therapeutic by virtue of its ability to terminate fibrillation by passing a current of electricity through the heart's critical mass.

6. Cardioversion or synchronous defibrillation is the delivery of an electrical shock to the heart delivered to coincide with the R wave of the cardiac cycle.

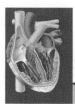

Review Questions
CHAPTER 15

1. The goal of managing the patient with symptomatic chest pain is to attempt to:
   a. administer prehospital fibrinolytics.
   b. stop the infarction process.
   c. reverse the infarction process.
   d. alleviate the patient's symptoms.

2. The maximum benefit of fibrinolytic therapy is best achieved when the agent is administered within ___ hour(s) after onset of symptoms.

   a. 2

   b. 10

   c. 6

   d. 1

3. The most commonly utilized tool to indicate the presence of myocardial damage that may lead to infarction is:

   a. ST segment depression.

   b. ST segment elevation.

   c. pathologic Q wave.

   d. prolonged PR interval.

4. The major complication of fibrinolytic therapy is:

   a. urticaria.

   b. thrombosis.

   c. dysrhythmia.

   d. hemorrhage.

5. All of the following clinical presentations may indicate the need for fibrinolytic therapy EXCEPT:

   a. pallor.

   b. diaphoresis.

   c. ventricular fibrillation.

   d. chest pain unrelieved by rest.

6. Criteria for fibrinolytic therapy include all of the following EXCEPT:

   a. age of less than 75 years.

   b. onset of chest pain occurring within 12 hours.

   c. most benefit from fibrinolysis if given within 6 hours.

   d. ST-segment elevation greater than or equal to 1 mm in three contiguous limb leads.

7. External cardiac pacing (TCP) is sometimes indicated for the treatment of certain reperfusion dysrhythmias, such as:

   a. asymptomatic bradycardia.

   b. symptomatic bradycardia.

   c. asymptomatic tachycardia.

   d. symptomatic tachycardia.

8. One of the more common complications of transcutaneous pacing is:

    a. pain.

    b. burns.

    c. electrocution.

    d. muscle damage.

9. There are many factors that can determine the amount of transthoracic resistance to current flow. These factors include all of the following EXCEPT:

    a. room temperature.

    b. electrode size.

    c. energy-level selection.

    d. electrode position.

10. In the emergent setting, you must determine whether your patient is perfusing, as evidenced by the presence of a:

    a. pulse.

    b. heart rhythm.

    c. heart rate.

    d. blood pressure.

11. Synchronized cardioversion is designed to deliver the shock approximately 10 milliseconds after the peak of the ___ wave of the cardiac cycle.

    a. Q

    b. R

    c. S

    d. P

12. Energy requirements for synchronized cardioversion are based on the:

    a. number of QRS complexes in a 6-second strip.

    b. type of dysrhythmia being treated.

    c. defibrillator capacity.

    d. manufacturer's guidelines.

13. In biphasic waveforms, energy is delivered through the heart, traveling in one direction from one paddle to the other in one phase.

    a. True

    b. False

14. Certain dysrhythmias, notably those of atrial origin, can be treated with as little as ___ joules.

    a. 10

    b. 5

    c. 15

    d. 20

15. If a dysrhythmia appears to be ventricular in origin, the initial energy setting should be ___ joules or equivalent biphasic energy level.

a. 200

b. 100

c. 300

d. 360

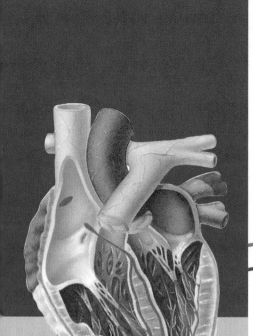

Cardiovascular Pharmacology

objectives

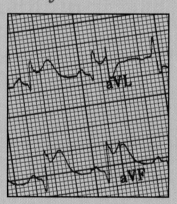

Upon completion of this chapter, the student will be able to:

➤ Explain the drug known as oxygen

➤ Describe and list the indications, precautions, side effects, adjuncts, contraindications, and dosages for oxygen

➤ Discuss the class of drugs known as sympathomimetics

➤ Describe and list the indications, precautions, side effects, contraindications, and dosages for epinephrine, isoproterenol, dopamine, and amrinone

➤ Explain the class of drugs known as sympatholytics

➤ Describe and list the indications, precautions, side effects, contraindications, and dosages for beta blockers

➤ Explain the class of drugs known as antidysrhythmics

➤ Describe and list the indications, precautions, side effects, contraindications, and dosages for lidocaine, procainamide, amiodarone, magnesium sulfate, atropine sulfate, adenosine, verapamil, diltiazem, and digitalis

➤ Discuss the class of drugs known as analgesics

➤ Describe and list the indications, precautions, side effects, contraindications, and dosages for morphine sulfate and meperidine

➤ Explain the class of drugs known as antianginals

➤ Describe and list the indications, precautions, side effects, contraindications, and dosages for nitroglycerin

➤ Explain the class of drugs known as alkalinizing agents

➤ Describe and list the indications, precautions, side effects, contraindications, and dosages for sodium bicarbonate

➤ Explain the class of drugs known as anticoagulants

➤ Describe and list the indications, precautions, side effects, contraindications, and dosages for heparin, Lovenox, and Fragmin

pharmacology
the study of drugs and their effects on living organisms

cardiovascular pharmacological agents drugs aimed at the specialized treatment of the heart and blood vessels

drugs agents used in the cure, treatment, or prevention of disease

mechanism of action interaction at the cellular level between a drug and cellular components

side effects undesirable effects of a drug

contraindications signs or symptoms that indicate an inappropriate response to a form of treatment

dosages determination of the amount, number, and frequency of medication for a patient

INTRODUCTION

Pharmacological therapy is an essential component of the overall treatment and care of the patient who may be experiencing an acute MI. In addition, the frequency of the occurrence of reperfusion dysrhythmias that are encountered as a result of fibrinolytic therapy dictates that the health-care provider must be knowledgeable in the area of cardiovascular **pharmacology.**

Throughout this text, and in the companion textbook, *Understanding EKGs: A Practical Approach,* 2nd ed., we have repeatedly stressed to you the importance of quality patient care. In this chapter, we will discuss the pharmacological components that you will utilize in your care and treatment of patients who are or may be experiencing an acute MI. Just as observing your patient's clinical condition is a must when administering fibrinolytic agents, you must also be diligent in your observation of the patient who has received a pharmacological agent. You must question whether the drug administered had the desired effect, as well as whether your patient's overall condition has improved as a result of the pharmacological agent that was administered.

The drugs discussed in this chapter are among the most commonly used **cardiovascular pharmacological agents.** Take the time required to study and learn the **drugs** listed in this chapter. When you, as a health-care provider, are in an emergent situation, you will often be a key team member (or perhaps a team leader). In order for you to be comfortable in this role, your knowledge level must continually be heightened and refreshed. We have thus elected to conclude the content of this text with the pharmacological agents that you will most commonly encounter in your management of the patient who is receiving fibrinolytic therapy.

We believe that the presentation of this particular subject can initially be a bit overwhelming. Consequently, we have chosen to present the pharmacologic agents in a simple, straightforward, and specific format. Each agent is discussed within its specific classification. We will then briefly discuss the most important aspects of each agent, namely, the **mechanism of action,** indications, precautions, **side effects, contraindications,** and **dosages.**

OXYGEN

The drug that is most often used and whose importance cannot be overemphasized is oxygen. We are well aware that you have read and heard that statement numerous times; however, it is a vital component of emergency cardiac care that must never be forgotten or overlooked. Oxygen is a colorless, odorless, tasteless gas that is absolutely necessary to sustain life.

Mechanism of action

Oxygen rapidly circulates across the alveolar walls and attaches to hemoglobin molecules in the red blood cells. During the process of systemic circulation, oxygen is distributed throughout the body to achieve adequate tissue perfusion. Oxygen is essential for the body to maintain its normal metabolic activities. Metabolism that occurs in the absence of oxygen is termed **anaerobic metabolism.** The end product of anaerobic metabolism is lactic acid, which, in combination with increased carbon dioxide levels, will lead to respiratory and metabolic acidoses. It is for this reason that proper oxygenation of body cells is so critical.

anaerobic metabolism
metabolism that occurs in the absence of oxygen

Indications

➤ Hypoxia, secondary to trauma or illness.

Precautions

➤ Chronic obstructive pulmonary disease (COPD).

Side effects

➤ Oxygen toxicity.
➤ **Epistaxis,** if prolonged administration of nonhumidified oxygen.

epistaxis
nosebleed

Contraindications

➤ None, in the emergent situation.

Dosage

➤ Based on the patient's clinical condition.
➤ In the emergent situation, 100% oxygen is usually administered.

This is the perfect time to mention an adjunct that can be used with oxygen. It is **capnography.** Capnography involves a device that measures the expiratory CO_2 partial pressures and allows you to ensure a near-normal alveolar level. Normal expiratory CO_2 levels run between 35 mmHg and 40 mmHg and should not drop below 30 mmHg. A CO_2 level above 40 is usually indicative of hypoventilation. The presence of hypoventilation indicates a need for faster and/or deeper ventilations. The device has attachments that can be utilized either on the end of an endotracheal tube or with a nasal cannula. These devices also are becoming widely accepted accessories on several prehospital and in-hospital cardiac monitoring systems, as well as in stand-alone units.

capnography
involves a device that measures the expiratory CO_2 partial pressures

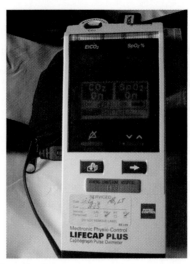

Figure 16–1. CO_2 detection devices

Another variation of CO_2 monitoring is the colorimetric end-tidal CO_2 detection device. This is a disposable device that is placed on the end of an endotracheal tube and measures exhaled CO_2 by changing color when CO_2 is detected (see Figure 16–1).

SYMPATHOMIMETICS

sympathomimetics agents that mimic the actions of the sympathetic nervous system

Sympathomimetics are agents that mimic the actions of the sympathetic nervous system (Figure 16–2). These agents either directly or indirectly stimulate the sympathetic nervous system. As a result, hormones called *catecholamines* are released within the body. The subsequent result is an increase in sympathetic tone, which ultimately leads to an increase in heart rate or *positive chronotropic effects,* and myocardial contractility, or a *positive inotropic effect.* It also may lead to an increase of the electrical conduction velocity through the heart's conduction system, or a *positive dromotropic effect.*

For the purposes of this chapter, we will primarily discuss information that is relative to the effects of cardiovascular pharmacological agents, as well as to the patients who are treated as a result of cardiac disorders.

Epinephrine

Mechanism of action

Epinephrine is a naturally occurring catecholamine that acts to stimulate both the alpha- and beta-adrenergic receptor sites. At this point, you may wish to refer to Chapter 2 of the companion textbook, *Understanding EKGs: A Practical Approach,* in order to refresh your knowledge of the autonomic nervous system. The stimulation of the beta 1 and beta 2 receptor sites increases the activity of the heart and dilates the bronchioles. The stimulation of the alpha receptor sites increases vascular tone, which assists in increasing blood pressure.

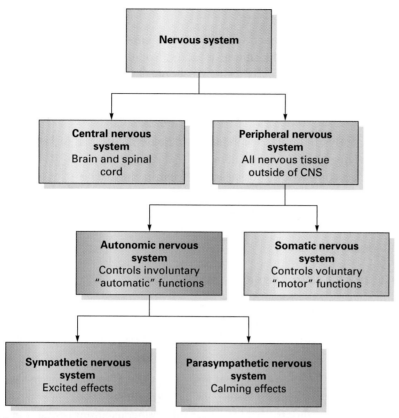

Figure 16–2.   Nervous system components

Cardiac effects

➤ Increased heart rate (positive chronotropic effect from beta 1).
➤ Increased contractility (positive inotropic effect from beta 1).
➤ Increased activity of the electrical conduction system (positive dromotropic effect from beta 1).
➤ Increased systemic vascular resistance (mixed beta and alpha effects).

Indications

➤ Management of cardiac arrest.
➤ Severe **anaphylaxis.**

anaphylaxis
severe allergic
reaction

In the emergent setting, the administration of epinephrine can convert asystole to fine V-fib and can convert fine V-fib to coarse V-fib. The chance of successful defibrillation is enhanced by administration of epinephrine and proper oxygenation.

Recent research has suggested the use of another drug, vasopression (to be discussed later in this chapter), as a possible alternative to the administration of epinephrine. Vasopression may now be given as the first drug of choice after the initial stacked defibrillation attempts in ventricular fibrillation. As always, be sure to follow your local protocols.

Precautions

alkaline agents
agents used to buffer the acids present in the body

➤ Can be deactivated if mixed with **alkaline agents;** the IV line should be flushed prior to and following the administration of sodium bicarbonate.
➤ Should be protected from light.

Side effects

➤ May create dysrhythmias secondary to increased workload of the heart.
➤ Increased myocardial oxygen demand.
➤ Anxiety, nervousness, restlessness, tachycardia, headache.
➤ Hypertension.
➤ May increase ventricular ectopy in patients who are receiving digitalis.

Contraindications

➤ In the face of severe cardiovascular compromise, there are no absolute contraindications.

Dosage

It is important to note that epinephrine is packaged in two strengths. The common packaging for intravenous administration yields 1 milligram of epinephrine in 10 milliliters of solution (1:10,000) in a prefilled syringe. In addition, epinephrine comes packaged for intramuscular (IM), endotracheal (ET), or subcutaneous administration in a solution of 1:1,000 or 1 milligram of drug in 1 milliliter of solution. The latter of these two solutions is much more concentrated (more drug, less solution). Certain enzymes in the body constantly degrade epinephrine, consequently decreasing the effects of the drug. For this reason, it is necessary to administer frequent doses. Current research in the utilization of high-dose epinephrine (HDE) continues. Whether HDE may or may not be beneficial in the cardiac-arrest state is still to be determined.

➤ Cardiac arrest
  ➤ 1 milligram every 3 to 5 minutes via IV push or via ET; utilize 1:10,000 solution.
  ➤ The utilization of HDE may be considered if the traditional doses have proved ineffective following numerous attempts. If utilized, escalating epinephrine administration is typically initiated at a dosage of 1, 3, or 5 milligrams 3 to 5 minutes apart. However, you should understand that HDE is *not* recommended in ACLS 2000 due to the lack of documented research associated with improved survival to hospital discharge. Always follow local protocols as well as medical direction.
➤ Anaphylaxis
  ➤ 0.3 to 0.5 milligrams of a 1:1,000 solution, administered subcutaneously.
  ➤ Repeat same dose every 5 to 15 minutes.

Vasopressin

Mechanism of Action Vasopressin is a naturally occurring antidiuretic hormone. In higher doses (than when utilized for its antidiuretic action), the drug is a vasoconstrictor. It causes vasoconstriction by directly stimulating smooth muscle V_1 receptors, which results in the elevation of systemic vascular resistance. Vasopressin has been shown to be beneficial in maintaining coronary blood flow during CPR in cardiac-arrest patients.

Indications Vasopressin may be effective in the initial management of ventricular fibrillation in the cardiac-arrest patient. It is to be used as an *alternative* pressure agent instead of epinephrine. The two drugs should not be used concurrently during cardiac-arrest management. The half-life of vasopressin is 10 to 20 minutes, which is longer than the half-life of epinephrine (3 to 4 minutes during CPR). Vasopressin may also be effective in patients with asystole or pulseless electrical activity, although studies are insufficient at this time to indicate its use in either of these dysrhythmias. Remember, vasopressin is used as an *alternative* to epinephrine in the cardiac-arrest patient in shock refractory ventricular fibrillation. When vasopressin is utilized as the first-line drug, it should be followed with the utilization of epinephrine 10 to 20 minutes after administration of vasopressin in the absence of any clinical response to the drug.

Precautions

➤ With patients who are pregnant, vasopressin can cause uterine contractions.

Side Effects

➤ Nausea and possible vomiting.
➤ Potential bronchial vasoconstriction.
➤ Intestinal cramps.

Contraindications

➤ Hypersensitivity, no other contraindications exist in present usage in cardiac arrest.

Dosage

➤ For cardiac arrest, with presenting rhythm of ventricular fibrillation or pulseless ventricular tachycardia: a single dose of 40 units via intravenous push. After 10 to 20 minutes without clinical change, follow with the administration of epinephrine, 1 milligram IV push, every 3 to 5 minutes until condition warrants change.

Isoproterenol (Isuprel)

Mechanism of Action Isoproterenol primarily acts on beta-adrenergic receptors. This drug is a synthetic catecholamine and primarily stimulates the beta 1 and beta 2 receptors of the sympathetic nervous system. Isuprel produces an overall increase in heart rate and myocardial contractility. It promotes vasodilation and relaxation of the pulmonary bronchioles. This drug is used in cardiac emergency situations to increase heart rate in bradycardias that are refractory to atropine, dopamine, and epinephrine. Because transcutaneous cardiac pacing (TCP) has become available, as well as newer drugs such as dobutamine and other drugs with fewer side effects, Isuprel should never be used as the first-line drug in hemodynamically significant bradycardia.

Indications

➤ Hemodynamically significant bradycardias resulting from high-degree heart blocks (second-degree Mobitz II and third-degree blocks), especially when TCP is unavailable.
➤ Hemodynamically significant bradycardias refractory to atropine and other medications, as well as when TCP is not available.

Precautions

➤ Increased myocardial oxygen demands.
➤ Patient should be continually monitored for signs of ventricular irritability, such as premature ventricular contractions (PVCs), V-tach, or even V-fib.
➤ Can be deactivated by alkaline solutions (sodium bicarbonate).
➤ Should be used cautiously in patients with digitalis toxicity as it may exacerbate **tachydysrhythmias.**

tachydysrhyth-mias irregular rhythms in combination with a rapid heart rate

Side Effects

➤ Myocardial ischemia.
➤ Hypokalemia (decreased potassium level).
➤ Hypertension (high blood pressure).
➤ Tremor, tachycardia, restlessness, nervousness.

Contraindications

cardiogenic shock condition that is the result of inadequate pumping of the heart

➤ **Cardiogenic shock.**
➤ Cardiac arrest.
➤ Not recommended for use as a first-line drug for the treatment of bradydysrhythmias in the hemodynamically unstable patient.

Dosage

➤ Administered via IV infusion (utilize mini-drip set or infusion pump) by mixing 1 milligram of Isuprel in 250 cubic centimeters D5W; mixture yields 4 micrograms per cubic centimeter; administer 2 to 10 micrograms per minute, titrated to desired hemodynamic effect (heart rate 60 beats per minute or systolic blood pressure 90 or above). You should not use more than 10 micrograms per minute.

Dopamine (Intropin)

Mechanism of Action   Dopamine is a naturally occurring catecholamine that is a chemical precursor of norepinephrine. Dopamine acts on alpha-, beta-, and dopaminergic adrenergic receptors. This drug promotes vasoconstriction and increases myocardial contractility without much effect on heart rate. The effect of this drug depends directly upon the amount administered.

Indications

➤ Nonhypovolemic hypotension.
➤ Cardiogenic shock.
➤ Hemodynamically significant bradycardia unresponsive to atropine and TCP.

Precautions

➤ Increases heart rate.
➤ Can worsen supraventricular and ventricular dysrhythmias.
➤ Must be discontinued if tachydysrhythmia or ventricular fibrillation develops.

Side Effects

➤ Hypokalemia.
➤ Development of dysrhythmias.
➤ Nausea, vomiting, tachycardia, restlessness, nervousness.

Contraindications

➤ Never used as a first-line or single agent in the management of hypovolemic shock unless fluid resuscitation is well underway.

➤ Should not be used in patients with known pheochromocytoma (tumor of the adrenal glands).

Dosage

➤ Mix 800 milligrams of dopamine in 500 cubic centimeters D5W; mixture yields 1,600 micrograms per cubic centimeter.

➤ Renal dose: 2 to 5 micrograms per kilogram per minute; renal output greatly increased. (Due to current research, dopamine is no longer recommended for treatment of renal failure.)

➤ Cardiac dose: 5 to 10 micrograms per kilogram per minute; interacts with mostly cardiac beta receptors to cause an increase in cardiac output and blood pressure.

➤ Vasopressor dose: 10 to 20 micrograms per kilogram per minute; interacts with mostly alpha receptors, thereby causing an increase in blood pressure.

Dobutamine

Mechanism of Action Dobutamine is a synthetic catecholamine that stimulates beta 1 receptors and alpha receptors in the myocardium. It also stimulates the beta 2 receptors in the smooth muscle of the bronchioles and peripheral blood vessels, but has little effect on peripheral vascular resistance. Dobutamine may also increase mesenteric blood flow by increasing cardiac output.

Indications

➤ Acute pulmonary edema.

➤ Hypotension when no other signs or symptoms of shock are present but the systolic pressure is around 70 to 100 mmHg.

➤ Patients with left-sided heart failure who cannot tolerate the use of vasodilators.

Precautions

➤ May cause tachydysrhythmias and provoke myocardial ischemia.

Side Effects

➤ Nervousness.
➤ Nausea and vomiting.
➤ Hypertension.
➤ Headache.
➤ Tremor.

Contraindications

➤ Symptomatic hypotension until other interventions to treat underlying cause have been performed.

Dosage

➤ An infusion rate of 2 micrograms to 20 micrograms per kilogram per minute after mixing one ampule (250 milligrams) with 250 cubic centimeters D5W or normal saline.

➤ Titrate so that heart rate does not increase more than 10% of baseline rate.
➤ Must utilize an infusion pump to ensure accurate flow rate.
➤ To adjust therapy, use hemodynamic monitoring and hemodynamic end points rather than a specific dose. (This is why this drug is not often used in the prehospital setting.)

Amrinone (Inocor)

Mechanism of Action   Inocor is a rapidly acting positive inotropic agent. An inotropic agent is an agent that affects contractility or force. A **positive inotropic agent** increases contractility, whereas a **negative inotropic agent** decreases contractility. This drug increases vasodilation and consequently decreases the workload of the heart. Inocor is helpful when there is fluid in the pulmonary vessels and lung fields because it improves myocardial output.

Indications

➤ Congestive heart failure (CHF) refractory to **diuretics** and **vasodilators** or severe left ventricular dysfunction.

Precautions

➤ Increased myocardial ischemia.
➤ Due to chemical incompatibility, Inocor should not be diluted in solutions containing dextrose.
➤ Lasix should not be administered in an IV line delivering Inocor, as **precipitates** will form due to chemical incompatibilities.

Side Effects

➤ May cause dysrhythmias, hypotension, nausea, vomiting.
➤ May cause thrombocytopenia (decreased platelets).

Contraindications

➤ Sensitivity to sulfur compounds.
➤ Should not be used as a first-line agent in CHF or left ventricular failure (LVF).

Dosage

➤ Therapy should be initiated with an IV bolus (loading dose) of 0.75 milligrams per kilogram over a period of 2 to 5 minutes.
➤ Follow with an infusion prepared with 100 milligrams mixed into 500 cubic centimeters of normal saline; mixture yields 0.2 milligrams per cubic centimeter.
➤ Maintenance infusion of 2 to 5 micrograms per kilogram per minute.

SYMPATHOLYTICS

Beta blockers

Mechanism of Action   **Beta blockers** antagonize (oppose) adrenergic receptor sites. In simpler terms, the beta blockers obstruct the receptor site and serve to prevent

positive inotropic agent an agent that increases contractility

negative inotropic agent an agent that decreases contractility

diuretics agents that increase urine secretion

vasodilators agents that cause dilation of blood vessels

precipitates deposits formed as a result of reaction with a reagent

sympatholytics agents that inhibit adrenergic nerve function; agents that antagonize or oppose adrenergic receptor sites

beta blockers agents that antagonize (oppose) adrenergic receptor sites or inhibit stimulation. This action produces effects such as slowed conduction impulses and decreased heart rate and contractility.

Indications

➤ Used to control recurrent ventricular fibrillation, ventricular tachycardia, or paroxysmal supraventricular tachycardia (PSVT).
➤ Long-term treatment of myocardial infarction by decreasing the overall workload of the heart and myocardial oxygen consumption.

Precautions

➤ Can precipitate serious bronchospasm; should be used with caution in patients with history of COPD, asthma, or CHF.
➤ May decrease heart rate to unacceptable level.

Side Effects

➤ Hypotension secondary to decreased heart rate and contractility.
➤ Pulmonary congestion secondary to bronchodilation.

Contraindications

➤ Preexisting bradycardia.
➤ History of COPD, asthma.
➤ CHF.

Dosages

Atenolol (Tenormin)

➤ IV administration: 5 milligrams IV push over 5 minutes.
➤ Same dosage repeated 10 minutes later, if needed.
➤ Oral dosing should begin 10 minutes after second IV dose (50 milligrams).

Metoprolol (Lopressor)

➤ 5 milligrams IV push over 2 to 5 minutes.
➤ Readminister two times at 5-minute intervals, not to exceed 15 milligrams total.
➤ Oral administration following IV dosing should range between 180 and 300 milligrams daily.

Propranolol (Inderal)

➤ For IV administration, 1 to 3 milligrams IV push over 2 to 5 minutes.
➤ Can be repeated after 2 minutes, for a total dose of 0.1 milligram per kilogram.

Esmolol (Brevibloc)

➤ IV administration, 0.5 milligram per kilogram (500 micrograms per kilogram) over one minute followed by a continuous infusion of 0.05 milligram per kilogram per minute (50 micrograms per kilogram per minute).
➤ Can repeat loading infusion as above until maximum of 0.3 milligram per kilogram per minute (300 micrograms per kilogram per minute) or resolution of ectopy or desired effect.
➤ Mix 2.5 grams (10 milliliter ampule) of the drug into a 250-milliliter bag of D5W. Gives a concentration of 10 milligrams per milliliter.

Labetalol (Normodyne, Trandate)

➤ IV administration of 10 milligrams push over 1 to 2 minutes.
➤ May repeat initial dose or double the initial dose every 10 minutes to a maximum dose of 150 milligrams.
➤ Then can start an infusion at 2 to 8 milligrams per minute after initial dose by mixing 200 milligrams in 250 milliliters of D5W (0.8 milligram per milliliter).

ANTIDYSRHYTHMICS

The general classification of drugs that serve to remedy disturbances in the heart's electrical activity is **antidysrhythmics.** If, for example, a patient's heart rate becomes too fast or too slow, the physician may choose to prescribe an antidysrhythmic. In addition, antidysrhythmics may be used to correct disruptions in cardiac conduction.

antidysrhythmics agents that serve to remedy disturbances in the heart's electrical activity

Lidocaine

Mechanism of Action   The mechanisms of action of lidocaine are numerous. The more commonly recognized ones include:

➤ Depresses depolarization and automaticity in the ventricles.
➤ Suppresses ventricular **ectopy** rhythm in the setting of myocardial infarction.
➤ Increases ventricular fibrillation **threshold.**
➤ Does not affect myocardial contractility or conduction of the SA or AV nodes.

ectopy out of place

threshold refers to a point at which a stimulus will produce a cell response

Indications
➤ Lidocaine is one of the drugs of choice in the treatment of dysrhythmias that are a result of ventricular irritability—specifically, ventricular tachycardia and ventricular fibrillation.
➤ Suppression of malignant PVCs; that is, more than six PVCs per minute, multifocal PVCs, couplet PVCs, or R-on-T phenomenon.

Precautions
➤ Depressed liver function (delay in removing lidocaine from the body).
➤ Central nervous system depression (decreased level of consciousness, irritability, confusion, eventual seizures).

Side Effects
➤ Drowsiness.
➤ Bradycardia, heart block, cardiac arrest.
➤ Respiratory arrest.
➤ Hypoxia.
➤ Nausea and vomiting.

Contraindications
➤ Second-degree, Type II, and infranodal heart blocks.
➤ Bradycardia with PVCs. (PVCs may be the body's attempt to maintain cardiac perfusion; abolishing them with lidocaine can lead to cardiac arrest.)
➤ Lidocaine sensitivity.

Dosage

➤ Administer 1 to 1.5 milligrams per kilogram via IV bolus. (If ET administration, give 2 to 2.5 milligrams per kilogram.) If abnormality is suppressed, maintenance infusion should be initiated as follows:
  ➤ Place 2 grams in 500 cubic centimeters D5W or normal saline; infuse at a rate of 30 gtt per minute using a mini-drip set (60 microgtt set), which will yield 2 milligrams per minute, and titrate (slowly change rate of administration) to desired effect (until PVCs are suppressed). If using an IV pump with a standard set, reference the specific pump recommendations.
  ➤ Second dose should be decreased by 50% with geriatric patients.

Procainamide

Mechanism of Action   In cases where lidocaine has not proven effective or in cases of lidocaine sensitivity, procainamide may prove effective in the suppression of ventricular ectopies. In addition, it is important to understand that procainamide reduces the automaticity of the various pacemaker sites in the heart, as well as slows intraventricular conduction to a much greater degree than does lidocaine.

Indications

➤ Ventricular dysrhythmias refractory to lidocaine; that is, persistent malignant PVCs, persistent ventricular tachycardia with a pulse, persistent ventricular fibrillation/pulseless ventricular tachycardia.

Precautions

➤ Bradycardia with PVCs.
➤ Should be used with caution in the hypotensive patient.
➤ Should be discontinued if QRS widens by more than 50% from pretreatment width.
➤ Should not exceed maximum dose of 17 milligrams per kilogram.

Side Effects

➤ Drowsiness, confusion.
➤ Hypersensitivity.
➤ Seizures.
➤ Hypotension, bradycardia, heart blocks.
➤ Nausea and vomiting.

Contraindications

➤ Should not be administered to patients with severe conduction system disturbances, especially second- and third-degree heart blocks.
➤ Profound hypotension (less than 80 mmHg systolic).

Dosage

➤ Administer 1 gram in 50 milliliters of D5W (20 milligrams per milliliter) at a rate of 20 to 30 milligrams per minute, until maximum dose of 17 milligrams per kilogram, followed by a maintenance infusion of 1 gram in 500 milliliters D5W, which equals a 2:1 ratio; begin by administering 15 gtt per minute and titrate to effect or 2 grams in 500 milliliters of D5W for a 4:1 ratio.

Amiodarone (Cordarone)

Mechanism of Action   Amiodarone prolongs the refractory period of the myocardial cells. In addition, this agent causes systemic vasodilation. The primary therapeutic effect of amiodarone is the suppression of dysrhythmias.

Indications

➤ Management of life-threatening ventricular dysrhythmias unresponsive to electrical therapy.
➤ Recurring ventricular fibrillation.
➤ Hemodynamically unstable ventricular tachycardia or pulseless ventricular tachycardia.
➤ Wide complex tachycardia.
➤ Supraventricular dysrhythmias.

Precautions

➤ History of CHF.
➤ Severe pulmonary or liver disease.

Side Effects

➤ Headache.
➤ Bradycardia.
➤ Hypotension.

Contraindications

➤ Known hypersensitivity.
➤ Should not be administered to patients with severe conduction system disturbances, especially second- and third-degree heart blocks.
➤ Profound hypotension (less than 80 mmHg systolic).

Dosage   If the patient is in cardiac arrest:

➤ Administer 300 milligrams in 20 to 30 milliliters of saline rapid infusion.
➤ Repeat at 150 milligrams via IVP in 3 to 5 minutes, if condition unchanged.

If the patient is in ventricular tachycardia, wide complex tachycardia, or supraventricular tachycardia, and if the patient is hemodynamically stable:

➤ Administer 150 milligrams (3 milliliters) IV over a 10-minute period, which equals 15 milligrams per minute.
➤ Add 150 milligrams to 100 cubic centimeters D5W to equal 1.5 milligrams per milliliter.
➤ Infusion: add 900 milligrams to 500 milliliters D5W (concentration of 1.8 milligrams per milliliter). Slowly administer 360 milligrams over the next 6 hours at 1 milligram per minute.

If the patient is in ventricular tachycardia, wide complex tachycardia, or supraventricular tachycardia and is hemodynamically unstable following cardioversion:

➤ 360 milligrams mixed in 500 milliliters D5W (concentration of 1.8 milligrams per milliliter). Slowly administer 360 milligrams over the next 6 hours at 1 milligram per minute.

Magnesium Sulfate

Mechanism of Action   Magnesium sulfate is associated with cardiac dysrhythmias such as refractory VF and sudden cardiac death. Its actions are related to hypomagnesemia because it hinders the replenishment of intracellular potassium and has been associated with many life-threatening cardiac emergencies.

Indications

➤ Seizures of eclampsia (toxemia of pregnancy).
➤ Torsades de pointes.
➤ Heart blocks.
➤ Persistent or recurrent VF/pulseless VT, if associated with known hypomagnesemic state.
➤ Dysrhythmias secondary to a tricyclic antidepressant overdose or digitalis toxicity.
➤ Refractory ventricular fibrillation and ventricular tachycardia after administration of other antidysrhythmics.

Precautions

➤ Hypotension may occur with rapid administration.
➤ Use with caution if renal failure present.

Side Effects

➤ Hypotension (treat with calcium gluconate 500 milligrams to 1 gram).
➤ Severe flushing, sweating, heat sensation.
➤ PR interval prolongation, AV block.

Contraindications

➤ Should not be given to patients in shock or with a heart block.

Dosage   For a patient in cardiac arrest:

➤ 1 to 2 grams (2 to 4 milliliters of a 50% solution) diluted in 10 milliliters of D5W, IV push over 1 to 2 minutes.

For a patient in torsades de pointes:

➤ 1 to 2 grams mixed in 50 to 100 milliliters of D5W over 5 to 60 minutes and titrate dose to control torsades.

For a patient with seizure activity associated with pregnancy:

➤ 1 to 4 grams IVP with a maximum dose of 1.5 milliliters per minute, usually followed by 2 to 4 grams over 1 hour. Mixed with 40 grams in 1,000 milliliters (OB standard mix).

Atropine sulfate

parasympatholytics
agents that block the effects of the parasympathetic nervous system

Mechanism of Action   Atropine is classified further as a rate-control antidysrhythmic, as well as a **parasympatholytic.** Atropine increases the heart rate by blocking vagal tone (parasympathetic reduction in heart rate).

Indications

➤ Hemodynamically unstable (symptomatic) bradycardia.
➤ Asystole.

Precautions

➤ Maximum dose should not exceed 0.04 milligrams per kilogram.
➤ Use with caution in patients who present with a symptomatic Type II or third-degree block; may cause paradoxical slowing of the ventricular rate.
➤ Be prepared to artificially pace the patient should conduction defect deteriorate.

Side Effects

➤ Blurred vision.
➤ Dry mouth.
➤ Dilation of the pupils.
➤ Tachycardia.
➤ Drowsiness and confusion.
➤ Increase in myocardial oxygen demand.

Contraindications

➤ Hypersensitivity.
➤ Tachycardia.
➤ Third-degree block.

Dosage

➤ 0.5 to 1 milligram IV push (if administered via ET tube, 1 to 2 milligrams).
➤ Repeat dose every 3 to 5 minutes, to a maximum dose of 0.04 milligrams per kilogram.

Adenosine

Mechanism of Action   Adenosine works to interrupt reentry pathways in the AV node and slows conduction time through the AV node. This agent also produces coronary artery vasodilation and thus enhances myocardial perfusion.

Indications

➤ Symptomatic PSVT.
➤ Atrial dysrhythmias resulting in a rapid ventricular response.
➤ Wide complex tachycardia of unknown etiology.

Precautions

➤ Hypersensitivity.
➤ Use cautiously in patients with history of unstable angina or asthma.
➤ Effects may be decreased by theophylline (methylxanthine) or caffeine.

➤ Effects may be increased by dipyridamole (Persantine), so dosage may need to be decreased.

Side Effects

➤ Transient dysrhythmias.
➤ Facial flushing.
➤ Nausea, dyspnea.
➤ Headache.
➤ Chest pain, palpitations, and hypotension.

Contraindications

➤ Hypersensitivity.
➤ Second- or third-degree heart block.

Dosage

➤ 6-milligram rapid IV bolus over 1 to 2 seconds.
➤ After 2 minutes, 12-milligram rapid IV bolus over 1 to 2 seconds; may consider third dose after waiting another 2 minutes.
➤ Total dose not to exceed 30 milligrams.

Verapamil (Isoptin, Calan)

Mechanism of Action   Verapamil is a calcium channel blocker. **Calcium channel blockers** relax vascular smooth muscle, cause vascular dilation, and consequently act to slow conduction through the AV node. This agent also serves to reduce myocardial oxygen demand, while at the same time inhibiting dysrhythmias that are secondary to reentry, such as PSVT.

calcium channel blockers agents that relax vascular smooth muscle, cause vascular dilation, and consequently act to slow conduction through the AV node

Indications

➤ PSVT refractory to adenosine.

Precautions

➤ May cause systemic hypotension; blood pressure must be monitored vigilantly.

Side Effects

➤ Nausea and vomiting.
➤ Dizziness.
➤ Headache.
➤ Tachycardia.
➤ Hypotension.
➤ Heart block and asystole.

Contraindications

➤ Should not be administered to patients with severe hypotension.
➤ Cardiogenic shock.
➤ Should not be administered in the prehospital arena to patients with ventricular tachycardia.
➤ **Wolfe-Parkinson-White syndrome.**

Wolfe-Parkinson-White syndrome a cardiac rhythm disturbance that is characterized by a delta wave, or a slur of the R wave on a QRS complex

Dosage

➤ In PSVT, initial dosage is 2.5 to 5 milligrams IV push over a 2- to 3-minute interval.
➤ Repeat dosage of 5 to 10 milligrams can be given over 15- to 30-minute period if PSVT persists and the patient has demonstrated no adverse effects.
➤ Total dose should not exceed 30 milligrams in 30 minutes.

Diltiazem (Cardizem)

Mechanism of Action Diltiazem is a calcium channel blocker that slows conduction and prolongs refractoriness by interfering with the movement of calcium across the cellular membrane. Diltiazem has a mild negative inotropic effect (contractile force) but has a potent negative chronotropic effect (rate). It lessens myocardial oxygen demand and also causes coronary artery dilation.

Indications

➤ PSVT refractory to adenosine.
➤ Atrial fibrillation or atrial flutter that does not require electrical cardioversion.

Precautions

➤ May cause systemic hypotension; blood pressure must be monitored vigilantly.
➤ Do not use with digitalis, beta blockers, or Lasix, as may potentiate the seriousness of the side effects.

Side Effects

➤ Nausea and vomiting.
➤ Dizziness.
➤ Headache.
➤ Tachycardia.
➤ Hypotension.
➤ Heart block and asystole.

Contraindications

➤ Severe hypotension.
➤ Cardiogenic shock.
➤ Should not be administered in the prehospital arena to patients with ventricular tachycardia.
➤ Wolfe-Parkinson-White syndrome.

Dosage

➤ For PSVT, administer initial dose of 20 to 25 milligrams as an initial bolus IVP over 1 to 2 minutes. After 15 minutes, can repeat once at 20 to 25 milligrams IVP over 2 minutes if desired effect not produced.
➤ After positive response, initiate a maintenance infusion at 5 to 15 milligrams per hour titrated to heart rate.

cardiac glycosides agents that increase the force of cardiac contraction, as well as cardiac output

Digitalis (Digoxin, Lanoxin)

Mechanism of Action Digitalis is a **cardiac glycoside** that increases the force of cardiac contraction, as well as cardiac output. This agent slows impulse conduction through the AV node. The administration of digitalis serves to decrease the ventricular response to certain supraventricular dysrhythmias such as PSVT, atrial flutter, and atrial fibrillation.

Indications

- ➤ CHF.
- ➤ PSVT.
- ➤ Atrial fibrillation.
- ➤ Atrial flutter.

Precautions

- ➤ Patients require constant monitoring for signs and symptoms of digitalis toxicity.
- ➤ Should not be given to a patient with a heart rate less than 60 beats per minute.
- ➤ Use cautiously in patients with documented electrolyte imbalances.

Side Effects

- ➤ Digitalis toxicity (yellow vision, nausea, vomiting, drowsiness, new-onset heart blocks).
- ➤ Dysrhythmias.

Contraindications   Lanoxin should not be administered to patients:

- ➤ In ventricular fibrillation.
- ➤ Showing any of the signs or symptoms of digitalis toxicity.
- ➤ With evidence of heart blocks.

Dosage

- ➤ Initial IV dose is 0.6 to 1 milligram at 4- to 8-hour intervals.
- ➤ Initial oral dose is 0.75 to 1.25 milligrams.

ANALGESICS

Morphine sulfate (Morphine, MS)

Mechanism of Action   Morphine sulfate is classified as a narcotic analgesic. In fact, this agent is one of the most potent analgesics on the market. MS is a central nervous system depressant that has hemodynamic properties, making it quite useful in the field of emergency medicine.

Indications

- ➤ Pulmonary edema (with or without associated pain).
- ➤ Severe chest pain associated with myocardial infarction.
- ➤ Severe pain associated with kidney stones.

Precautions

- ➤ Tendency for abuse and addiction.
- ➤ In high doses, may cause severe respiratory depression.
- ➤ Narcotic **antagonist** (such as Narcan) should be immediately available when this agent is administered.
- ➤ This agent is a controlled substance and must be kept in a locked cabinet or drug bag.

antagonist an agent that prevents a response from occurring

Side Effects

➤ Nausea and vomiting.
➤ Blurred vision.
➤ Pupillary constriction.
➤ Altered mental status.
➤ Headache.
➤ Respiratory depression.

Contraindications

hypersensitivity
abnormal sensitivity
to a stimulus of any
kind

➤ **Hypersensitivity.**
➤ Should not be administered to volume-depleted patients.
➤ Should not be administered to severely hypotensive patients.

Dosage

➤ Initial dose of 2 to 10 milligrams slow IV push, titrated to effect.
➤ Additional doses of 2 milligrams IV may be administered every few minutes until pain is relieved.

Meperidine (Demerol)

Mechanism of Action   Meperidine is classified as a narcotic analgesic. This agent is a central nervous system depressant that is widely used in medicine for the treatment of moderate to severe pain. Although meperidine is a potent analgesic, it is not as potent as morphine sulfate. Also, the rate of onset of this agent is slightly faster than morphine, yet its effects are much shorter in duration.

Indications

➤ Moderate to severe pain.

Precautions

➤ May cause respiratory distress.
➤ Narcan should always be available to reverse the effects of the drug if respiratory depression ensues.
➤ This agent is a controlled substance and must be kept in a locked cabinet or drug bag.

Side Effects

➤ Nausea and vomiting.
➤ Abdominal cramps.
➤ Blurred vision.
➤ Constricted pupils.
➤ Altered mental status, headache, hallucinations.
➤ Respiratory depression.

Contraindications

➤ Hypersensitivity.
➤ Should not be administered to patients with undiagnosed abdominal pain or head injury.

Dosage

➤ Initial dose for treatment of severe pain is 25 to 50 milligrams IV.

➤ Standard dose is 50 to 100 milligrams IM; however, when dealing with cardiac patients, IM injections should be avoided due to the effects of cardiac enzyme levels.

➤ Often administered with **antiemetic agent** due to its tendency to cause nausea/vomiting.

antiemetic agent an agent that prevents or relieves nausea and vomiting

ANTIANGINALS

Nitroglycerin (Nitrostat)

Mechanism of Action Nitroglycerin is a powerful smooth-muscle relaxant and is often used in the treatment of angina pectoris. Because of the relaxant properties of this agent, it can drastically reduce preload and cardiac workload. This agent also dilates coronary arteries, resulting in an increase in coronary blood flow. Consequently, the perfusion of the compromised myocardial muscle is increased. As the ischemia of the myocardial cells is alleviated, the patient will report a decrease in the intensity of chest pain. If, indeed, the patient's chest pain was caused by myocardial ischemia, the administration of nitroglycerin will generally minimize the pain within 1 to 3 minutes following the dosage.

Indications

➤ Chest pain associated with angina pectoris.

➤ Chest pain associated with acute MI.

➤ Acute pulmonary edema (unless accompanied by hypotension).

➤ CHF.

Precautions

➤ Development of **tolerance** to the drug may necessitate increased dosages.

➤ Drug rapidly deteriorates after the bottle is opened.

➤ Must be protected from light.

➤ Blood pressure and all vital signs should be closely monitored. Discontinue use if systolic blood pressure falls below 90 mmHg.

tolerance progressive decrease in effectiveness of a drug

Side Effects

➤ Headaches are common as a result of cerebral vasodilation.

➤ Dizziness, weakness.

➤ Tachycardia and hypotension.

➤ Dry mouth.

➤ Nausea and vomiting.

Contraindications

➤ Hypotension (systolic blood pressure is less than 90 mmHg).

➤ Increased intracranial pressure.

➤ Shock.

➤ Recent Viagra use. If a patient has used Viagra within the previous 24 hours, nitrates may cause severe hypotension refractory to vasopressor agents. This includes males and females.

Dosage

➤ For angina pectoris, initial dose is 1 tablet (0.4 milligram) sublingually.
➤ May be repeated in 3 to 5 minutes as required.
➤ In the prehospital setting, no more than three tablets should be administered.
➤ Agent is also available in spray, ointment, and patch forms.
➤ May be administered IV in the emergency department or intensive care unit setting or may be administered during intrafacility transfers.

ALKALINIZING AGENTS

Sodium bicarbonate

alkalinizing agent an agent that causes blood to become alkaline; an agent utilized in the treatment of metabolic acidosis

Mechanism of Action   Sodium bicarbonate is an **alkalinizing agent** that is sometimes utilized in the treatment of metabolic acidosis. This drug is a salt that provides bicarbonate to serve as a buffer in the management of metabolic acidosis. It is also used in the treatment of tricyclic antidepressant overdose to cause urine to be more alkaline by raising the pH and consequently to speed the excretion of urine.

Indications

➤ May be used in the treatment of cardiac arrest in documented cases of metabolic acidosis.
➤ Tricyclic antidepressant overdose.
➤ Severe acidosis refractory to hyperventilation.
➤ Phenobarbital overdose.

Precautions

➤ When administered in large doses, may produce metabolic alkalosis.
➤ Should not be administered in conjunction with calcium chloride, as a precipitate can form and lead to clogging of the IV line.

Side Effects

➤ Metabolic alkalosis.
➤ Few when administered in the emergent setting.

Contraindications

➤ No absolute contraindication.

Dosage

➤ Should be administered only by IV bolus.
➤ Initial dose is 1 milliequivalent per kilogram of body weight, followed by 0.5 milliequivalent per kilogram every 10 minutes.
➤ Whenever possible, dosage should be guided by arterial blood gas studies.

ANTICOAGULANTS

anticoagulant an agent that delays or prevents blood coagulation

Heparin

Mechanism of Action   Heparin is classified as an **anticoagulant** and is often used in conjunction with certain fibrinolytic (thrombolytic) agents. It may also be used after thrombolysis (*thrombo* = clot, *lysis* = dissolve) has occurred. In simpler terms, heparin increases the length of time required for clots to reform.

Indications
➤ Given in conjunction with thrombolytic (fibrinolytic) therapy.
➤ Pulmonary embolus.

Precautions
➤ Severe liver disease.
➤ Severe kidney disease.
➤ Risk of bleeding increases when administered in conjunction with aspirin and nonsteroidal antiinflammatory drugs.
➤ Must obtain Prothrombin Time (PT) and Partial Thromboplastin Time (PTT) prior to administration. Keep doses in the range to keep PTT at 1.5 to 2 times control values for 48 hours.

Side Effects
➤ Allergic reactions.
➤ Bruising.
➤ Epistaxis.
➤ **Hematuria.**

hematuria
presence of blood in urine

Contraindications
➤ Presence of active bleeding.
➤ Severe hypotension.
➤ Recent intracranial surgery.
➤ Hypersensitivity.

Dosage
➤ 5,000 units IV push, followed by infusion of 1,000 units per hour for 24 to 48 hours (25,000 units in 500 cubic centimeters D5W at a rate of 10 cubic centimeters per hour).

If acute reversal of heparin is necessary due to major bleeding complications, use protamine sulfate. Protamine binds with heparin to form an inactive complex without anticoagulant activity. Dosage is as follows:

➤ Less than 30 minutes after heparin bolus, 1 to 1.5 milligrams protamine per 100 units of heparin.
➤ 30 to 60 minutes after heparin bolus, 0.5 to 0.75 milligrams protamine per 100 units of heparin.
➤ 2 hours after heparin bolus, 0.25 to 0.375 milligrams per 100 units heparin.

Also, a newer generation of heparins is being used more and more often. They are known as low-molecular-weight heparins. They have fewer side effects, a lower number of contraindications, and can be given to the patient subcutaneously. Two examples are Lovenox (enoxaparin) and Fragmin (dalteparin). For these two drugs, doses are the same: 1 milligram per kilogram to be given subcutaneously twice a day.

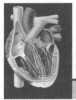

Summary

CHAPTER 16

Pharmacology is an ever-evolving field of study. Because research continues to identify new drugs and new uses for well-established drugs, you must be diligent in your continuing education efforts in order to remain current and competent as a health-care provider.

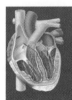

Key Points to Remember

CHAPTER 16

1. The drug that is most often used is oxygen.
2. Sympathomimetics are agents that mimic the actions of the sympathetic nervous system.
3. Sympatholytics antagonize or oppose adrenergic receptor sites.
4. Antidysrhythmics serve to remedy disturbances in the heart's electrical activity.
5. Analgesics are medications that reduce pain.
6. Antianginals are smooth-muscle relaxants.
7. Alkalinizing agents are agents utilized in the treatment of metabolic acidosis.
8. Anticoagulants are agents that prolong clotting times.

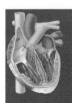

Review Questions

CHAPTER 16

1. Atropine 1.0 milligram may:
   1. be given via the ET tube.
   2. be useful in third-degree AV block.
   3. result in undesirable heart block.
   4. increase the rate of a sinus bradycardia.

   a. 1, 2, 3   c. 2, 3, 4

   b. 1, 2, 4   d. 1, 3

2. External pacing may be indicated for which one of the following rhythms when the rhythms are refractory to atropine?

   a. pulseless electrical activity

   b. first-degree atrioventricular block

   c. symptomatic bradycardia

   d. symptomatic ventricular tachycardia

3. An adult weighing 72 kilograms presents with ventricular tachycardia and a palpable pulse. Which one of the following schedules of lidocaine is preferred?

   a. IV bolus of 75 milligrams, followed by infusion at 2 to 4 milligrams per minute.

   b. IV bolus of 150 milligrams every 5 minutes to a total of 300 milligrams.

   c. 150 milligrams IV bolus followed by infusion of 4 to 6 milligrams per minute.

   d. 200 milligrams IV bolus followed by infusion of 1 to 2 milligrams per minute.

4. Lidocaine may be administered by:

   a. IV only.

   b. ET only.

   c. IV or IM.

   d. IV, ET, or IO.

5. Which one of the following statements regarding procainamide administration is FALSE?

   a. Administration of this agent should be discontinued if the patient becomes hypotensive.

   b. Administration of this agent should be discontinued when 2 grams have been delivered.

   c. Procainamide is never administered via the endotracheal tube route.

   d. Discontinue administration of this agent if the original QRS width has widened by 50% or more.

6. Verapamil is an:

   a. analgesic.

   b. alkalinizer.

   c. antidysrhythmic.

   d. antihypertensive.

7. Epinephrine may be administered:

   a. to relieve the pain of angina pectoris.

   b. via direct epicardial injection.

   c. by intraosseous injection.

   d. only via the intravenous route.

8. Which one of the following drugs increases heart rate?

   a. atropine

   b. adenosine

   c. verapamil

   d. sodium bicarbonate

9. The trade name for dopamine hydrochloride is:

   a. Amiorone.

   b. Intropin.

   c. Dobutamine.

   d. Diazepam.

10. The administration of an IV solution by regulating its flow rate based upon observation or desired or undesired effects is called:

    a. estimation.

    b. titration.

    c. approximation.

    d. calculation.

11. The mechanisms of action of Isuprel include:

    1. increased heart rate.
    2. increased cardiac output.
    3. increased myocardial oxygen consumption.
    4. production of secondary bronchodilation.

    a. 1, 2

    b. 3, 4

    c. 2, 3, 4

    d. 1, 2, 3, 4

12. A 66-year-old female weighing 132 pounds requires a bolus of sodium bicarbonate. The bicarbonate should be administered in a 1-milliequivalent-per-kilogram bolus. How many milliequivalents should be administered to this patient?

    a. 20

    b. 40

    c. 60

    d. 80

13. Diltiazem is utilized in which one of the following rhythms when the rate is stable and does not need electrical cardioversion?

    a. wide QRS tachycardia

    b. atrial fibrillation and atrial flutter

    c. ventricular tachycardia with a pulse

    d. sick sinus syndrome

14. Nitroglycerin is contraindicated when:
    a. Viagra has been taken within 24 hours.
    b. systolic blood pressure is more than 90 mmHg.
    c. there is chest pain associated with angina pectoris.
    d. there is acute pulmonary edema.

15. One of the side effects of digitalis toxicity is:
    a. green vision.
    b. anxiety and restlessness.
    c. new-onset heart blocks.
    d. decreased cardiac contractions.

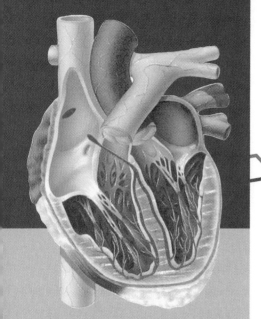

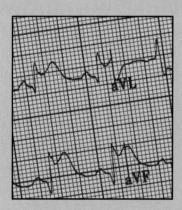

chapter 17

More Review Questions

1. Most cardiac dysrhythmias are caused by ischemia secondary to hypoxia. There-fore, the most appropriate drug to give a patient with any dysrhythmia is:

    a. oxygen.

    b. D5W.

    c. lidocaine.

    d. morphine.

2. The fibrous sac covering of the heart, which is in contact with the pleura, is the:

    a. epicardium.

    b. myocardium.

    c. pericardium.

    d. endocardium.

3. Mr. Young is a 56-year-old male patient who is experiencing crushing chest pain. Immediately after an IV has been established, Mr. Young becomes apneic and pulse-less. During resuscitation, the physician orders sodium bicarbonate and calcium chlo-ride to be administered. After the administration of the sodium bicarbonate, you must:

    a. immediately proceed to administer the calcium chloride.

    b. flush the IV line before administering the calcium chloride.

    c. wait 15 minutes before administering the calcium chloride.

    d. administer magnesium sulfate prior to the calcium chloride bolus.

4. The heart ventricle with the thickest myocardium is the:

    a. right.

    b. left.

5. The pulmonic and aortic valves are open during:

    a. systole.

    b. diastole.

6. The large blood vessel that returns deoxygenated blood from the head and neck to the right atrium is called the:

    a. jugular vein.

    b. carotid artery.

    c. superior vena cava.

    d. inferior vena cava.

7. Accepted uses of sodium bicarbonate include:

    a. severe acidosis.

    b. complete heart block.

    c. multifocal PVCs.

    d. atrial flutter.

8. The coronary sinus, which opens into the right atrium, allows venous return from the:

    a. azygos.

    b. pleura.

    c. myocardium.

    d. endocardium.

9. The saw-tooth pattern is indicative of which one of the following rhythms?

    a. atrial fibrillation

    b. atrial asystole

    c. ventricular flutter

    d. atrial flutter

10. The mitral valve is located between the:

    a. right and left atrium.

    b. right and left ventricle.

    c. left atrium and left ventricle.

    d. right atrium and right ventricle.

11. When dealing with inferior and inferoposterior MIs, the appearance of high-degree AV blocks may be present upon admission to the hospital. Examples of high-degree blocks include:

    a. first-degree block.

    b. second-degree Type I.

    c. third-degree block.

    d. Wenckebach, Mobitz I.

12. Sodium bicarbonate should be administered:

    a. intravenously.

    b. intraosseously.

    c. intradermally.

    d. endotracheally.

13. The QRS waves of all premature complexes are usually 0.10 second or less in duration:

    a. False

    b. True

14. Which one of the following is the most appropriate initial setting for defibrillating ventricular fibrillation in an adult?

    a. 400 joules

    b. 200 joules

    c. 1 joule per kilogram

    d. 20 to 25 joules per kilogram

15. A common cardiac drug encountered frequently in patient homes as oral medication is:

   a. bretylium.

   b. prednisone.

   c. penicillin.

   d. digitalis.

16. When preparing to defibrillate a patient who presents with ventricular fibrillation, the health-care provider should do all the following *except:*

   a. check pulses and lead wires.

   b. order all personnel to stand clear.

   c. perform CPR.

   d. ensure that the synchronization button is on.

17. The most appropriate treatment of uncomplicated acute MI is:

   a. IV D5W only.

   b. oxygen by mask, IV lactated Ringer solution.

   c. IV D50W, monitor, oxygen.

   d. IV normal saline, cardiac monitor, oxygen.

18. The coronary arteries receive oxygenated blood from the:

   a. aorta.

   b. coronary sinus.

   c. pulmonary veins.

   d. pulmonary arteries.

19. IV fluids are administered to cardiac patients primarily in order to:

   a. provide a lifeline.

   b. allow oxygen to the brain

   c. keep the patient well hydrated.

   d. prevent incipient pump failure.

20. EKG leads that record the electrical impulse formation in uninvolved myocardium directly opposite from the involved myocardium are called ___ leads.

   a. facing

   b. viewing

   c. reciprocal

   d. endocardial

21. The chambers of the heart that are thin-walled and pump against low pressure are the:

   a. apex.   c. atria.

   b. aorta.   d. ventricles.

22. Blood pressure is maintained by cardiac output and:
    a. alveoli.
    b. stroke volume.
    c. coronary arteries.
    d. peripheral resistance.

23. The sinoatrial (SA) node is located in the:
    a. right atrium.
    b. right ventricle.
    c. Purkinje fiber tract.
    d. atrioventricular septum.

24. The AV node is located in the:
    a. right ventricle.
    b. left ventricle.
    c. Purkinje fiber tract.
    d. atrioventricular septum.

25. The intrinsic firing rate of the AV node is ___ beats per minute.
    a. 60–100
    b. 25–35
    c. 35–45
    d. 40–60

26. EKG findings of infarction may occur in a single lead or in a combination of leads.
    a. True
    b. False

27. A sudden (paroxysmal) onset of tachycardia with a stimulus that arises above the AV node refers to a:
    a. sinus arrest.
    b. sinus tachycardia.
    c. sinus dysrhythmia.
    d. supraventricular dysrhythmia.

28. Oscilloscopic evidence of ventricular fibrillation can be mimicked by artifact.
    a. True
    b. False

29. Adenosine is a naturally occurring substance present in all body cells. Its mechanism of action is which one of the following?
    a. It increases conduction of the electrical impulse through the AV node.
    b. It decreases conduction of the electrical impulse through the AV node.
    c. It increases conduction of the electrical impulse through the Purkinje network.
    d. It increases conduction of the electrical impulse through the sinoatrial node.

30. Administration routes for atropine include:

   a. IV only.

   b. ET only.

   c. IV, ET, or IO.

   d. IV or ET.

31. The intrinsic rate of the SA node in the adult is ___ beats per minute.

   a. 20–60

   b. 40–80

   c. 60–100

   d. 80–100

32. The electrocardiogram is used to:

   a. determine cardiac output.

   b. detect valvular dysfunction.

   c. evaluate electrical activity in the heart.

   d. determine whether the heart muscle is contracting.

33. The PR interval should normally be ___ second or smaller.

   a. 0.10

   b. 0.12

   c. 0.08

   d. 0.20

34. Defined as "death of the myocardial tissue," a myocardial infarction commonly results from:

   a. myocardial necrosis.

   b. myocardial injury.

   c. myocardial ischemia.

   d. muscle oxygenation.

35. EKG changes that can be anticipated as a result of myocardial ischemia, injury, and/or necrosis of the myocardial tissues include all of the following *except:*

   a. PR interval prolongation.

   b. ST segment elevation.

   c. ST segment depression.

   d. pathologic Q wave.

36. The development of the pathologic Q waves often begins within the first 2 hours after an MI and, in most cases, is complete within:

   a. 60 minutes.

   b. 30 minutes.

   c. 24 hours.

   d. 48 hours.

37. The QRS interval should normally be ___ second or smaller.

   a. 0.20

   b. 0.12

   c. 0.18

   d. 0.36

38. The heart has four chambers. The upper chambers are called:

   a. atria.

   b. ventricles.

   c. septa.

   d. branches.

39. A sinus rhythm with cyclic variation caused by alterations in the respiratory pattern is:

   a. sinus arrest.

   b. sinus tachycardia.

   c. sinus dysrhythmia.

   d. supraventricular dysrhythmia.

40. In the presence of ventricular fibrillation, ineffective countershock attempts might be caused by:

   a. the presence of metabolic acidosis.

   b. ventricular irritability.

   c. inadequate oxygenation.

   d. all of the above.

41. Prior to performing carotid sinus massage, you should do all of the following *except:*

   a. monitor the EKG.

   b. ensure that the carotid pulses are present.

   c. have the patient perform Valsalva's maneuver.

   d. establish a secure airway by intubating the trachea.

42. The QRS complex is produced when the:

   a. ventricles repolarize.

   b. ventricles depolarize.

   c. ventricles contract.

   d. both b and c.

43. Most atrial fibrillation waves are NOT followed by a QRS complex because:

   a. the impulses are initiated in the left ventricle.

   b. the stimuli are not strong enough to be conducted.

   c. the ventricle can receive only 120 stimuli in one minute.

   d. the AV junction is unable to conduct all the excitation impulses.

44. What is the normal impulse flow of the heart's electrical conduction system?

    1. SA node
    2. Purkinje fibers
    3. bundle of His
    4. AV node
    5. bundle branches
    6. internodal pathways

  a. 1, 5, 2, 4, 6, 3

  b. 1, 6, 4, 3, 5, 2

  c. 1, 4, 3, 6, 5, 2

  d. 1, 2, 3, 4, 5, 6

45. When the EKG shows there is no relationship between the P wave and the QRS complex, you should suspect:

  a. first-degree block.

  b. second-degree block.

  c. third-degree block.

  d. electromechanical dissociation.

46. A 65-year-old man presents at the emergency department with severe chest pain. His weight is 75 kilograms. His heart rate is 40 and his blood pressure is 70/50. The cardiac monitor shows sinus bradycardia with an occasional premature ventricular complex. Which one of the following drugs is indicated first?

  a. atropine 0.5 milligram IV

  b. isuprel infusion

  c. lidocaine 75 milligrams IV bolus

  d. morphine 10 to 15 milligrams IV

47. Administration routes for Narcan include:

  a. IV only.   c. IO only.

  b. ET only.   d. IV or ET.

48. The pain of stable angina pectoris is:

  a. predictable.

  b. not predictable.

  c. never very severe.

  d. usually undetectable.

49. Signs and symptoms that can be observed in a patient with necrotic heart tissue could include:

  a. dysrhythmias.

  b. congestive heart failure.

  c. cardiogenic shock (severe).

  d. all of the above.

50. The term *supraventricular* indicates a stimulus arising above the ventricles.
    a. True
    b. False

51. Wenckebach differs from complete heart block in that complete heart block has a:
    a. faster rate.
    b. normal QRS.
    c. constant PR interval.
    d. regular RR interval.

52. Paroxysmal atrial tachycardia (PAT) is a sudden onset of atrial tachycardia.
    a. True
    b. False

53. The T wave on the EKG strip represents:
    a. rest period.
    b. bundle of His.
    c. atrial contraction.
    d. ventricular contraction.

54. The coronary circulation has ___ MAIN arteries?
    a. 2
    b. 6
    c. 4
    d. 8

55. Starling's law may be expressed as which one of the following?
    a. An increase in systolic filling does not alter cardiac output.
    b. A decrease in systolic filling will decrease the force of contraction.
    c. An increase in diastolic filling will increase the force of contraction.
    d. An increase in filling time yields greater cardiac output regardless of peripheral resistance.

56. Inferior wall infarctions are associated with the:
    a. right coronary artery.
    b. left coronary artery.
    c. bundle of His.
    d. coronary sinus.

57. Myocardial infarctions may be classified as either transmural or:
    a. supraendocardial.
    b. subendocardial.
    c. endocardial.
    d. precardial.

58. Subendocardial infarctions are commonly referred to as:

a. full-thickness.

b. transmural.

c. nontransmural.

d. transdermal.

59. Pulseless electrical activity may be manifested by:

a. normal EKG, normal pulse.

b. normal or abnormal EKG, absent pulse.

c. abnormal EKG, normal pulse.

d. normal or abnormal EKG, absent blood pressure.

60. The function of the chordae tendineae and papillary muscles is to:

a. prevent backflow of blood into the ventricles.

b. protect the coronary orifices when the aortic valve opens.

c. prevent backflow of blood into the atrium.

d. facilitate backflow of blood from the aorta.

61. A 50-year-old man is complaining of chest pain that began while he was clearing underbrush on a vacant lot. He describes the pain as a "heavy pressure" that has lasted 5 to 10 minutes. Vital signs are blood pressure 140/95, heart rate 82, respirations 16. He has no previous cardiac history. EKG shows normal sinus rhythm. The chest pain is most probably due to:

a. dysrhythmias.

b. pulmonary embolus.

c. coronary insufficiency.

d. congestive heart failure.

62. Lead II is the lead most commonly used in the prehospital arena because it:

a. is easier to apply.

b. shows good T waves.

c. illustrates good P waves.

d. is faster to apply.

63. The ability of certain cardiac cells to initiate excitation impulses spontaneously is called:

a. automaticity.   c. conductivity.

b. contractility.   d. excitability.

64. The keys to interpretation of second-degree heart block, Mobitz Type II, are the presence of constant PR intervals and the fact that there are more P waves present than QRS complexes.

a. True

b. False

65. The absence of electrical impulse results in the recording of a flat line on an EKG strip.

    a. False

    b. True

66. Your patient is a race car driver who was in a head-on automobile collision. Upon assessment, you immediately notice that the patient has multiple contusions on the chest area. You realize you are probably dealing with:

    a. angina pectoris.

    b. myocardial infarction.

    c. myocardial trauma.

    d. hypertensive crisis.

67. A person complains of substernal chest pain radiating to his left arm and jaw. He has vomited once and still feels nauseated. He is sitting up, appears to be short of breath, and is sweating profusely. Your patient's signs and symptoms most probably are related to:

    a. pacemaker failure.

    b. pulmonary edema.

    c. hypertensive crisis.

    d. acute myocardial infarction.

68. If a known coronary bypass patient suffers a cardiac arrest, the health-care provider should:

    a. not perform CPR due to the risk of further injury.

    b. deliver lighter compressions due to the risk of further injury.

    c. provide CPR as you would do for any other patient in arrest.

    d. provide CPR unless fracture of the sternum or ribs becomes apparent.

69. The expected rate of a junctional escape rhythm is ___ beats per minute.

    a. 20–40

    b. 60–100

    c. 40–60

    d. 60–80

70. When interpreting dysrhythmias, you should remember that the most important key is the:

    a. PR interval.

    b. rate and rhythm.

    c. presence of dysrhythmias.

    d. patient's clinical appearance.

71. In order to obtain a two-lead EKG strip, you should apply ___ leads to the patient's chest.

    a. three   c. five

    b. four   d. six

72. The uppermost portion of the heart is known as the:
   a. apex.
   b. base.
   c. atria.
   d. aorta.

73. The most common causes of poor EKG tracings are:
   a. patient movement.
   b. loose leads/electrodes.
   c. both a and b are true.
   d. none of the above are true.

74. "A graphic record of the electrical activity of the heart" describes a(n):
   a. echocardiogram.
   b. electrocardiogram.
   c. encephalogram.
   d. radiogram.

75. The initial treatment for multifocal PVCs should be:
   a. defibrillation.
   b. cardioversion.
   c. oxygen administration.
   d. pulse oximetry.

76. All of the following statements about verapamil are correct *except:*
   a. it may be used to treat PSVT.
   b. it causes peripheral vasodilation.
   c. it is contraindicated in hypotensive patients.
   d. it is indicated in patients with a history of Wolfe-Parkinson-White syndrome.

77. Atropine is indicated for all of the following situations *except:*
   a. asystole.
   b. symptomatic third-degree block.
   c. asymptomatic first-degree block.
   d. symptomatic bradycardia.

78. In cardiac arrest, atropine is administered in doses of:
   a. 1.0 milligram every 5 minutes, not to exceed 2 milligrams.
   b. 0.5 milligram every 5 minutes, not to exceed 3 milligrams.
   c. 1.0 milligram every 5 minutes, not to exceed 5 milligrams.
   d. 0.5 milligram every 10 minutes, not to exceed 3 milligrams.

79. The initial bolus of lidocaine should be:

    a. administered via IV infusion if the patient is complaining of chest pain.

    b. reduced by half if the patient is 70 years old or older.

    c. doubled if the patient is in cardiopulmonary arrest.

    d. titrated to effect if the patient is symptomatic.

80. Lidocaine is indicated in all of the following situations *except:*

    a. atrial fibrillation with a ventricular rate of 100.

    b. malignant premature ventricular contractions.

    c. ventricular tachycardia (with palpable pulse).

    d. symptomatic multifocal premature ventricular contractions.

81. Which one of the following medications decreases automaticity of the heart?

    a. isoproterenol

    b. atropine

    c. lidocaine

    d. naloxone

82. A patient may experience side effects of blurred vision, dilated pupils, dry mouth, and flushing of the skin when which drug is administered?

    a. adenosine

    b. Narcan

    c. atropine

    d. morphine

83. In order to accurately calculate heart rate by the R-to-R interval method, the patient must have a regular rhythm.

    a. True

    b. False

84. Second-degree heart block, Type I, may be transient and self-correcting.

    a. True

    b. False

85. Cardiovascular disease is the number one cause of death in the United States.

    a. False

    b. True

86. Prompt, definitive intervention has proven effective in preventing many cardio-vascular-related deaths.

    a. True

    b. False

87. The innermost lining of the heart is contiguous with the visceral pericardium and is called the:

a. endocardium.

b. pericardium.

c. myocardium.

d. epicardium.

88. The right and left atria are separated anatomically by the:

a. interatrial septum.

b. bundle of Kent.

c. interventricular septum.

d. endocardial mass.

89. The right atrium receives blood from the myocardium via the:

a. left marginal branch.

b. inferior vena cavae.

c. great cardiac vein.

d. internal carotid artery.

90. Two examples of atrioventricular valves are the:

1. pulmonic valve
2. tricuspid valve
3. papillary valve
4. bicuspid valve

a. 1 and 2

b. 2 and 4

c. 1 and 3

d. 3 and 4

91. Deoxygenated blood enters the heart through the:

1. coronary sinus.
2. pulmonary artery.
3. superior vena cava.
4. inferior vena cava.

a. 1, 2, and 3

b. 2, 3 and 4

c. 2 and 3 only

d. 1, 3, and 4

92. In EKG strips representing dysrhythmias originating in the AV junction, the P wave, if present, will be inverted or absent.

a. True

b. False

93. The amount of blood ejected by the heart in one cardiac contraction is known as:

   a. preload.

   b. afterload.

   c. cardiac cycle.

   d. stroke volume.

94. The pressure in the ventricle at the end of diastole is referred to as:

   a. preload.

   b. afterload.

   c. cardiac output.

   d. autonomic.

95. The parasympathetic nervous system is mediated by the 10th cranial nerve, which runs from the brainstem to the rectum. This nerve is called the:

   a. optic.   c. plexus.

   b. vagus.   d. ganglia.

96. The neurotransmitter for the parasympathetic nervous system is acetylcholine. Release of acetylcholine:

   1. slows the heart rate.
   2. increases the heart rate.
   3. slows atrioventricular conduction.
   4. increases atrioventricular conduction.

   a. 1 and 3

   b. 2 and 3

   c. 3 and 4

   d. 1 and 4

97. Hyperkalemia refers to an increased level of potassium in the blood and can result in decreased automaticity and conduction.

   a. False

   b. True

98. Cardiac function, both electrical and mechanical, is strongly influenced by electrolyte imbalance.

   a. True

   b. False

99. An EKG strip illustrates a regular rhythm, a heart rate of 70, and QRS complexes that are within normal limits. P waves are variable in configuration across the strip. This rhythm is identified as a:

   a. wandering atrial pacemaker.

   b. first-degree heart block.

   c. third-degree heart block.

   d. second-degree heart block, Mobitz Type I.

100. Ventricular irritability in the presence of myocardial infarction is:

a. a precursor to respiratory involvement.

b. very dangerous and should be treated.

c. to be expected and not a cause for alarm.

d. highly unlikely if oxygen is administered.

101. Prolonged episodes of supraventricular tachycardia may increase myocardial oxygen demand and may thus increase the need for supplemental oxygen therapy.

a. False

b. True

102. A progressing PR interval until such time that a QRS is dropped is considered to be:

a. third-degree block.

b. atrial fibrillation.

c. second-degree AV block, Mobitz Type I.

d. second-degree AV block, Mobitz Type II.

103. *Artifact* is defined as EKG waveforms produced from sources outside the heart.

a. True

b. False

104. Parasympathetic stimulation controls cardiac action by reducing the heart rate, the speed of impulse through the AV node, and the force of atrial contraction. This response is known as the:

a. nodal response.

b. sinoatrial node.

c. neurotransmitter.

d. vagal response.

105. An abnormality in conduction through the ventricles may be identified on the EKG tracing by a(n):

a. distorted, varying P wave pattern.

b. prolonged P R interval.

c. wide and bizarre QRS complex.

d. elevated S T segment.

106. Lidocaine should be considered for suppressing premature ventricular contractions (PVCs) in acute MI in which one of the following situations?

a. when PVCs are more frequent than six per minute or are multifocal

b. in second- or third-degree heart block

c. in the presence of sinus bradycardia

d. in patients who are known to be allergic to local anesthetics

107. The faster discharging rate of the AV junction in an accelerated junctional rhythm may be due to:

   a. increased automaticity of the AV junction.

   b. blockage of the parasympathetic nervous system response.

   c. increased excitation of the internodal pathways.

   d. increased excitation of the sinoatrial node.

108. Paroxysmal junctional tachycardia is often more appropriately called paroxysmal supraventricular tachycardia because it may be difficult to distinguish this rhythm from paroxysmal atrial tachycardia due to the rapid rate.

   a. True

   b. False

109. Defibrillation is the treatment of choice for:

   1. asystole.
   2. pulseless ventricular tachycardia.
   3. ventricular fibrillation.
   4. idioventricular rhythms.

   a. 1, 2, and 3

   b. 2 and 3

   c. 1, 3, and 4

   d. 3 and 4

110. Because unifocal PVCs imply uniform irritability of the entire myocardium, they are generally considered more life-threatening than multifocal PVCs.

   a. True

   b. False

111. A 69-year-old male is experiencing mild chest pain. Physical exam reveals no other significant findings. Vital signs are: blood pressure 160/88, pulse 84 and irregular, respirations 24. The cardiac monitor reveals a normal sinus rhythm with 5 unifocal PVCs per minute. The most appropriate treatment is:

   a. monitor patient only, as no treatment is indicated.

   b. oxygen via nonrebreathing mask, IV, cardiac monitor.

   c. oxygen at 6 liters per nasal cannula, IV with D5W normal saline at keep-vein-open (KVO) rate, cardiac monitor.

   d. oxygen at 10 liters per endotracheal tube, rapid IV infusion of lactated Ringer solution, cardiac monitor.

112. Which one of the following is NOT a trait of malignant or dangerous PVCs?

   a. unifocal premature complexes

   b. R-on-T phenomenon

   c. greater than 6 per minute

   d. runs of ventricular tachycardia

113. What is the CORRECT sequence of treatment for ventricular fibrillation?

   1. Defibrillate at 200–300 joules.
   2. Intubate.
   3. Defibrillate at 200 joules.
   4. Begin CPR.
   5. Defibrillate at 360 joules.
   6. Establish IV access.

   a. 4, 3, 1, 5, 2, 6

   b. 4, 2, 5, 1, 3, 6

   c. 4, 2, 3, 1, 5, 6

   d. 3, 1, 5, 4, 2, 6

114. Your patient is an 82-year-old woman with a history of coronary artery disease. She is alert and complaining of substernal chest pain, radiating to the left arm. She is diaphoretic and short of breath. Vital signs are: blood pressure 120/64, pulse 56 and irregular, respirations 32, shallow and congested. You connect the cardiac monitor and it shows ventricular fibrillation. Your immediate action is to:

   a. begin CPR.

   b. prepare to defibrillate at 200 joules.

   c. check the monitor leads.

   d. defibrillate at 200 joules.

115. Because pacemakers are prone to damage from strong electrical stimuli, you should never defibrillate a patient who has an implanted pacemaker at a setting over 300 joules.

   a. True

   b. False

116. Second-degree AV block (Mobitz Type II) is usually associated with acute MI and septal necrosis and is considered to be more serious than Wenckebach.

   a. True

   b. False

117. The point at which the QRS complex meets the ST segment is known as the:

   a. delta wave.

   b. end point.

   c. J point.

   d. vector.

118. How many cardiac monitor pads are utilized when obtaining a 12-lead EKG?

   a. 10

   b. 12

   c. 3

   d. 6

119. The 12-lead EKG is used to evaluate all of the following *except:*

    a. pulse rate.

    b. valvular dysfunction.

    c. electrical activity in the heart.

    d. waveforms indicative of acute MI.

120. The right and left coronary arteries branch off of the:

    a. ventricular artery.

    b. myocardial fossa.

    c. proximal portion of the aorta.

    d. distal portion of the aorta.

121. Collateral circulation allows for:

    a. alternate path of blood flow in the event of occlusion.

    b. circulation continuum during diastole.

    c. maintaining artery patency during spasms.

    d. the ability of blood flow continuum during systole.

122. Myocardial infarction is:

    a. always temporary.

    b. not treatable.

    c. age limited in most patients.

    d. due to myocardial cell necrosis.

123. The most common cause of the majority of acute MIs is:

    a. coronary vasospasms.

    b. atherosclerotic lesions.

    c. thrombus formation.

    d. arteriosclerotic blebs.

124. In acute MIs, chest pain is _____ relieved by nitroglycerin.

    a. short in duration and

    b. short in duration but NOT

    c. long in duration and

    d. long in duration and NOT

125. The primary goal of management of the patient with symptomatic chest pain is to:

    a. interrupt the infarction process.

    b. enhance the infarction process.

    c. institute fibrinolytic therapy.

    d. increase myocardial oxygen consumption.

126. Management of a patient who is suspected of having sustained a myocardial contusion should:

    a. focus primarily on the associated and isolated chest injury.

    b. be similar to the treatment administered to a suspected MI patient.

    c. only be initiated at the definitive care facility following transport.

    d. completed in the prehospital arena, prior to transport to the hospital.

127. Signs and symptoms the health-care provider may expect to observe in a patient with necrotic heart tissue could include:

    a. dysrhythmias.

    b. congestive heart failure.

    c. cardiogenic shock (severe).

    d. all of the above.

128. The right atrium receives blood from the myocardium via the:

    a. left marginal branch.

    b. inferior vena cavae.

    c. great cardiac vein.

    d. internal carotid artery.

129. ST segment depression may be evident on a 12-lead EKG strip, following both angina and strenuous exercise.

    a. False

    b. True

130. EKG changes of significance with myocardial ischemia include ST segment depression, T wave inversion, or _____ wave.

    a. depressed T   c. peaked P

    b. peaked T   d. inverted P

131. Chest pain should be considered cardiac in origin and managed accordingly until proven otherwise.

    a. True

    b. False

132. Leads that record electrical impulses generated from the heart's electrical conduction system and "look at" specific areas of damaged myocardium are called ___ leads.

    a. reciprocal

    b. facing

    c. viewing

    d. specific

133. The most important diagnostic tool that you can use when assessing and treating a patient with a suspected inferior MI is the:

    a. 12-lead EKG machine.

    b. cardiac enzymes

    c. patient's clinical appearance.

    d. patient's presenting vital signs.

134. If ST segment elevation is noted in the lower limb leads, Leads II, III, and aVF, this finding is indicative of _____ myocardial infarction.

    a. anterior

    b. lateral

    c. superior

    d. inferior

135. If your patient is hypotensive and is exhibiting EKG changes consistent with an inferior myocardial infarction, you should consider the possibility of _____ infarction.

    a. right atrial

    b. left atrial

    c. right ventricular

    d. left ventricular

136. Any patient who complains of chest pain must be thoroughly evaluated and management continued until the possibility of acute MI is ruled out by the physician.

    a. True

    b. False

137. In the two-lead method of axis determination, a normal axis is determined by:

    a. negative QRS deflection in Leads I and aVF.

    b. positive QRS deflection in Leads I and aVF.

    c. negative QRS deflection in Lead I and positive QRS deflection in aVF.

    d. negative QRS deflection in Lead I and positive QRS deflection in aVL.

138. In the two-lead method of axis determination, a left axis deviation is determined by:

    a. negative QRS deflection in Leads I and aVF.

    b. positive QRS deflection in Leads I and aVF.

    c. negative QRS deflection in Lead I and positive QRS deflection in aVF.

    d. positive QRS deflection in Lead I and negative QRS deflection in aVF.

139. In the two-lead method of axis determination, a right axis deviation is determined by:

    a. negative QRS deflection in Leads I and aVF.

    b. positive QRS deflection in Leads I and aVF.

    c. negative QRS deflection in Lead I and positive QRS deflection in aVF.

    d. positive QRS deflection in Lead I and negative QRS deflection in aVF.

140. In the two-lead method of axis determination, an indeterminate right axis deviation is determined by:

a. negative QRS deflection in Leads I and aVF.

b. positive QRS deflection in Leads I and aVF.

c. negative QRS deflection in Lead I and positive QRS deflection in aVF.

d. positive QRS deflection in Lead I and negative QRS deflection in aVF.

141. Which one of the following disease processes can be expected in left axis deviation?

a. left bundle branch block

b. pulmonary hypertension

c. Wolfe-Parkinson-White syndrome

d. ischemic heart disease

142. Which one of the following disease processes can be expected in right axis deviation?

a. ischemic heart disease

b. chronic obstructive pulmonary disease

c. right bundle branch block

d. systemic hypertension

143. The right bundle branch runs down the right side of the interventricular septum and terminates at the ___ in the right ventricle.

a. Purkinje network

b. papillary muscles

c. anterior fascicle

d. posterior fascicle

144. To determine right bundle branch block, the primary EKG leads to observe are:

a. V1, V2.

b. V5, V6.

c. V2, V3.

d. V2, V4.

145. If ST segment elevation is noted in Leads V5 and V6, this finding is indicative of _____ myocardial infarction.

a. anterior

b. lateral

c. superior

d. inferior

146. If ST segment depression is noted in V1, V2, V3 and possibly V4, this finding is indicative of ___ myocardial infarction.

a. anterior   c. posterior

b. lateral   d. inferior

147. The combination of posterior wall injury evidence, in addition to evidence of
_____, indicates a more extensive infarction and a greater risk of complications.

a. anterior wall ischemia

b. inferior infarction

c. T wave inversion

d. prolonged PR interval

148. If ST segment elevation is noted in Leads V1 and V2, this finding is indicative of
___ myocardial infarction.

a. anterior

b. septal

c. superior

d. inferior

149. If ST segment elevation is noted in Leads V3 and V4, this finding is indicative of
_____ myocardial infarction.

a. anterior

b. septal

c. superior

d. inferior

150. The drug most commonly used in the treatment of symptomatic bradycardia is:

a. amiodarone.

b. adenosine.

c. atropine.

d. adrenalin.

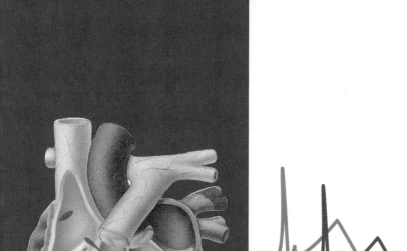

chapter 18

12-Lead EKG Review Strips

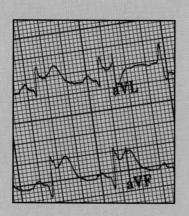

The review strips in this chapter are provided to enhance your ability to interpret 12-lead EKGs. Although the answers are provided at the end of the book, we strongly encourage you to apply the 5 + 3 approach to *each* review strip *before* you refer to the answer. We trust that this chapter will prove valuable to you. Good luck!

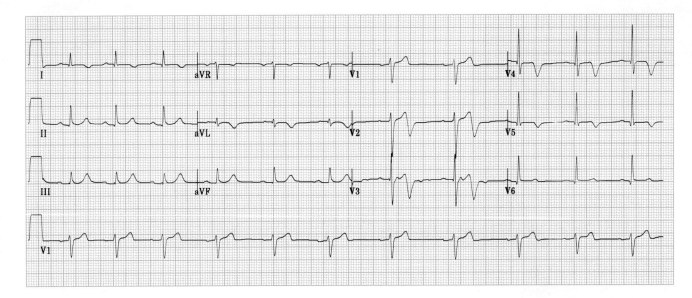

1

1. Rate: _____   2. Rhythm: _____   3. P wave: _____
4. PR Interval: _____   5. QRS complex: _____   +1. ST elevation: _____
+2. ST depression: _____   +3. Pathologic Q waves: _____   Interpretation: _____

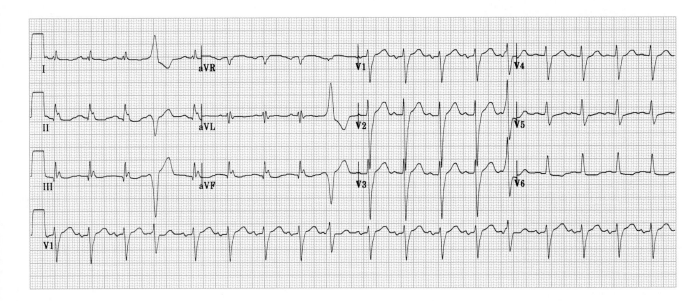

2

1. Rate: _____   2. Rhythm: _____   3. P wave: _____
4. PR Interval: _____   5. QRS complex: _____   +1. ST elevation: _____
+2. ST depression: _____   +3. Pathologic Q waves: _____   Interpretation: _____

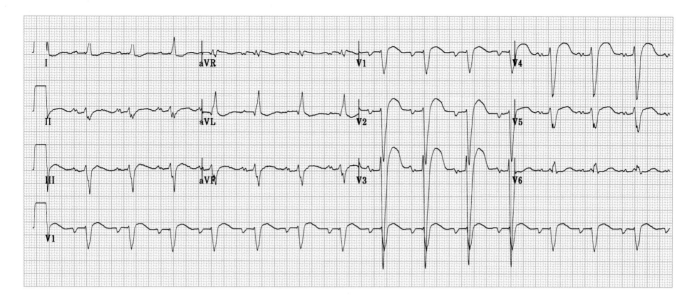

3

1. Rate: _____   2. Rhythm: _____   3. P wave: _____
4. PR Interval: _____   5. QRS complex: _____   +1. ST elevation: _____
+2. ST depression: _____   +3. Pathologic Q waves: _____   Interpretation: _____

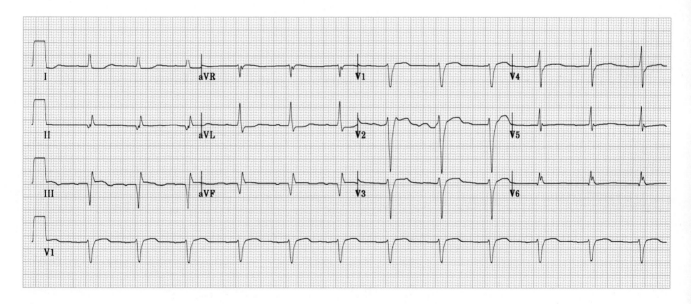

4

1. Rate: _____   2. Rhythm: _____   3. P wave: _____
4. PR Interval: _____   5. QRS complex: _____   +1. ST elevation: _____
+2. ST depression: _____   +3. Pathologic Q waves: _____   Interpretation: _____

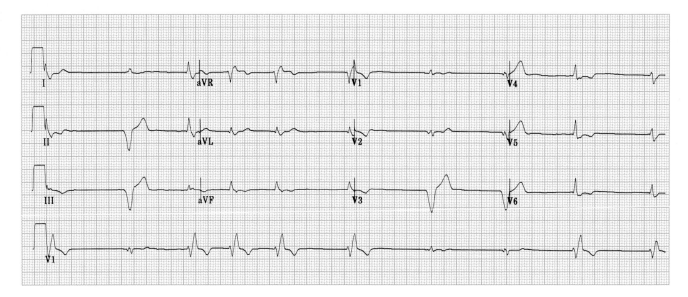

5

1. Rate: _____   2. Rhythm: _____   3. P wave: _____
4. PR Interval: _____   5. QRS complex: _____   +1. ST elevation: _____
+2. ST depression: _____   +3. Pathologic Q waves: _____   Interpretation: _____

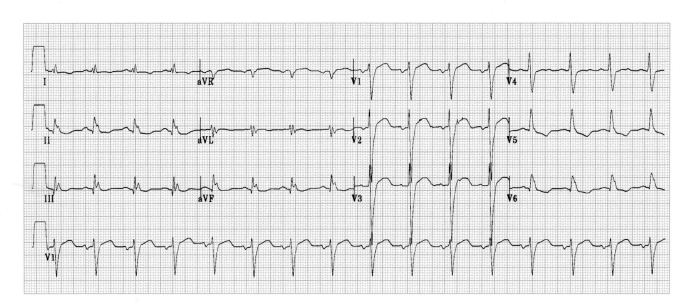

6

1. Rate: _____   2. Rhythm: _____   3. P wave: _____
4. PR Interval: _____   5. QRS complex: _____   +1. ST elevation: _____
+2. ST depression: _____   +3. Pathologic Q waves: _____   Interpretation: _____

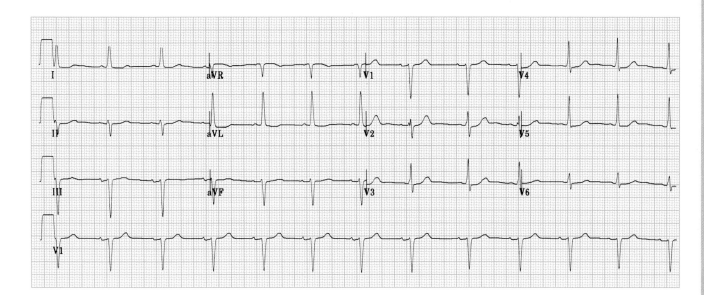

7

1. Rate: _____
4. PR Interval: _____
+2. ST depression: _____

2. Rhythm: _____
5. QRS complex: _____
+3. Pathologic Q waves: _____

3. P wave: _____
+1. ST elevation: _____
Interpretation: _____

8

1. Rate: _____
4. PR Interval: _____
+2. ST depression: _____

2. Rhythm: _____
5. QRS complex: _____
+3. Pathologic Q waves: _____

3. P wave: _____
+1. ST elevation: _____
Interpretation: _____

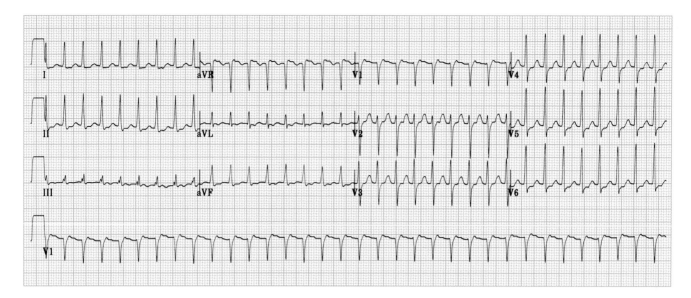

9

1. Rate: _____   2. Rhythm: _____   3. P wave: _____
4. PR Interval: _____   5. QRS complex: _____   +1. ST elevation: _____
+2. ST depression: _____   +3. Pathologic Q waves: _____   Interpretation: _____

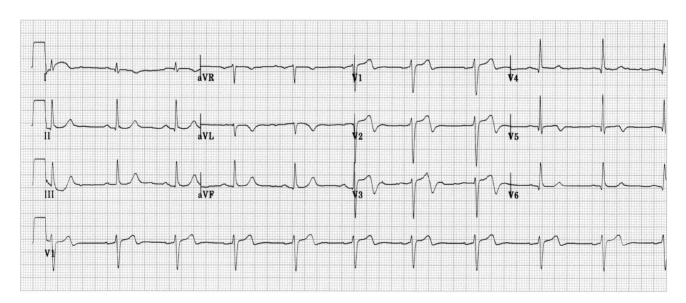

10

1. Rate: _____   2. Rhythm: _____   3. P wave: _____
4. PR Interval: _____   5. QRS complex: _____   +1. ST elevation: _____
+2. ST depression: _____   +3. Pathologic Q waves: _____   Interpretation: _____

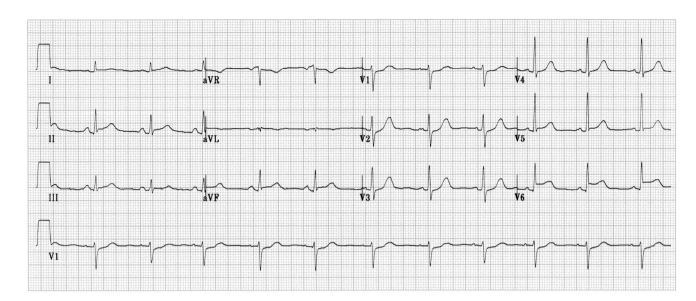

11

1. Rate: _____   2. Rhythm: _____   3. P wave: _____
4. PR Interval: _____   5. QRS complex: _____   +1. ST elevation: _____
+2. ST depression: _____   +3. Pathologic Q waves: _____   Interpretation: _____

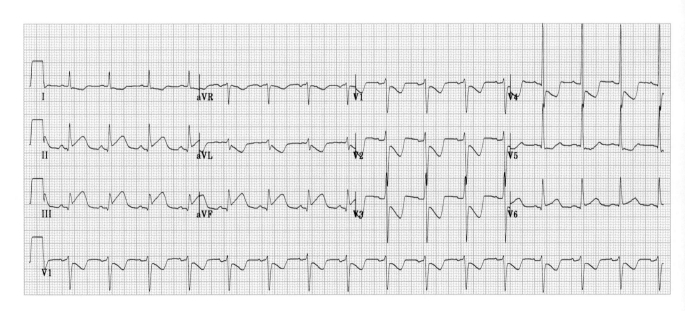

12

1. Rate: _____   2. Rhythm: _____   3. P wave: _____
4. PR Interval: _____   5. QRS complex: _____   +1. ST elevation: _____
+2. ST depression: _____   +3. Pathologic Q waves: _____   Interpretation: _____

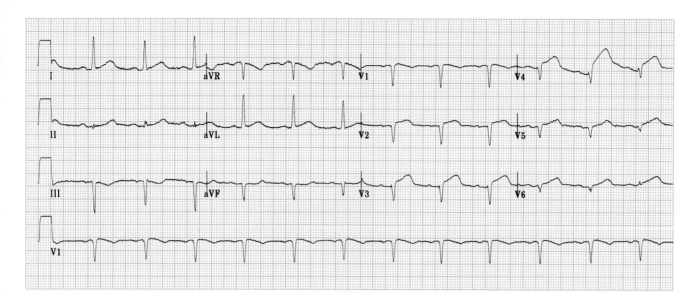

13

1. Rate: _____   2. Rhythm: _____   3. P wave: _____
4. PR Interval: _____   5. QRS complex: _____   +1. ST elevation: _____
+2. ST depression: _____   +3. Pathologic Q waves: _____   Interpretation: _____

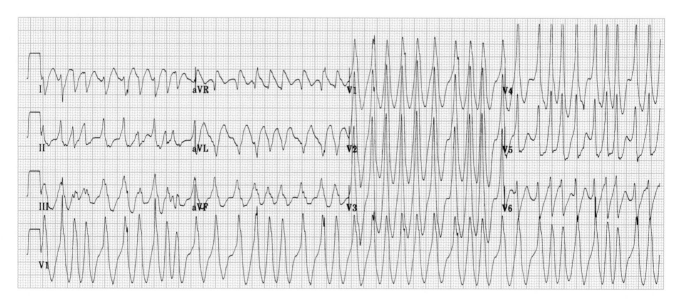

14

1. Rate: _____   2. Rhythm: _____   3. P wave: _____
4. PR Interval: _____   5. QRS complex: _____   +1. ST elevation: _____
+2. ST depression: _____   +3. Pathologic Q waves: _____   Interpretation: _____

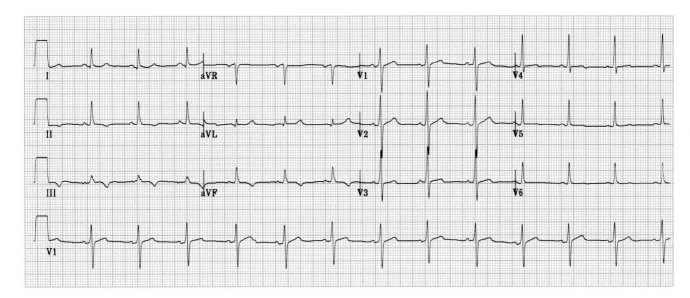

15

1. Rate: _____   2. Rhythm: _____   3. P wave: _____
4. PR Interval: _____   5. QRS complex: _____   +1. ST elevation: _____
+2. ST depression: _____   +3. Pathologic Q waves: _____   Interpretation: _____

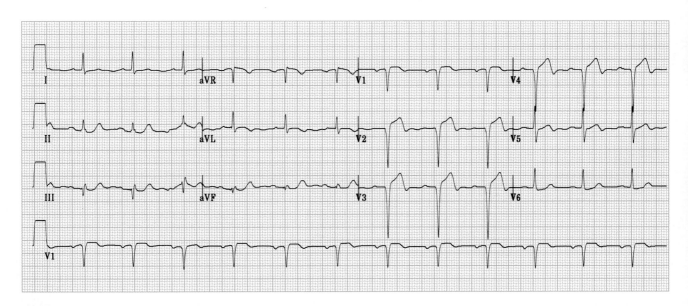

16

1. Rate: _____   2. Rhythm: _____   3. P wave: _____
4. PR Interval: _____   5. QRS complex: _____   +1. ST elevation: _____
+2. ST depression: _____   +3. Pathologic Q waves: _____   Interpretation: _____

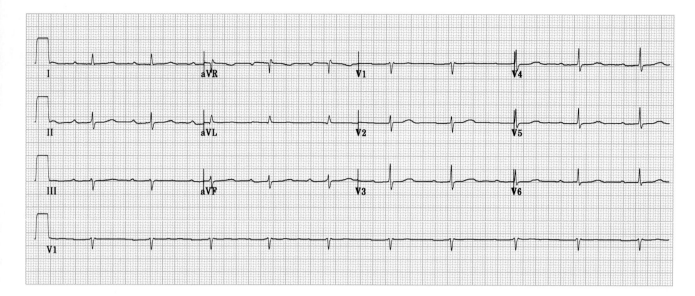

17

1. Rate: _____   2. Rhythm: _____   3. P wave: _____
4. PR Interval: _____   5. QRS complex: _____   +1. ST elevation: _____
+2. ST depression: _____   +3. Pathologic Q waves: _____   Interpretation: _____

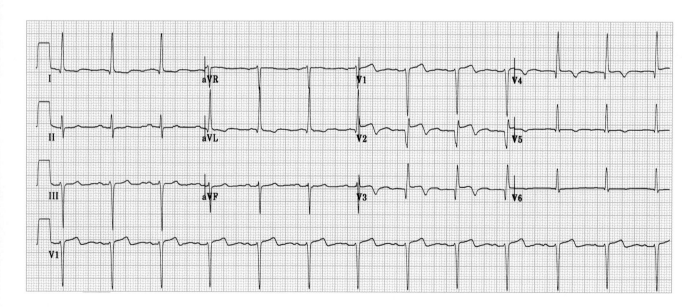

18

1. Rate: _____   2. Rhythm: _____   3. P wave: _____
4. PR Interval: _____   5. QRS complex: _____   +1. ST elevation: _____
+2. ST depression: _____   +3. Pathologic Q waves: _____   Interpretation: _____

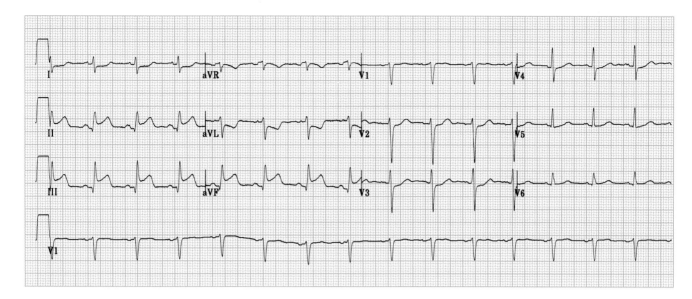

19

1. Rate: _____
2. Rhythm: _____
3. P wave: _____
4. PR Interval: _____
5. QRS complex: _____
+1. ST elevation: _____
+2. ST depression: _____
+3. Pathologic Q waves: _____
Interpretation: _____

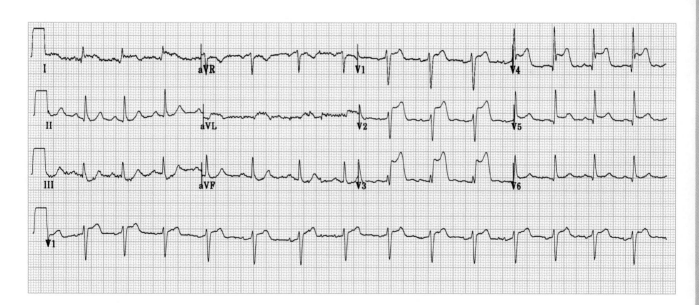

20

1. Rate: _____
2. Rhythm: _____
3. P wave: _____
4. PR Interval: _____
5. QRS complex: _____
+1. ST elevation: _____
+2. ST depression: _____
+3. Pathologic Q waves: _____
Interpretation: _____

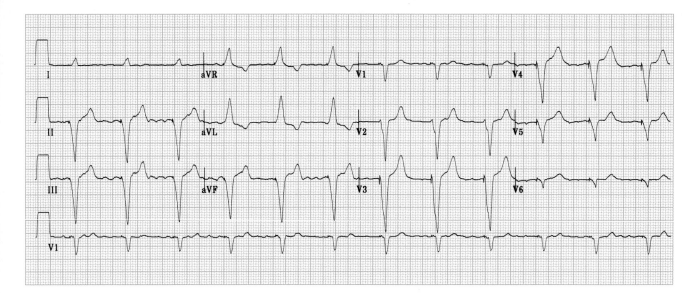

21

1. Rate: _____
4. PR Interval: _____
+2. ST depression: _____

2. Rhythm: _____
5. QRS complex: _____
+3. Pathologic Q waves: _____

3. P wave: _____
+1. ST elevation: _____
Interpretation: _____

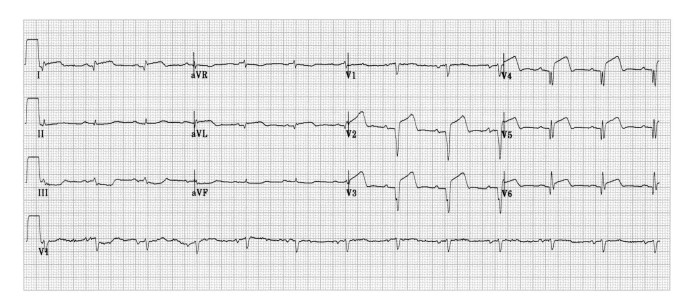

22

1. Rate: _____
4. PR Interval: _____
+2. ST depression: _____

2. Rhythm: _____
5. QRS complex: _____
+3. Pathologic Q waves: _____

3. P wave: _____
+1. ST elevation: _____
Interpretation: _____

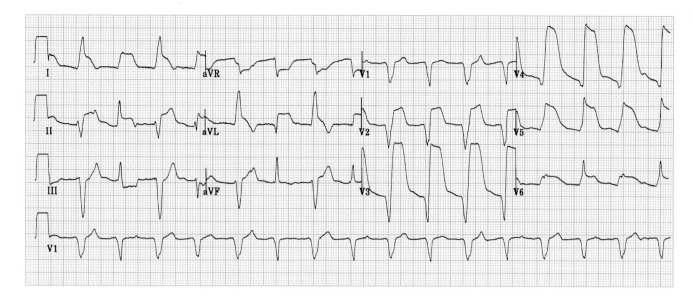

23

1. Rate: _____

4. PR Interval: _____

+2. ST depression: _____

2. Rhythm: _____

5. QRS complex: _____

+3. Pathologic Q waves: _____

3. P wave: _____

+1. ST elevation: _____

Interpretation: _____

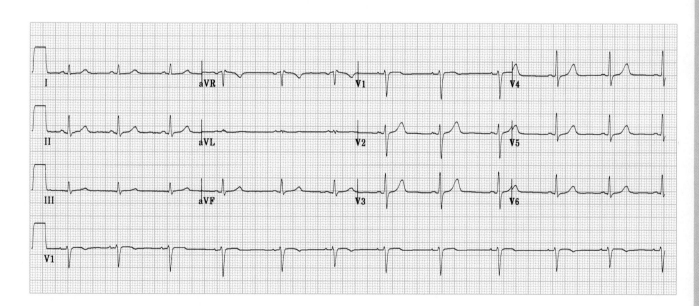

24

1. Rate: _____

4. PR Interval: _____

+2. ST depression: _____

2. Rhythm: _____

5. QRS complex: _____

+3. Pathologic Q waves: _____

3. P wave: _____

+1. ST elevation: _____

Interpretation: _____

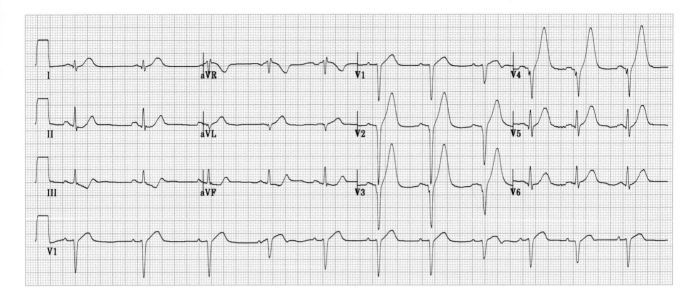

25

1. Rate: _____
4. PR Interval: _____
+2. ST depression: _____

2. Rhythm: _____
5. QRS complex: _____
+3. Pathologic Q waves: _____

3. P wave: _____
+1. ST elevation: _____
Interpretation: _____

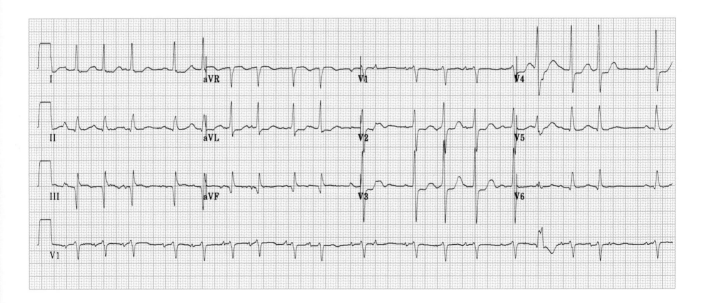

26

1. Rate: _____
4. PR Interval: _____
+2. ST depression: _____

2. Rhythm: _____
5. QRS complex: _____
+3. Pathologic Q waves: _____

3. P wave: _____
+1. ST elevation: _____
Interpretation: _____

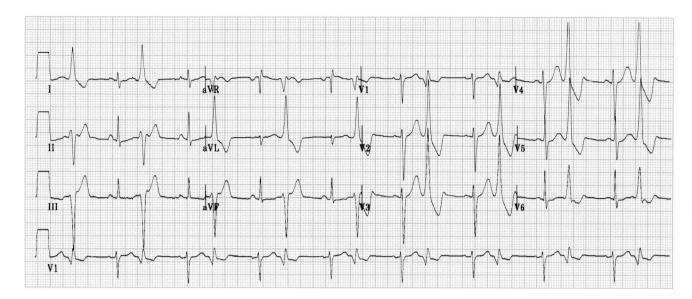

27

1. Rate: _____   2. Rhythm: _____   3. P wave: _____
4. PR Interval: _____   5. QRS complex: _____   +1. ST elevation: _____
+2. ST depression: _____   +3. Pathologic Q waves: _____   Interpretation: _____

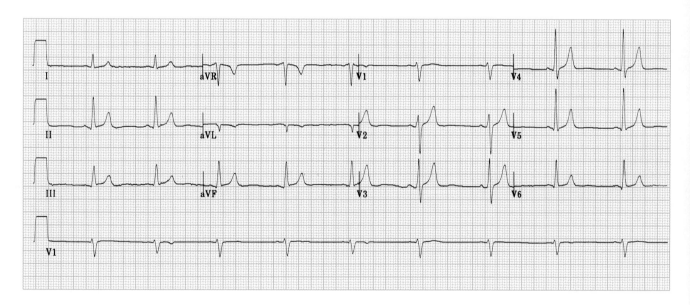

28

1. Rate: _____   2. Rhythm: _____   3. P wave: _____
4. PR Interval: _____   5. QRS complex: _____   +1. ST elevation: _____
+2. ST depression: _____   +3. Pathologic Q waves: _____   Interpretation: _____

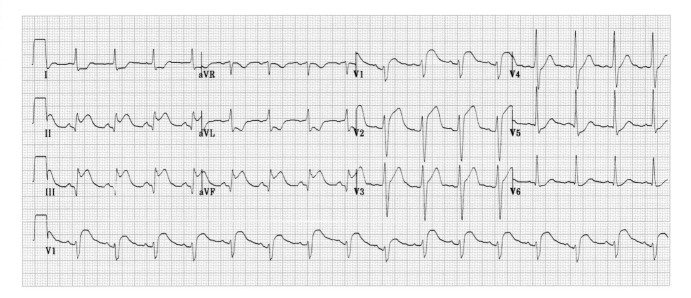

29

1. Rate: _____   2. Rhythm: _____   3. P wave: _____
4. PR Interval: _____   5. QRS complex: _____   +1. ST elevation: _____
+2. ST depression: _____   +3. Pathologic Q waves: _____   Interpretation: _____

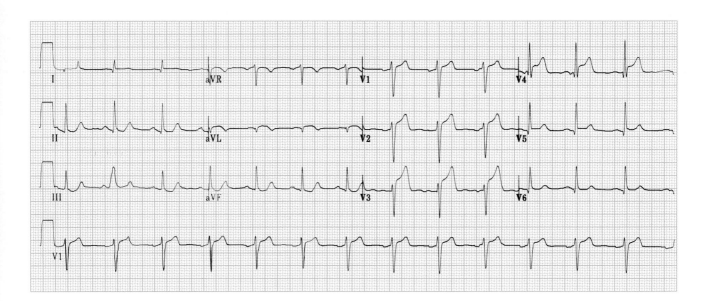

30

1. Rate: _____   2. Rhythm: _____   3. P wave: _____
4. PR Interval: _____   5. QRS complex: _____   +1. ST elevation: _____
+2. ST depression: _____   +3. Pathologic Q waves: _____   Interpretation: _____

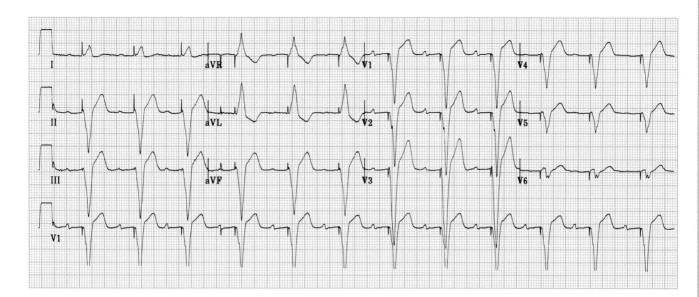

31

1. Rate: _____   2. Rhythm: _____   3. P wave: _____
4. PR Interval: _____   5. QRS complex: _____   +1. ST elevation: _____
+2. ST depression: _____   +3. Pathologic Q waves: _____   Interpretation: _____

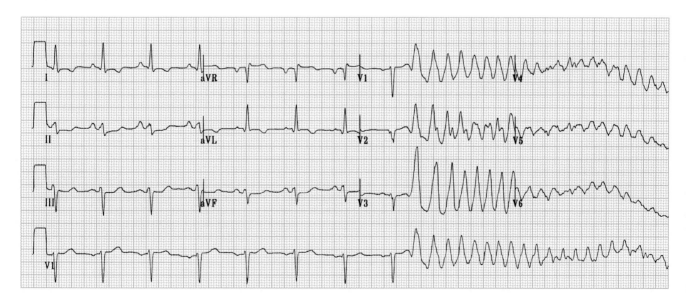

32

1. Rate: _____   2. Rhythm: _____   3. P wave: _____
4. PR Interval: _____   5. QRS complex: _____   +1. ST elevation: _____
+2. ST depression: _____   +3. Pathologic Q waves: _____   Interpretation: _____

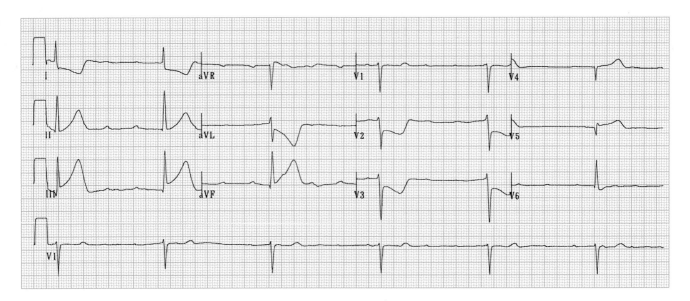

33

1. Rate: _____
4. PR Interval: _____
+2. ST depression: _____

2. Rhythm: _____
5. QRS complex: _____
+3. Pathologic Q waves: _____

3. P wave: _____
+1. ST elevation: _____
Interpretation: _____

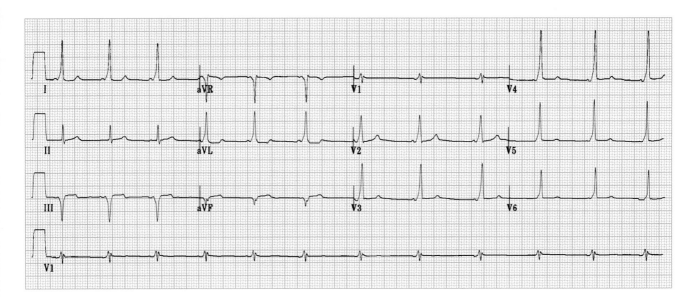

34

1. Rate: _____
4. PR Interval: _____
+2. ST depression: _____

2. Rhythm: _____
5. QRS complex: _____
+3. Pathologic Q waves: _____

3. P wave: _____
+1. ST elevation: _____
Interpretation: _____

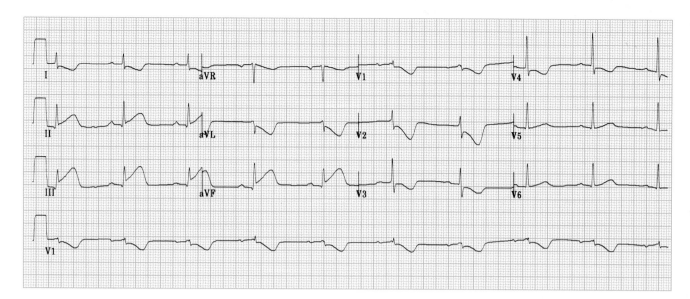

35

1. Rate: _____   2. Rhythm: _____   3. P wave: _____
4. PR Interval: _____   5. QRS complex: _____   +1. ST elevation: _____
+2. ST depression: _____   +3. Pathologic Q waves: _____   Interpretation: _____

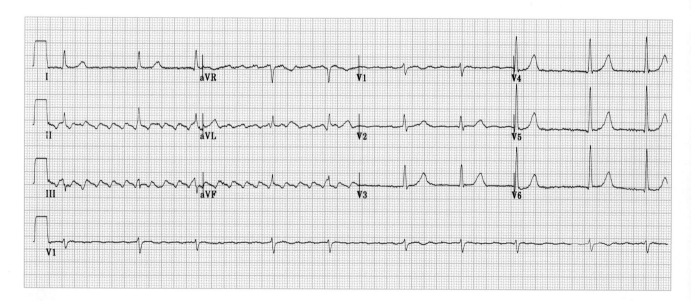

36

1. Rate: _____   2. Rhythm: _____   3. P wave: _____
4. PR Interval: _____   5. QRS complex: _____   +1. ST elevation: _____
+2. ST depression: _____   +3. Pathologic Q waves: _____   Interpretation: _____

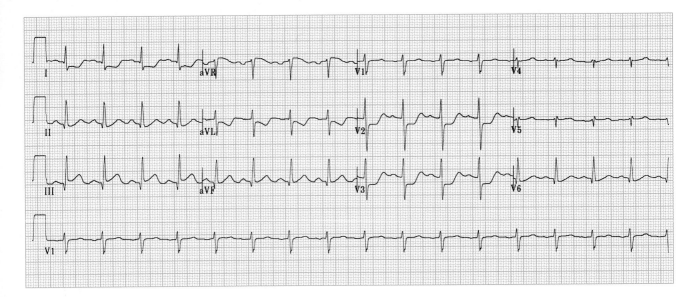

37

1. Rate: _____   2. Rhythm: _____   3. P wave: _____

4. PR Interval: _____   5. QRS complex: _____   +1. ST elevation: _____

+2. ST depression: _____   +3. Pathologic Q waves: _____   Interpretation: _____

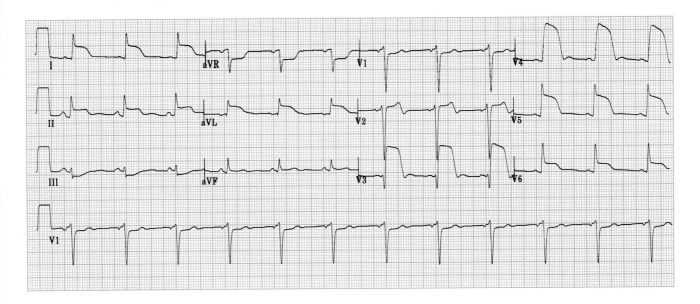

38

1. Rate: _____   2. Rhythm: _____   3. P wave: _____

4. PR Interval: _____   5. QRS complex: _____   +1. ST elevation: _____

+2. ST depression: _____   +3. Pathologic Q waves: _____   Interpretation: _____

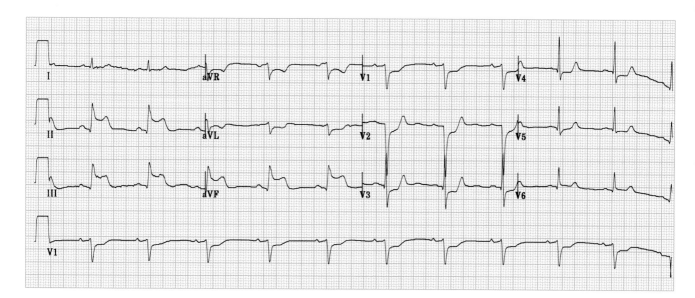

39

1. Rate: _____   2. Rhythm: _____   3. P wave: _____
4. PR Interval: _____   5. QRS complex: _____   +1. ST elevation: _____
+2. ST depression: _____   +3. Pathologic Q waves: _____   Interpretation: _____

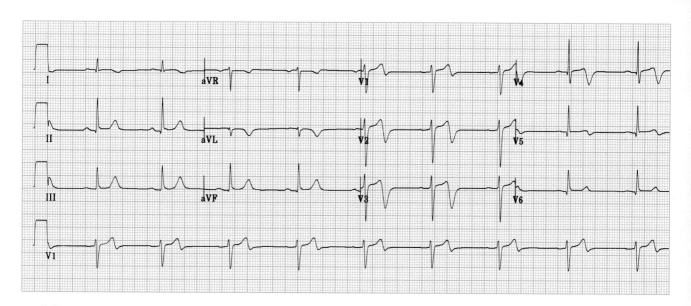

40

1. Rate: _____   2. Rhythm: _____   3. P wave: _____
4. PR Interval: _____   5. QRS complex: _____   +1. ST elevation: _____
+2. ST depression: _____   +3. Pathologic Q waves: _____   Interpretation: _____

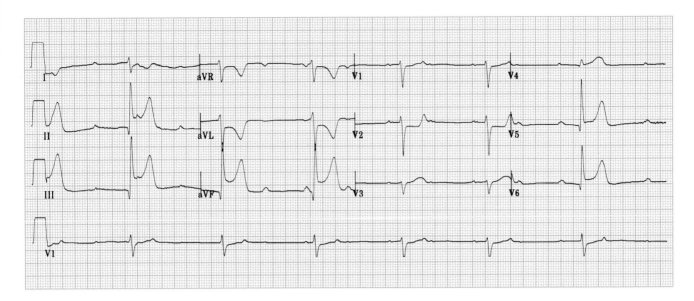

41

1. Rate: _____

2. Rhythm: _____

3. P wave: _____

4. PR Interval: _____

5. QRS complex: _____

+1. ST elevation: _____

+2. ST depression: _____

+3. Pathologic Q waves: _____

Interpretation: _____

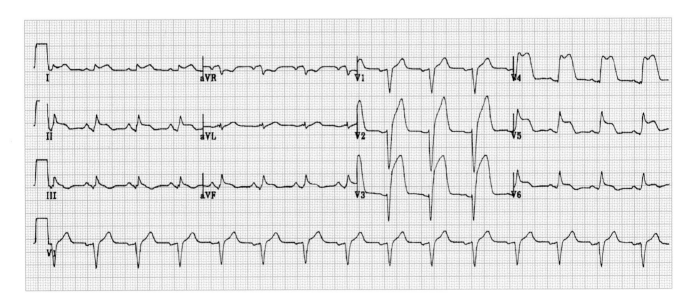

42

1. Rate: _____

2. Rhythm: _____

3. P wave: _____

4. PR Interval: _____

5. QRS complex: _____

+1. ST elevation: _____

+2. ST depression: _____

+3. Pathologic Q waves: _____

Interpretation: _____

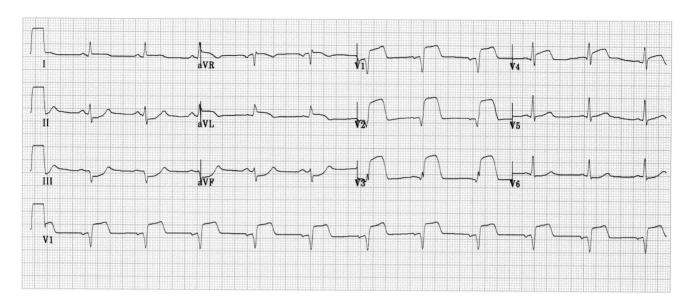

43

1. Rate: _____ 2. Rhythm: _____ 3. P wave: _____
4. PR Interval: _____ 5. QRS complex: _____ +1. ST elevation: _____
+2. ST depression: _____ +3. Pathologic Q waves: _____ Interpretation: _____

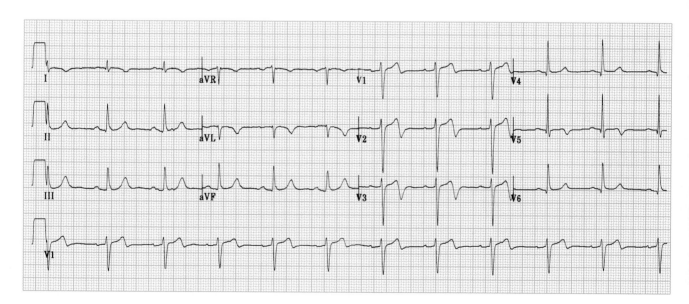

44

1. Rate: _____ 2. Rhythm: _____ 3. P wave: _____
4. PR Interval: _____ 5. QRS complex: _____ +1. ST elevation: _____
+2. ST depression: _____ +3. Pathologic Q waves: _____ Interpretation: _____

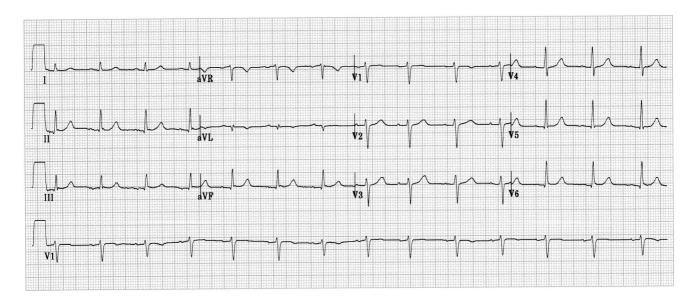

45

1. Rate: _____
4. PR Interval: _____
+2. ST depression: _____

2. Rhythm: _____
5. QRS complex: _____
+3. Pathologic Q waves: _____

3. P wave: _____
+1. ST elevation: _____
Interpretation: _____

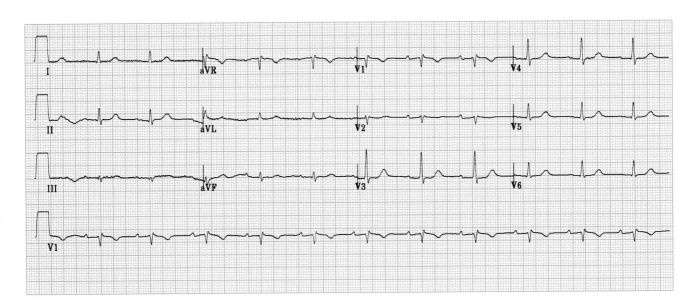

46

1. Rate: _____
4. PR Interval: _____
+2. ST depression: _____

2. Rhythm: _____
5. QRS complex: _____
+3. Pathologic Q waves: _____

3. P wave: _____
+1. ST elevation: _____
Interpretation: _____

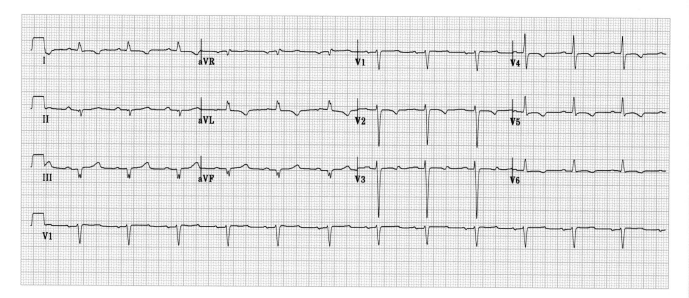

47

1. Rate: _____
4. PR Interval: _____
+2. ST depression: _____

2. Rhythm: _____
5. QRS complex: _____
+3. Pathologic Q waves: _____

3. P wave: _____
+1. ST elevation: _____
Interpretation: _____

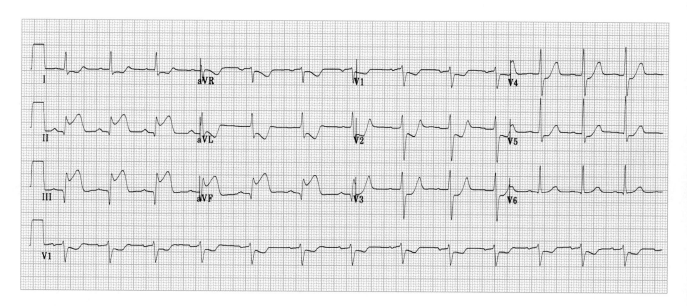

48

1. Rate: _____
4. PR Interval: _____
+2. ST depression: _____

2. Rhythm: _____
5. QRS complex: _____
+3. Pathologic Q waves: _____

3. P wave: _____
+1. ST elevation: _____
Interpretation: _____

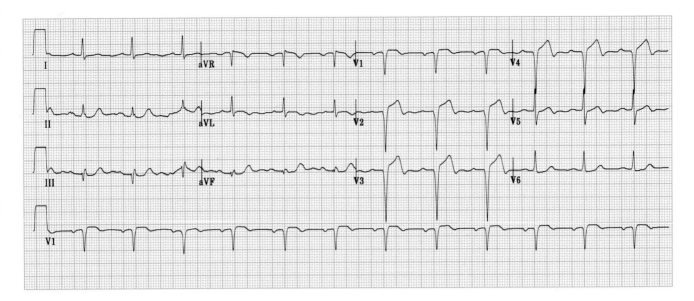

49

1. Rate: _____
4. PR Interval: _____
+2. ST depression: _____

2. Rhythm: _____
5. QRS complex: _____
+3. Pathologic Q waves: _____

3. P wave: _____
+1. ST elevation: _____
Interpretation: _____

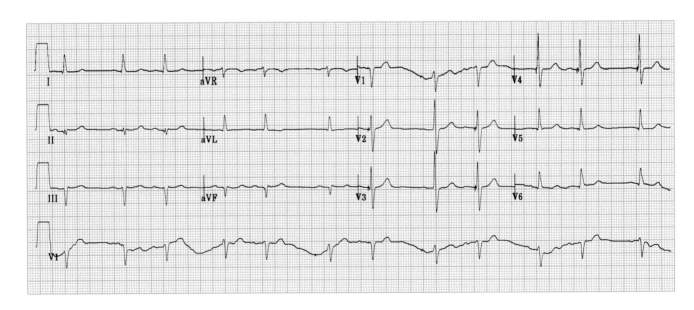

50

1. Rate: _____
4. PR Interval: _____
+2. ST depression: _____

2. Rhythm: _____
5. QRS complex: _____
+3. Pathologic Q waves: _____

3. P wave: _____
+1. ST elevation: _____
Interpretation: _____

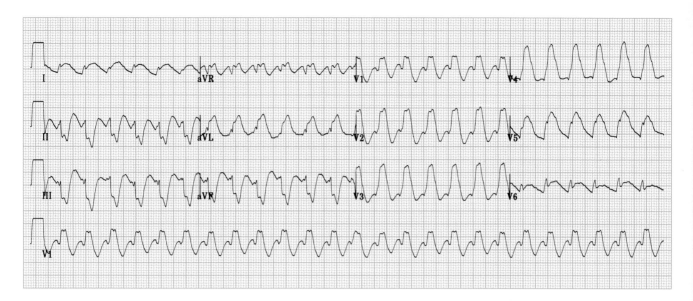

51

1. Rate: _____   2. Rhythm: _____   3. P wave: _____
4. PR Interval: _____   5. QRS complex: _____   +1. ST elevation: _____
+2. ST depression: _____   +3. Pathologic Q waves: _____   Interpretation: _____

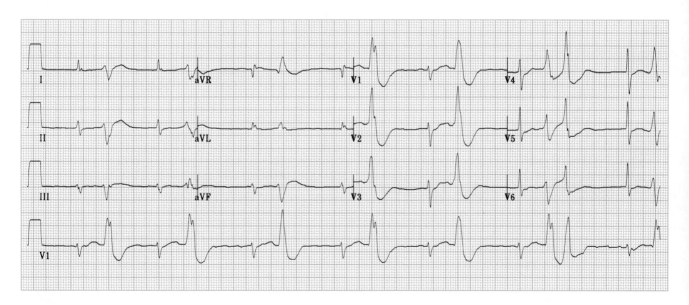

52

1. Rate: _____   2. Rhythm: _____   3. P wave: _____
4. PR Interval: _____   5. QRS complex: _____   +1. ST elevation: _____
+2. ST depression: _____   +3. Pathologic Q waves: _____   Interpretation: _____

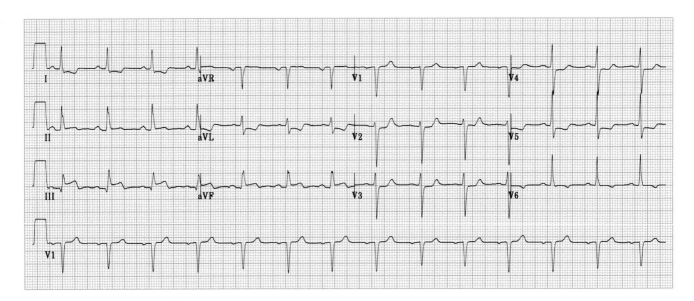

53

1. Rate: _____

4. PR Interval: _____

+2. ST depression: _____

2. Rhythm: _____

5. QRS complex: _____

+3. Pathologic Q waves: _____

3. P wave: _____

+1. ST elevation: _____

Interpretation: _____

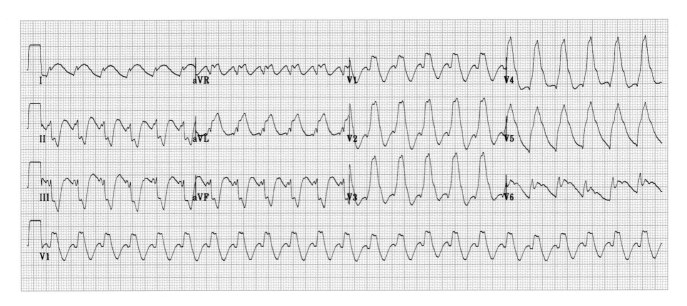

54

1. Rate: _____

4. PR Interval: _____

+2. ST depression: _____

2. Rhythm: _____

5. QRS complex: _____

+3. Pathologic Q waves: _____

3. P wave: _____

+1. ST elevation: _____

Interpretation: _____

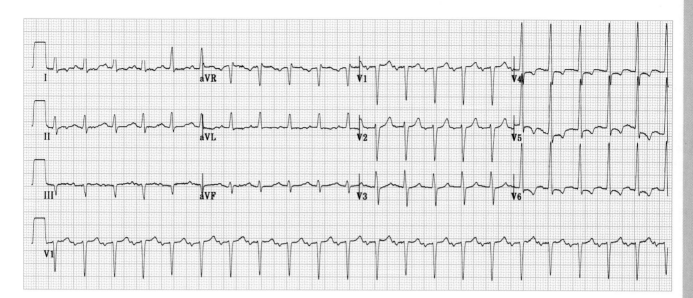

55

1. Rate: _____
4. PR Interval: _____
+2. ST depression: _____

2. Rhythm: _____
5. QRS complex: _____
+3. Pathologic Q waves: _____

3. P wave: _____
+1. ST elevation: _____
Interpretation: _____

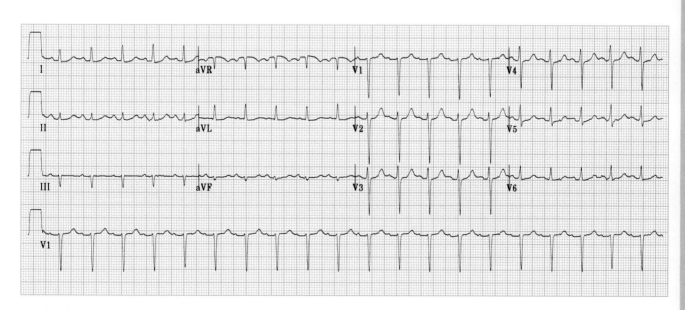

56

1. Rate: _____
4. PR Interval: _____
+2. ST depression: _____

2. Rhythm: _____
5. QRS complex: _____
+3. Pathologic Q waves: _____

3. P wave: _____
+1. ST elevation: _____
Interpretation: _____

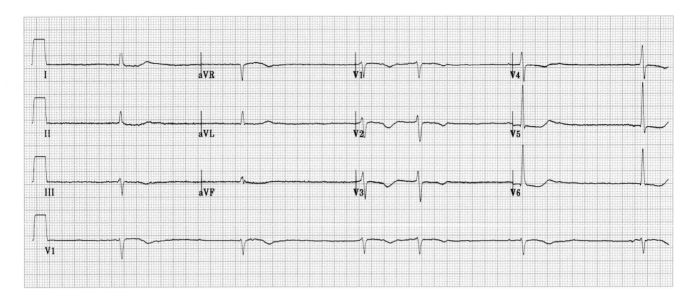

57

1. Rate: _____ 2. Rhythm: _____ 3. P wave: _____
4. PR Interval: _____ 5. QRS complex: _____ +1. ST elevation: _____
+2. ST depression: _____ +3. Pathologic Q waves: _____ Interpretation: _____

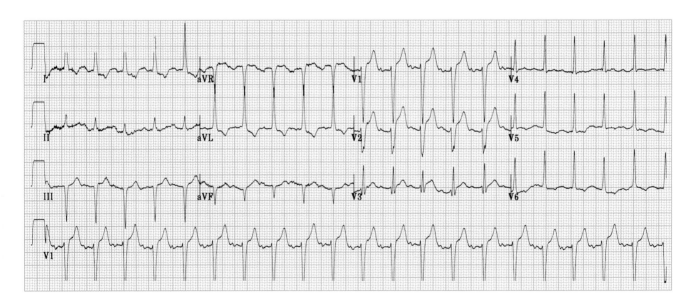

58

1. Rate: _____ 2. Rhythm: _____ 3. P wave: _____
4. PR Interval: _____ 5. QRS complex: _____ +1. ST elevation: _____
+2. ST depression: _____ +3. Pathologic Q waves: _____ Interpretation: _____

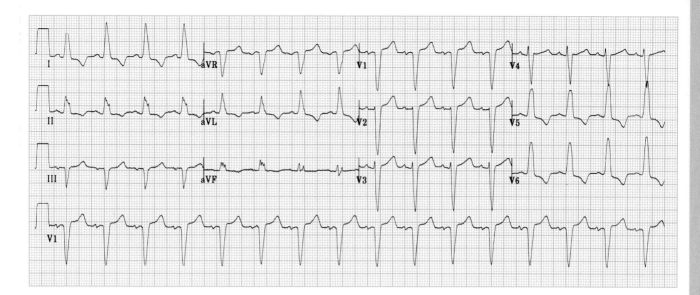

59

1. Rate: _____
2. Rhythm: _____
3. P wave: _____
4. PR Interval: _____
5. QRS complex: _____
+1. ST elevation: _____
+2. ST depression: _____
+3. Pathologic Q waves: _____
Interpretation: _____

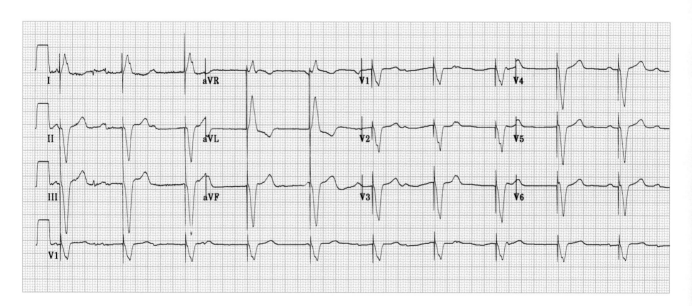

60

1. Rate: _____
2. Rhythm: _____
3. P wave: _____
4. PR Interval: _____
5. QRS complex: _____
+1. ST elevation: _____
+2. ST depression: _____
+3. Pathologic Q waves: _____
Interpretation: _____

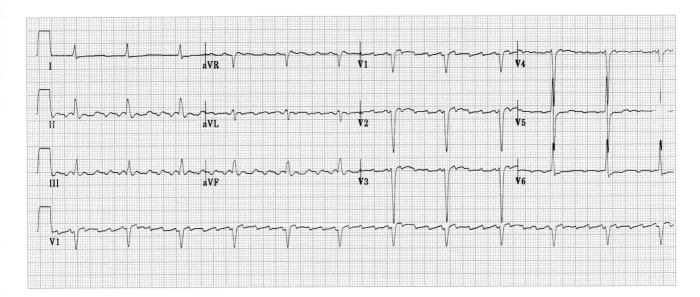

61

1. Rate: _____
4. PR Interval: _____
+2. ST depression: _____

2. Rhythm: _____
5. QRS complex: _____
+3. Pathologic Q waves: _____

3. P wave: _____
+1. ST elevation: _____
Interpretation: _____

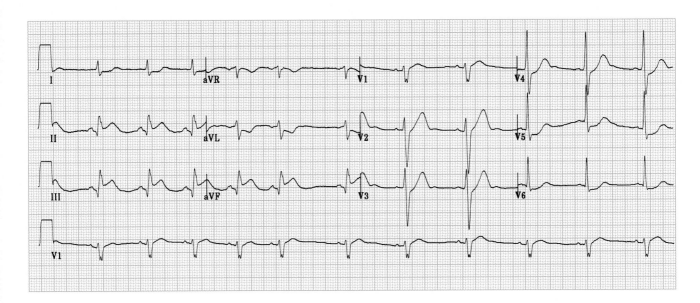

62

1. Rate: _____
4. PR Interval: _____
+2. ST depression: _____

2. Rhythm: _____
5. QRS complex: _____
+3. Pathologic Q waves: _____

3. P wave: _____
+1. ST elevation: _____
Interpretation: _____

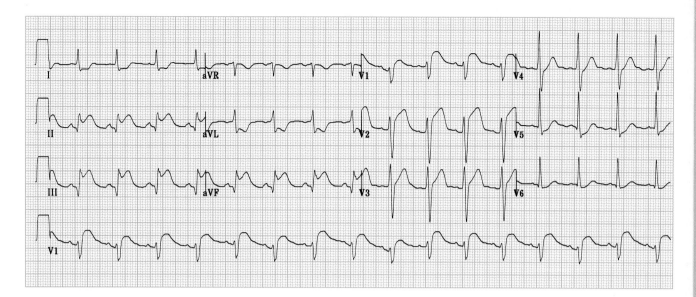

63

1. Rate: _____   2. Rhythm: _____   3. P wave: _____
4. PR Interval: _____   5. QRS complex: _____   +1. ST elevation: _____
+2. ST depression: _____   +3. Pathologic Q waves: _____   Interpretation: _____

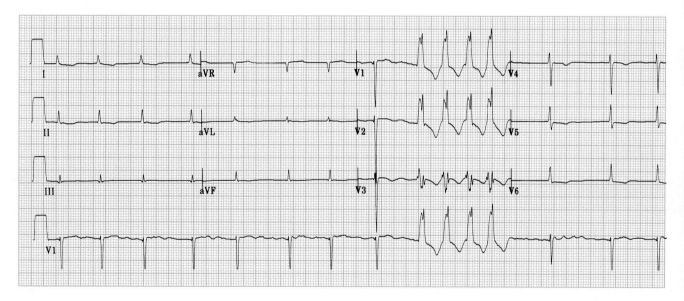

64

1. Rate: _____   2. Rhythm: _____   3. P wave: _____
4. PR Interval: _____   5. QRS complex: _____   +1. ST elevation: _____
+2. ST depression: _____   +3. Pathologic Q waves: _____   Interpretation: _____

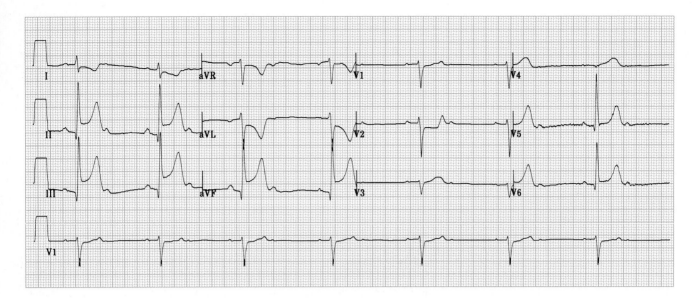

65

1. Rate: _____
4. PR Interval: _____
+2. ST depression: _____

2. Rhythm: _____
5. QRS complex: _____
+3. Pathologic Q waves: _____

3. P wave: _____
+1. ST elevation: _____
Interpretation: _____

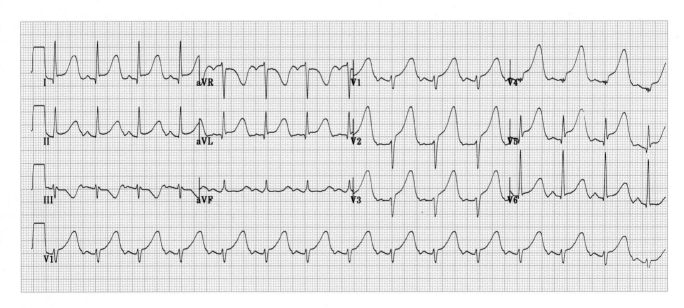

66

1. Rate: _____
4. PR Interval: _____
+2. ST depression: _____

2. Rhythm: _____
5. QRS complex: _____
+3. Pathologic Q waves: _____

3. P wave: _____
+1. ST elevation: _____
Interpretation: _____

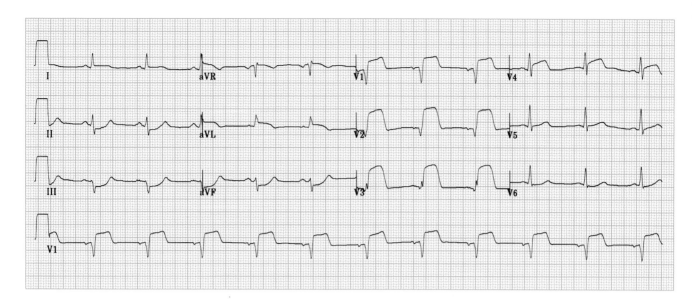

67

1. Rate: _____
2. Rhythm: _____
3. P wave: _____
4. PR Interval: _____
5. QRS complex: _____
+1. ST elevation: _____
+2. ST depression: _____
+3. Pathologic Q waves: _____
Interpretation: _____

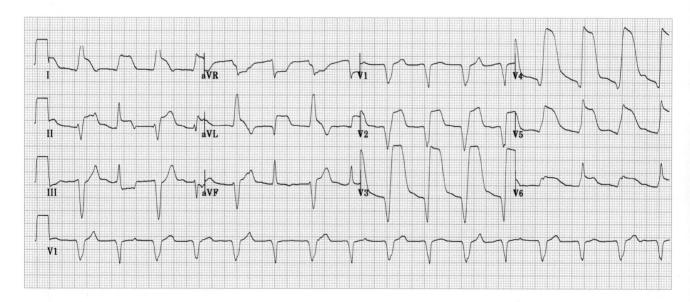

68

1. Rate: _____
2. Rhythm: _____
3. P wave: _____
4. PR Interval: _____
5. QRS complex: _____
+1. ST elevation: _____
+2. ST depression: _____
+3. Pathologic Q waves: _____
Interpretation: _____

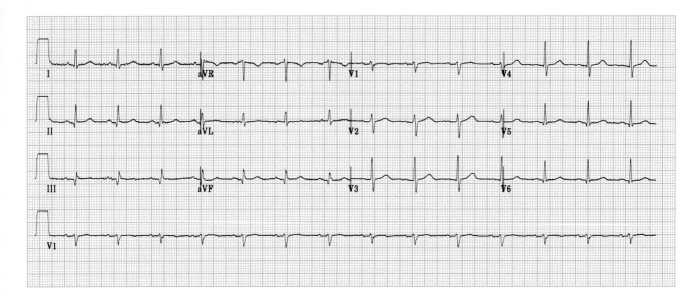

69

1. Rate: _____   2. Rhythm: _____   3. P wave: _____
4. PR Interval: _____   5. QRS complex: _____   +1. ST elevation: _____
+2. ST depression: _____   +3. Pathologic Q waves: _____   Interpretation: _____

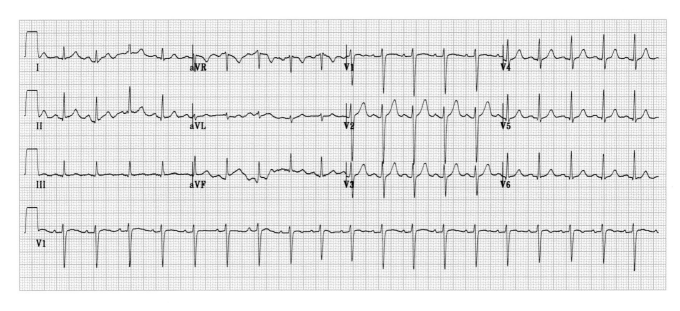

70

1. Rate: _____   2. Rhythm: _____   3. P wave: _____
4. PR Interval: _____   5. QRS complex: _____   +1. ST elevation: _____
+2. ST depression: _____   +3. Pathologic Q waves: _____   Interpretation: _____

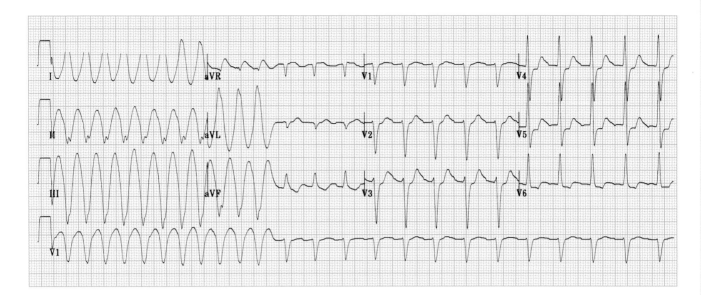

71

1. Rate: _____   2. Rhythm: _____   3. P wave: _____
4. PR Interval: _____   5. QRS complex: _____   +1. ST elevation: _____
+2. ST depression: _____   +3. Pathologic Q waves: _____   Interpretation: _____

72

1. Rate: _____   2. Rhythm: _____   3. P wave: _____
4. PR Interval: _____   5. QRS complex: _____   +1. ST elevation: _____
+2. ST depression: _____   +3. Pathologic Q waves: _____   Interpretation: _____

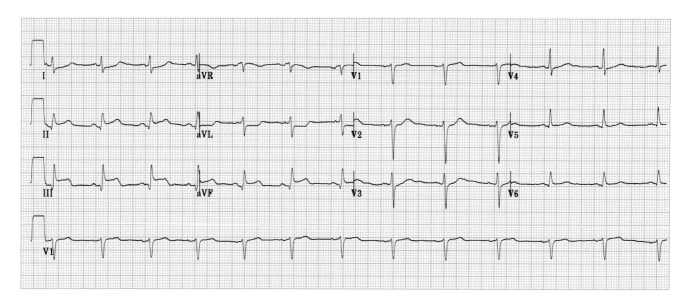

73

1. Rate: _____
4. PR Interval: _____
+2. ST depression: _____

2. Rhythm: _____
5. QRS complex: _____
+3. Pathologic Q waves: _____

3. P wave: _____
+1. ST elevation: _____
Interpretation: _____

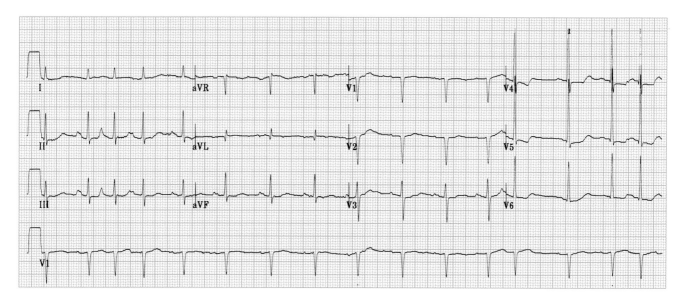

74

1. Rate: _____
4. PR Interval: _____
+2. ST depression: _____

2. Rhythm: _____
5. QRS complex: _____
+3. Pathologic Q waves: _____

3. P wave: _____
+1. ST elevation: _____
Interpretation: _____

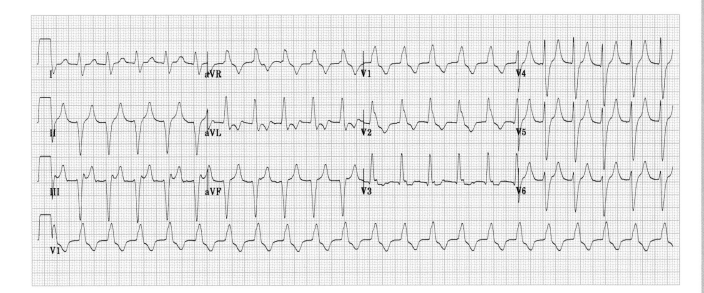

75

1. Rate: _____
4. PR Interval: _____
+2. ST depression: _____

2. Rhythm: _____
5. QRS complex: _____
+3. Pathologic Q waves: _____

3. P wave: _____
+1. ST elevation: _____
Interpretation: _____

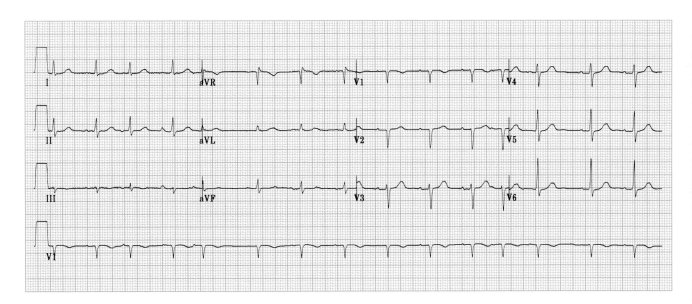

76

1. Rate: _____
4. PR Interval: _____
+2. ST depression: _____

2. Rhythm: _____
5. QRS complex: _____
+3. Pathologic Q waves: _____

3. P wave: _____
+1. ST elevation: _____
Interpretation: _____

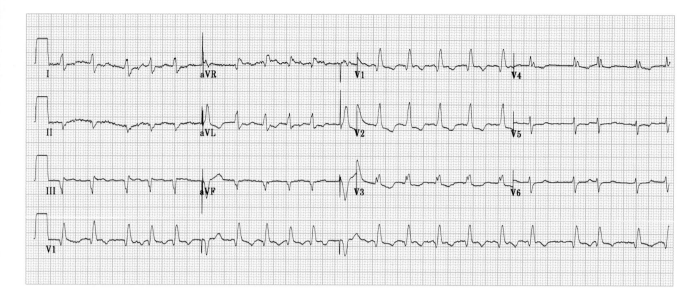

77

1. Rate: _____   2. Rhythm: _____   3. P wave: _____
4. PR Interval: _____   5. QRS complex: _____   +1. ST elevation: _____
+2. ST depression: _____   +3. Pathologic Q waves: _____   Interpretation: _____

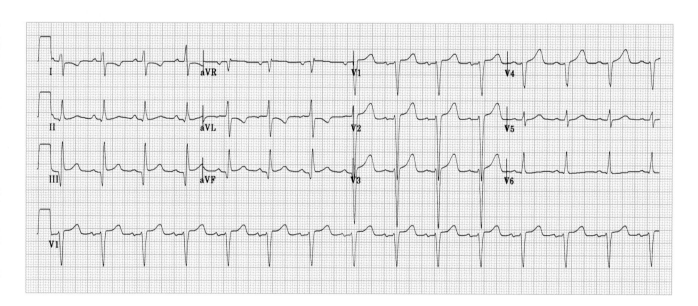

78

1. Rate: _____   2. Rhythm: _____   3. P wave: _____
4. PR Interval: _____   5. QRS complex: _____   +1. ST elevation: _____
+2. ST depression: _____   +3. Pathologic Q waves: _____   Interpretation: _____

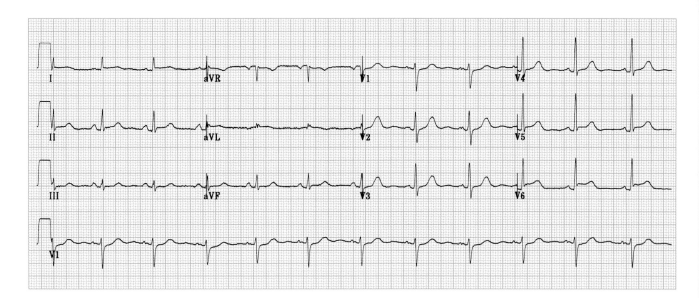

79

1. Rate: _____
2. Rhythm: _____
3. P wave: _____
4. PR Interval: _____
5. QRS complex: _____
+1. ST elevation: _____
+2. ST depression: _____
+3. Pathologic Q waves: _____
Interpretation: _____

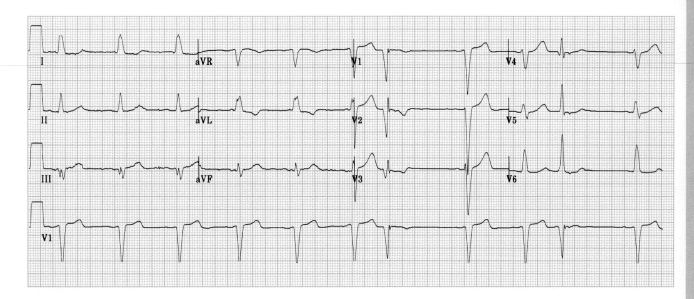

80

1. Rate: _____
2. Rhythm: _____
3. P wave: _____
4. PR Interval: _____
5. QRS complex: _____
+1. ST elevation: _____
+2. ST depression: _____
+3. Pathologic Q waves: _____
Interpretation: _____

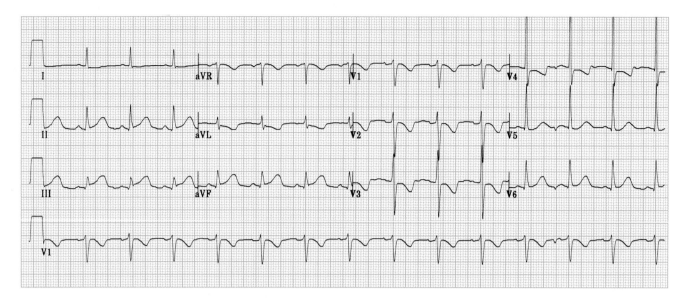

81

1. Rate: _____   2. Rhythm: _____   3. P wave: _____

4. PR Interval: _____   5. QRS complex: _____   +1. ST elevation: _____

+2. ST depression: _____   +3. Pathologic Q waves: _____   Interpretation: _____

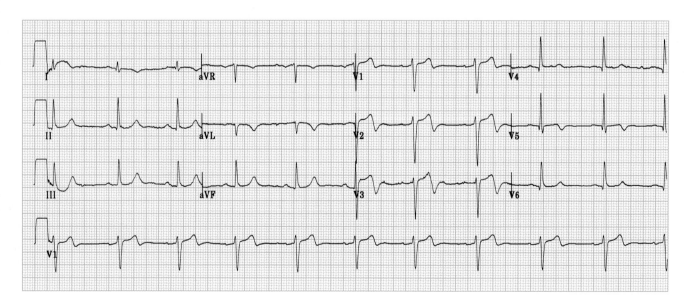

82

1. Rate: _____   2. Rhythm: _____   3. P wave: _____

4. PR Interval: _____   5. QRS complex: _____   +1. ST elevation: _____

+2. ST depression: _____   +3. Pathologic Q waves: _____   Interpretation: _____

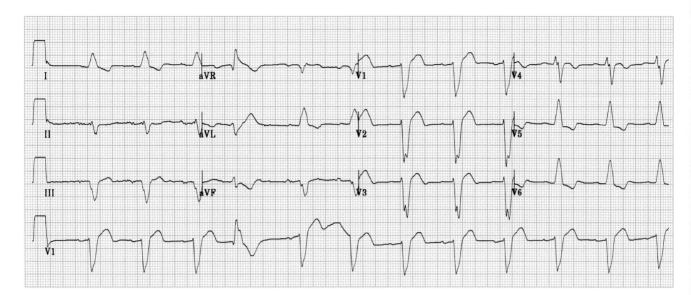

83

1. Rate: _____   2. Rhythm: _____   3. P wave: _____
4. PR Interval: _____   5. QRS complex: _____   +1. ST elevation: _____
+2. ST depression: _____   +3. Pathologic Q waves: _____   Interpretation: _____

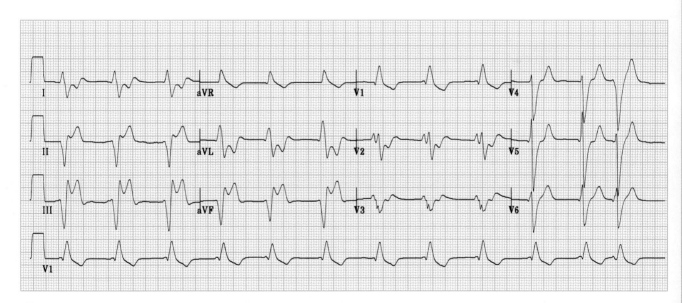

84

1. Rate: _____   2. Rhythm: _____   3. P wave: _____
4. PR Interval: _____   5. QRS complex: _____   +1. ST elevation: _____
+2. ST depression: _____   +3. Pathologic Q waves: _____   Interpretation: _____

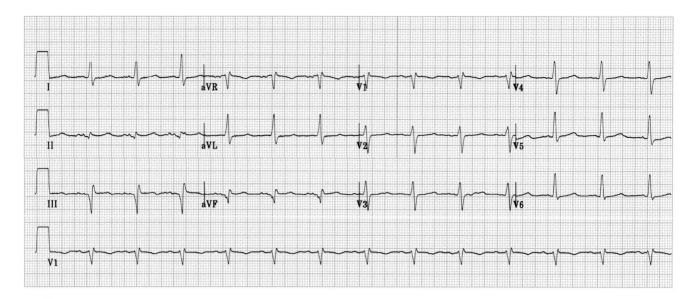

85

1. Rate: _____   2. Rhythm: _____   3. P wave: _____
4. PR Interval: _____   5. QRS complex: _____   +1. ST elevation: _____
+2. ST depression: _____   +3. Pathologic Q waves: _____   Interpretation: _____

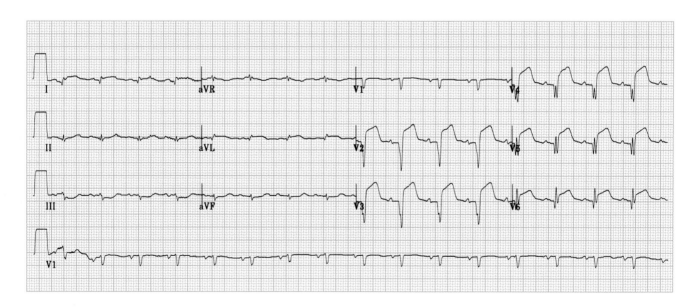

86

1. Rate: _____   2. Rhythm: _____   3. P wave: _____
4. PR Interval: _____   5. QRS complex: _____   +1. ST elevation: _____
+2. ST depression: _____   +3. Pathologic Q waves: _____   Interpretation: _____

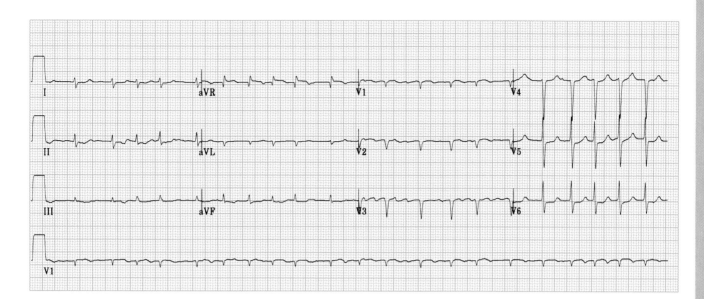

87

1. Rate: _____
4. PR Interval: _____
+2. ST depression: _____

2. Rhythm: _____
5. QRS complex: _____
+3. Pathologic Q waves: _____

3. P wave: _____
+1. ST elevation: _____
Interpretation: _____

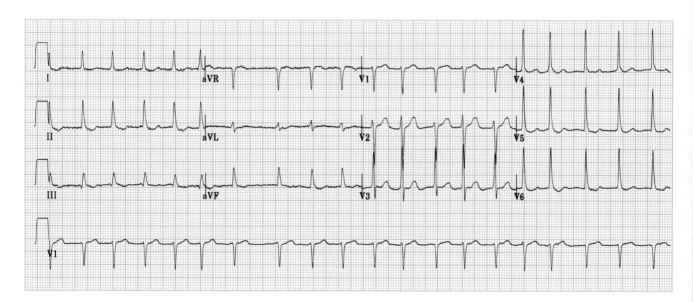

88

1. Rate: _____
4. PR Interval: _____
+2. ST depression: _____

2. Rhythm: _____
5. QRS complex: _____
+3. Pathologic Q waves: _____

3. P wave: _____
+1. ST elevation: _____
Interpretation: _____

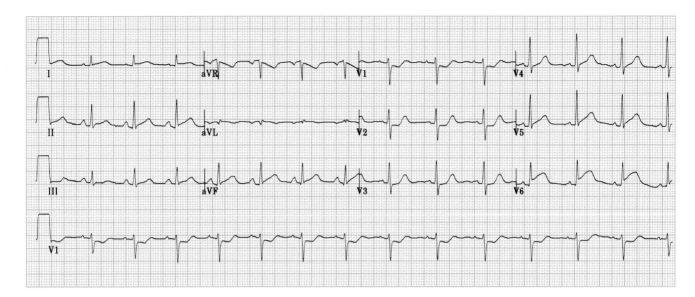

89

1. Rate: _____
2. Rhythm: _____
3. P wave: _____
4. PR Interval: _____
5. QRS complex: _____
+1. ST elevation: _____
+2. ST depression: _____
+3. Pathologic Q waves: _____
Interpretation: _____

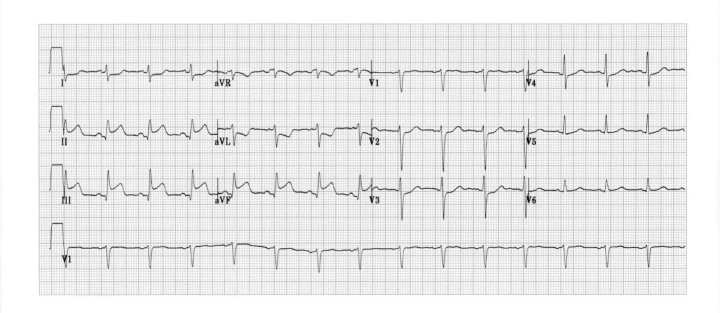

90

1. Rate: _____
2. Rhythm: _____
3. P wave: _____
4. PR Interval: _____
5. QRS complex: _____
+1. ST elevation: _____
+2. ST depression: _____
+3. Pathologic Q waves: _____
Interpretation: _____

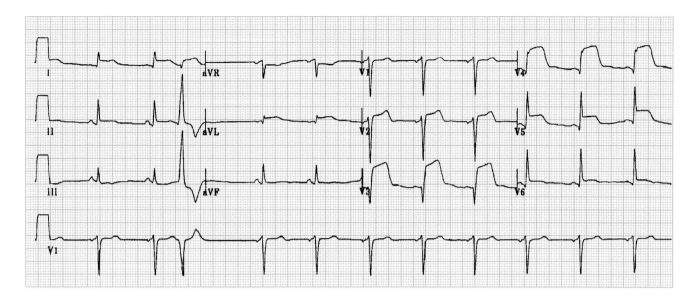

91

1. Rate: _____
2. Rhythm: _____
3. P wave: _____
4. PR Interval: _____
5. QRS complex: _____
+1. ST elevation: _____
+2. ST depression: _____
+3. Pathologic Q waves: _____
Interpretation: _____

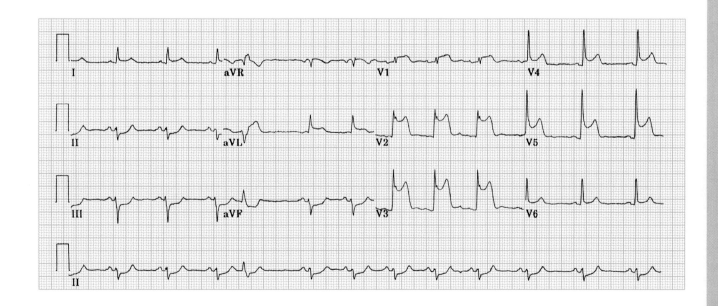

92

1. Rate: _____
2. Rhythm: _____
3. P wave: _____
4. PR Interval: _____
5. QRS complex: _____
+1. ST elevation: _____
+2. ST depression: _____
+3. Pathologic Q waves: _____
Interpretation: _____

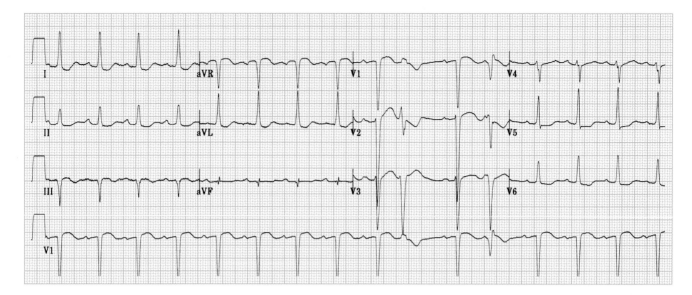

93

1. Rate: _____
2. Rhythm: _____
3. P wave: _____
4. PR Interval: _____
5. QRS complex: _____
+1. ST elevation: _____
+2. ST depression: _____
+3. Pathologic Q waves: _____
Interpretation: _____

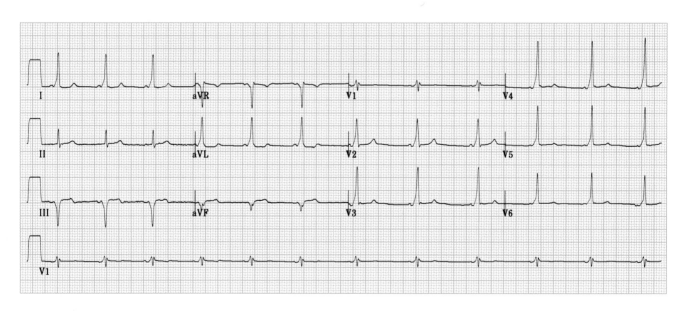

94

1. Rate: _____
2. Rhythm: _____
3. P wave: _____
4. PR Interval: _____
5. QRS complex: _____
+1. ST elevation: _____
+2. ST depression: _____
+3. Pathologic Q waves: _____
Interpretation: _____

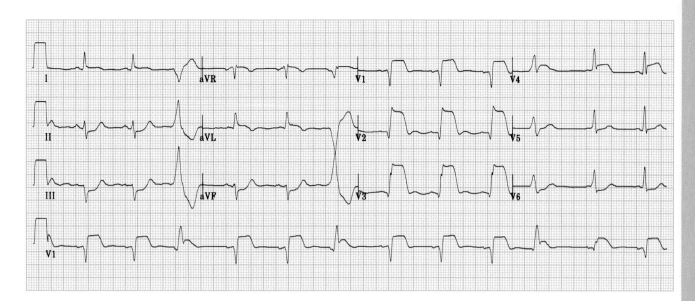

95

1. Rate: _____   2. Rhythm: _____   3. P wave: _____
4. PR Interval: _____   5. QRS complex: _____   +1. ST elevation: _____
+2. ST depression: _____   +3. Pathologic Q waves: _____   Interpretation: _____

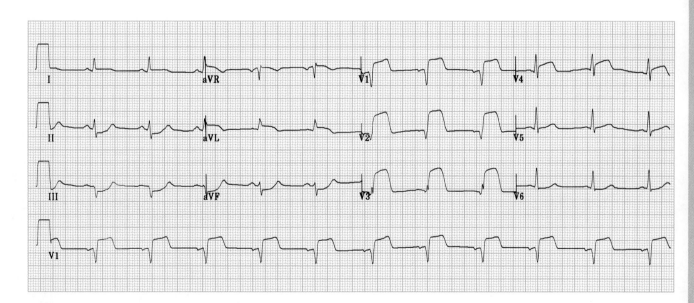

96

1. Rate: _____   2. Rhythm: _____   3. P wave: _____
4. PR Interval: _____   5. QRS complex: _____   +1. ST elevation: _____
+2. ST depression: _____   +3. Pathologic Q waves: _____   Interpretation: _____

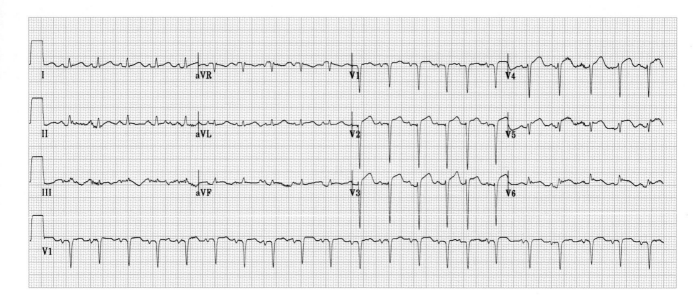

97

1. Rate: _____
2. Rhythm: _____
3. P wave: _____
4. PR Interval: _____
5. QRS complex: _____
+1. ST elevation: _____
+2. ST depression: _____
+3. Pathologic Q waves: _____
Interpretation: _____

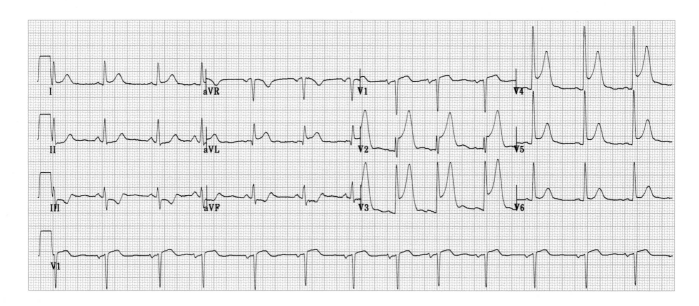

98

1. Rate: _____
2. Rhythm: _____
3. P wave: _____
4. PR Interval: _____
5. QRS complex: _____
+1. ST elevation: _____
+2. ST depression: _____
+3. Pathologic Q waves: _____
Interpretation: _____

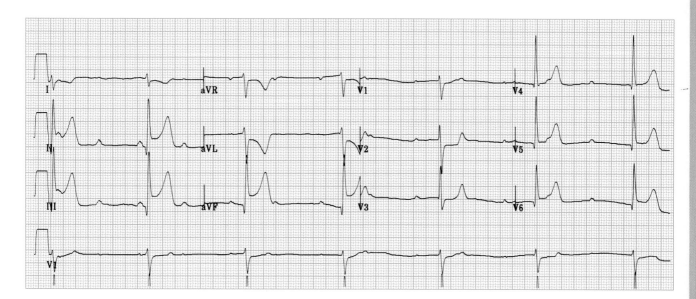

99

1. Rate: _____
2. Rhythm: _____
3. P wave: _____
4. PR Interval: _____
5. QRS complex: _____
+1. ST elevation: _____
+2. ST depression: _____
+3. Pathologic Q waves: _____
Interpretation: _____

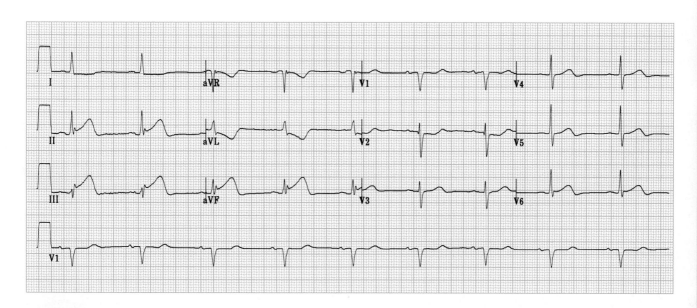

100

1. Rate: _____
2. Rhythm: _____
3. P wave: _____
4. PR Interval: _____
5. QRS complex: _____
+1. ST elevation: _____
+2. ST depression: _____
+3. Pathologic Q waves: _____
Interpretation: _____

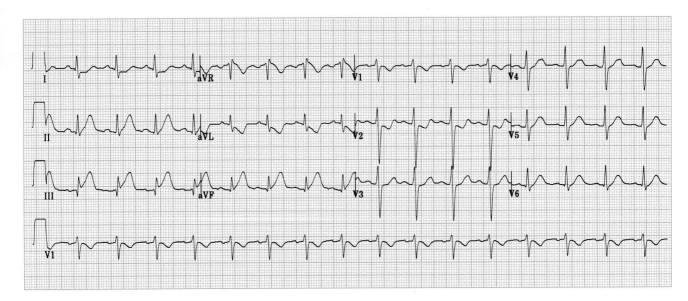

101

1. Rate: _____   2. Rhythm: _____   3. P wave: _____
4. PR Interval: _____   5. QRS complex: _____   +1. ST elevation: _____
+2. ST depression: _____   +3. Pathologic Q waves: _____   Interpretation: _____

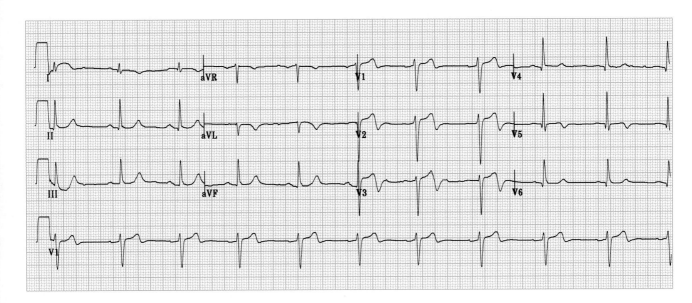

102

1. Rate: _____   2. Rhythm: _____   3. P wave: _____
4. PR Interval: _____   5. QRS complex: _____   +1. ST elevation: _____
+2. ST depression: _____   +3. Pathologic Q waves: _____   Interpretation: _____

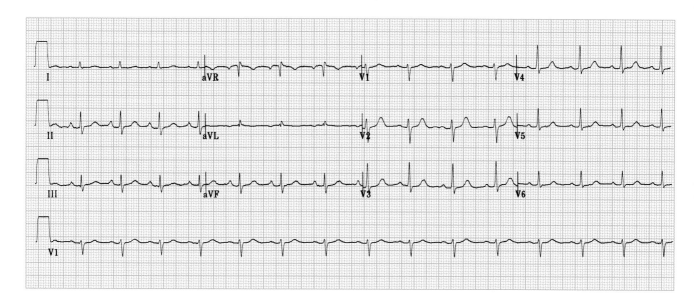

103

1. Rate: _____
4. PR Interval: _____
+2. ST depression: _____

2. Rhythm: _____
5. QRS complex: _____
+3. Pathologic Q waves: _____

3. P wave: _____
+1. ST elevation: _____
Interpretation: _____

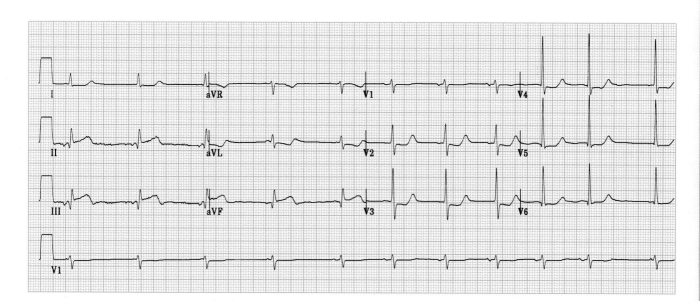

104

1. Rate: _____
4. PR Interval: _____
+2. ST depression: _____

2. Rhythm: _____
5. QRS complex: _____
+3. Pathologic Q waves: _____

3. P wave: _____
+1. ST elevation: _____
Interpretation: _____

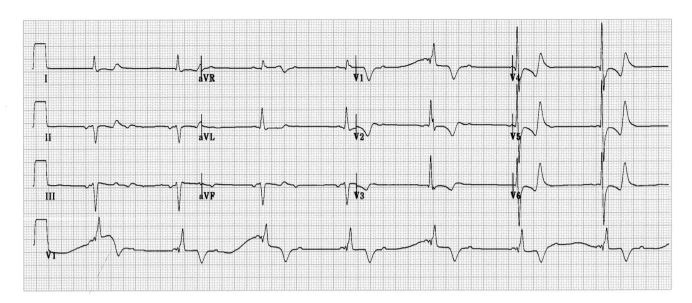

105

1. Rate: _____
2. Rhythm: _____
3. P wave: _____
4. PR Interval: _____
5. QRS complex: _____
+1. ST elevation: _____
+2. ST depression: _____
+3. Pathologic Q waves: _____
Interpretation: _____

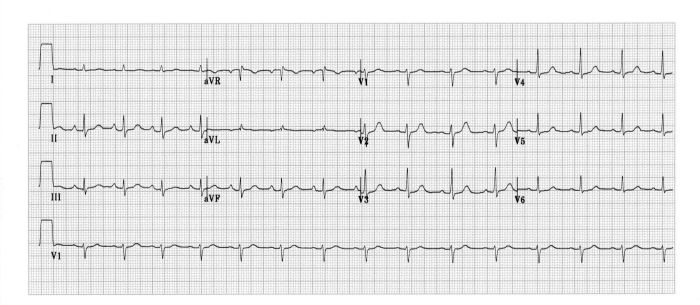

106

1. Rate: _____
2. Rhythm: _____
3. P wave: _____
4. PR Interval: _____
5. QRS complex: _____
+1. ST elevation: _____
+2. ST depression: _____
+3. Pathologic Q waves: _____
Interpretation: _____

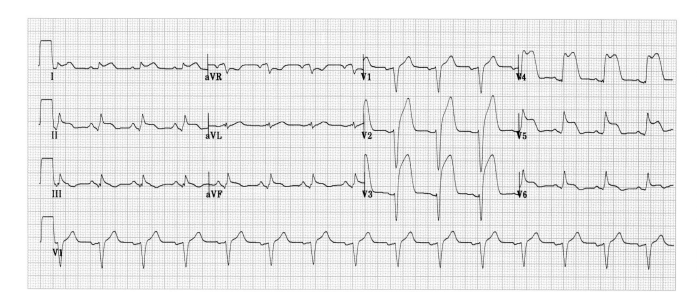

107

1. Rate: _____
4. PR Interval: _____
+2. ST depression: _____

2. Rhythm: _____
5. QRS complex: _____
+3. Pathologic Q waves: _____

3. P wave: _____
+1. ST elevation: _____
Interpretation: _____

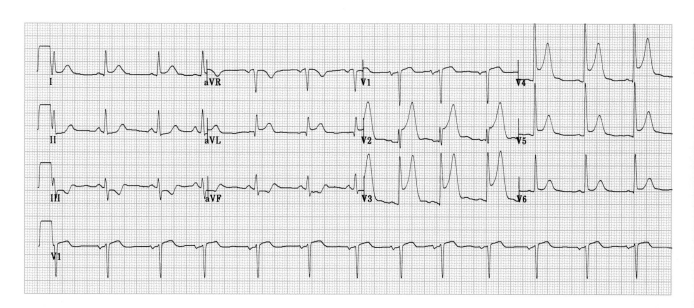

108

1. Rate: _____
4. PR Interval: _____
+2. ST depression: _____

2. Rhythm: _____
5. QRS complex: _____
+3. Pathologic Q waves: _____

3. P wave: _____
+1. ST elevation: _____
Interpretation: _____

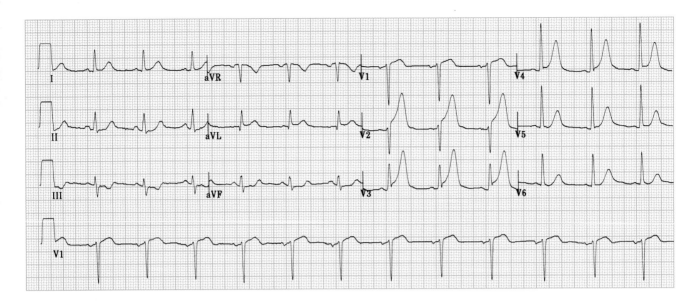

109

1. Rate: _____
4. PR Interval: _____
+2. ST depression: _____

2. Rhythm: _____
5. QRS complex: _____
+3. Pathologic Q waves: _____

3. P wave: _____
+1. ST elevation: _____
Interpretation: _____

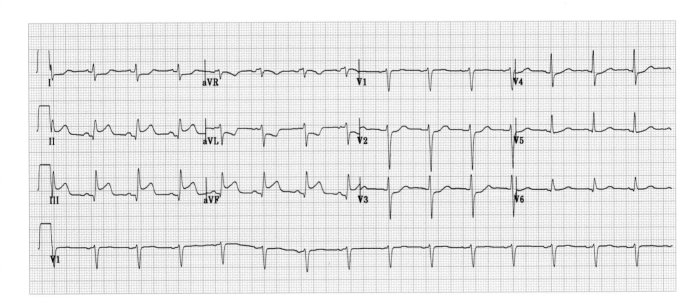

110

1. Rate: _____
4. PR Interval: _____
+2. ST depression: _____

2. Rhythm: _____
5. QRS complex: _____
+3. Pathologic Q waves: _____

3. P wave: _____
+1. ST elevation: _____
Interpretation: _____

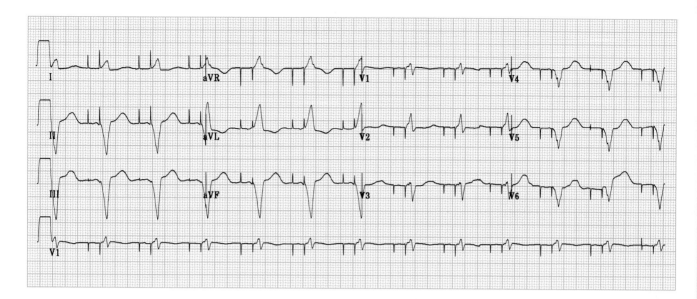

111

1. Rate: _____   2. Rhythm: _____   3. P wave: _____
4. PR Interval: _____   5. QRS complex: _____   +1. ST elevation: _____
+2. ST depression: _____   +3. Pathologic Q waves: _____   Interpretation: _____

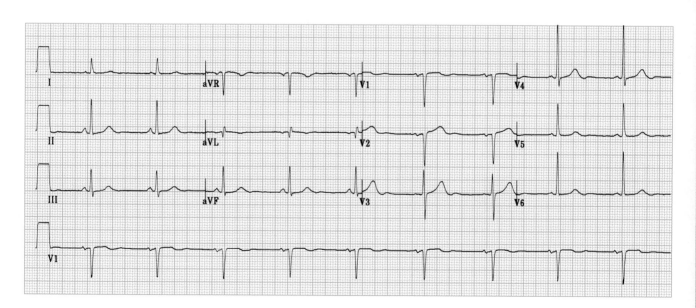

112

1. Rate: _____   2. Rhythm: _____   3. P wave: _____
4. PR Interval: _____   5. QRS complex: _____   +1. ST elevation: _____
+2. ST depression: _____   +3. Pathologic Q waves: _____   Interpretation: _____

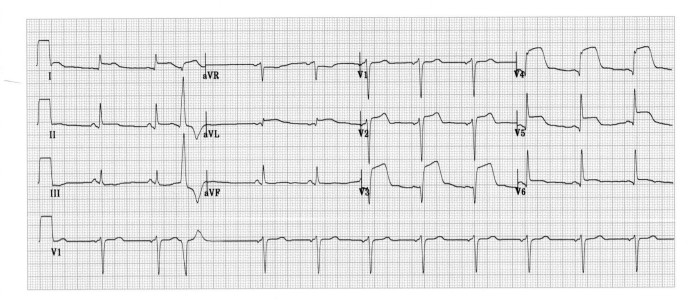

113

1. Rate: _____
2. Rhythm: _____
3. P wave: _____
4. PR Interval: _____
5. QRS complex: _____
+1. ST elevation: _____
+2. ST depression: _____
+3. Pathologic Q waves: _____
Interpretation: _____

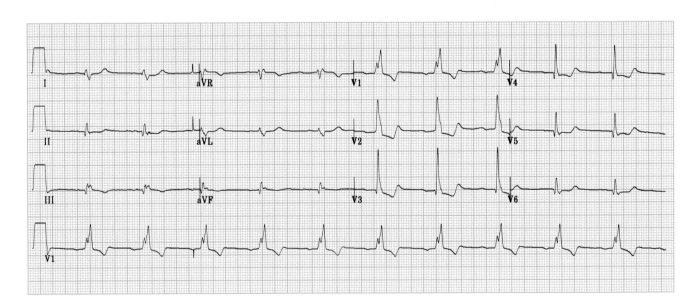

114

1. Rate: _____
2. Rhythm: _____
3. P wave: _____
4. PR Interval: _____
5. QRS complex: _____
+1. ST elevation: _____
+2. ST depression: _____
+3. Pathologic Q waves: _____
Interpretation: _____

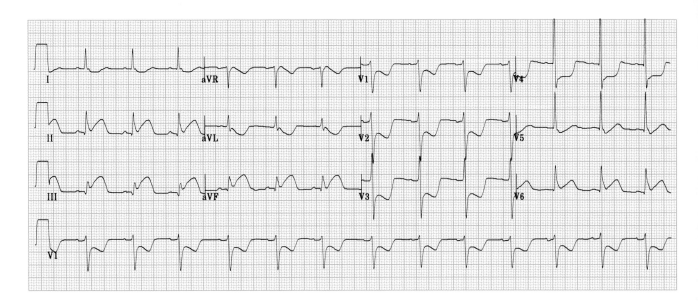

115

1. Rate: _____
2. Rhythm: _____
3. P wave: _____
4. PR Interval: _____
5. QRS complex: _____
+1. ST elevation: _____
+2. ST depression: _____
+3. Pathologic Q waves: _____
Interpretation: _____

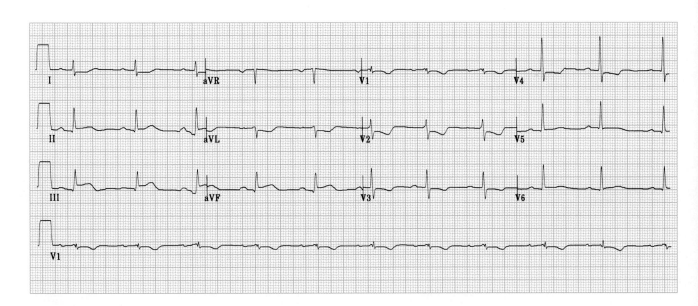

116

1. Rate: _____
2. Rhythm: _____
3. P wave: _____
4. PR Interval: _____
5. QRS complex: _____
+1. ST elevation: _____
+2. ST depression: _____
+3. Pathologic Q waves: _____
Interpretation: _____

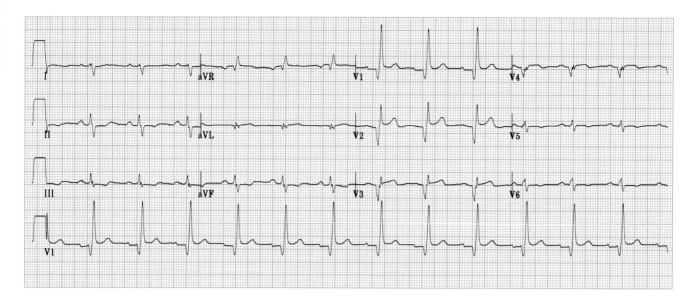

117

1. Rate: _____
2. Rhythm: _____
3. P wave: _____
4. PR Interval: _____
5. QRS complex: _____
+1. ST elevation: _____
+2. ST depression: _____
+3. Pathologic Q waves: _____
Interpretation: _____

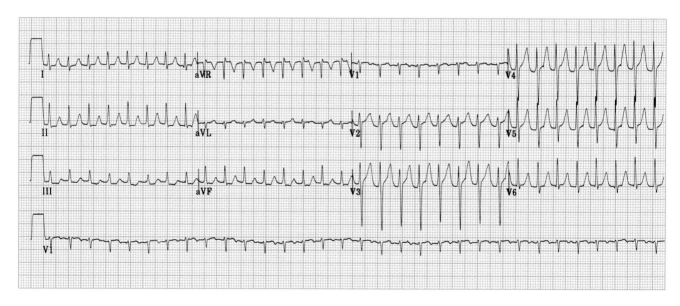

118

1. Rate: _____
2. Rhythm: _____
3. P wave: _____
4. PR Interval: _____
5. QRS complex: _____
+1. ST elevation: _____
+2. ST depression: _____
+3. Pathologic Q waves: _____
Interpretation: _____

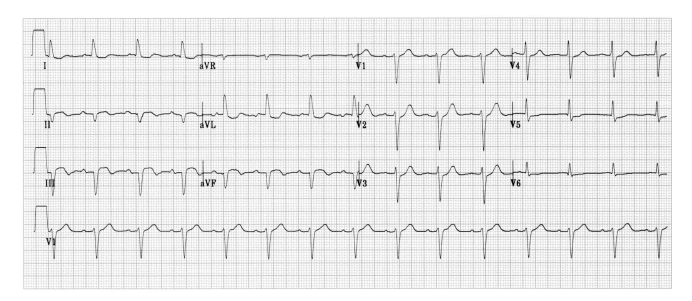

119

1. Rate: _____   2. Rhythm: _____   3. P wave: _____
4. PR Interval: _____   5. QRS complex: _____   +1. ST elevation: _____
+2. ST depression: _____   +3. Pathologic Q waves: _____   Interpretation: _____

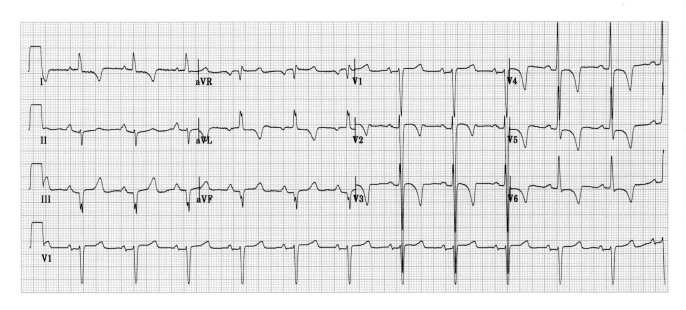

120

1. Rate: _____   2. Rhythm: _____   3. P wave: _____
4. PR Interval: _____   5. QRS complex: _____   +1. ST elevation: _____
+2. ST depression: _____   +3. Pathologic Q waves: _____   Interpretation: _____

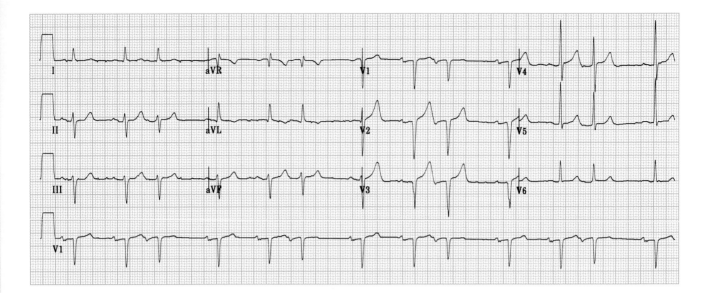

121

1. Rate: _____
4. PR Interval: _____
+2. ST depression: _____

2. Rhythm: _____
5. QRS complex: _____
+3. Pathologic Q waves: _____

3. P wave: _____
+1. ST elevation: _____
Interpretation: _____

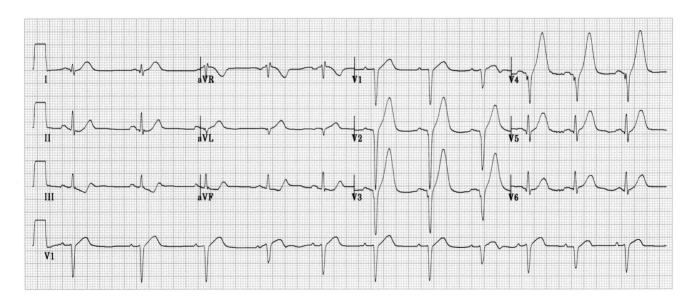

122

1. Rate: _____
4. PR Interval: _____
+2. ST depression: _____

2. Rhythm: _____
5. QRS complex: _____
+3. Pathologic Q waves: _____

3. P wave: _____
+1. ST elevation: _____
Interpretation: _____

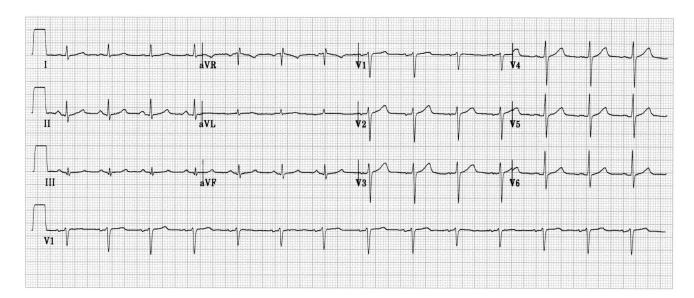

123

1. Rate: _____
4. PR Interval: _____
+2. ST depression: _____

2. Rhythm: _____
5. QRS complex: _____
+3. Pathologic Q waves: _____

3. P wave: _____
+1. ST elevation: _____
Interpretation: _____

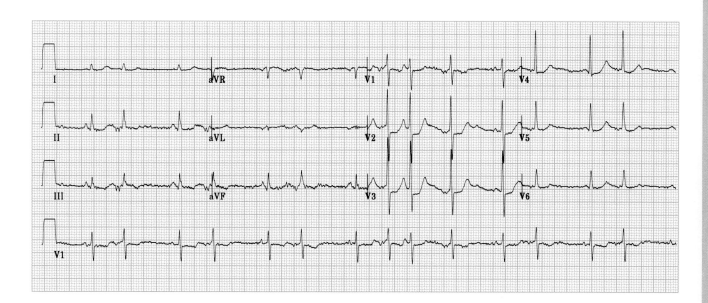

124

1. Rate: _____
4. PR Interval: _____
+2. ST depression: _____

2. Rhythm: _____
5. QRS complex: _____
+3. Pathologic Q waves: _____

3. P wave: _____
+1. ST elevation: _____
Interpretation: _____

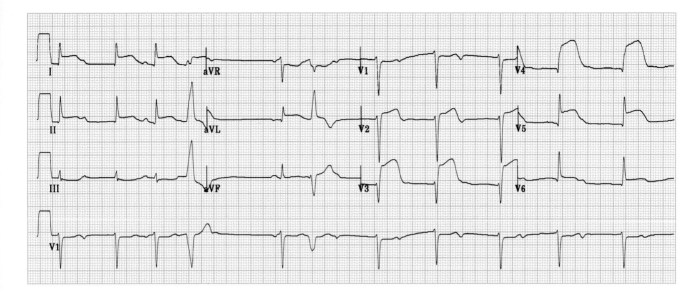

125

1. Rate: _____
4. PR Interval: _____
+2. ST depression: _____

2. Rhythm: _____
5. QRS complex: _____
+3. Pathologic Q waves: _____

3. P wave: _____
+1. ST elevation: _____
Interpretation: _____

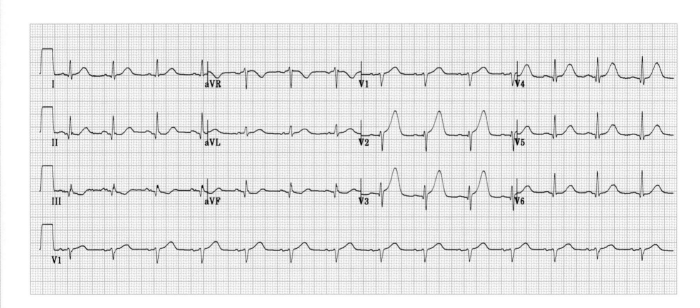

126

1. Rate: _____
4. PR Interval: _____
+2. ST depression: _____

2. Rhythm: _____
5. QRS complex: _____
+3. Pathologic Q waves: _____

3. P wave: _____
+1. ST elevation: _____
Interpretation: _____

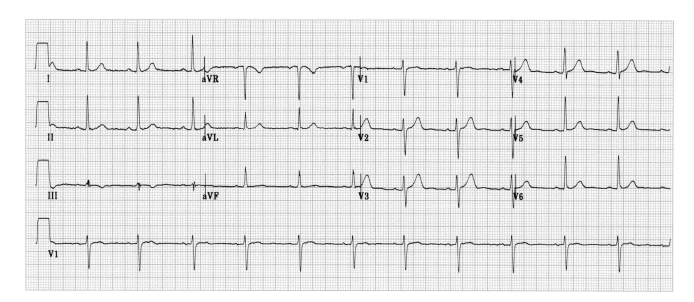

127

1. Rate: _____   2. Rhythm: _____   3. P wave: _____
4. PR Interval: _____   5. QRS complex: _____   +1. ST elevation: _____
+2. ST depression: _____   +3. Pathologic Q waves: _____   Interpretation: _____

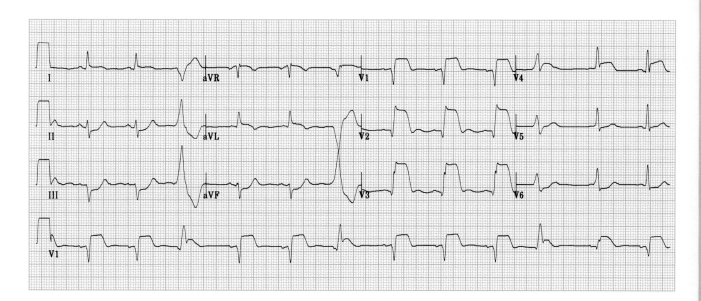

128

1. Rate: _____   2. Rhythm: _____   3. P wave: _____
4. PR Interval: _____   5. QRS complex: _____   +1. ST elevation: _____
+2. ST depression: _____   +3. Pathologic Q waves: _____   Interpretation: _____

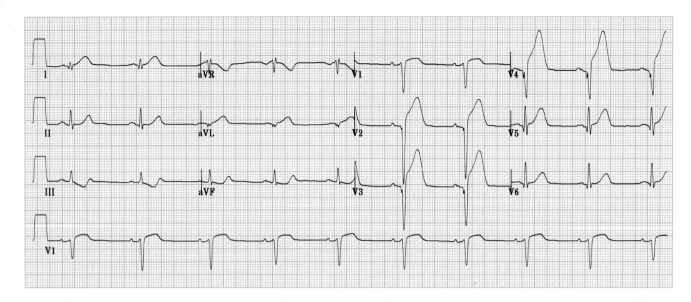

129

1. Rate: _____
4. PR Interval: _____
+2. ST depression: _____

2. Rhythm: _____
5. QRS complex: _____
+3. Pathologic Q waves: _____

3. P wave: _____
+1. ST elevation: _____
Interpretation: _____

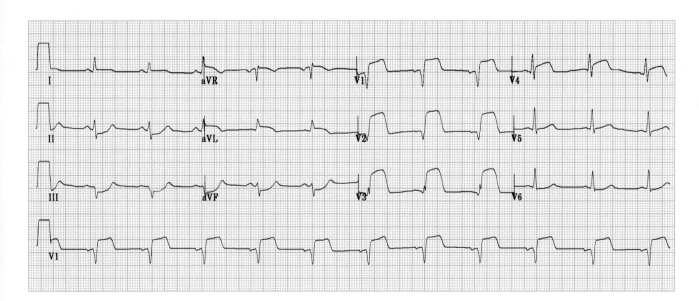

130

1. Rate: _____
4. PR Interval: _____
+2. ST depression: _____

2. Rhythm: _____
5. QRS complex: _____
+3. Pathologic Q waves: _____

3. P wave: _____
+1. ST elevation: _____
Interpretation: _____

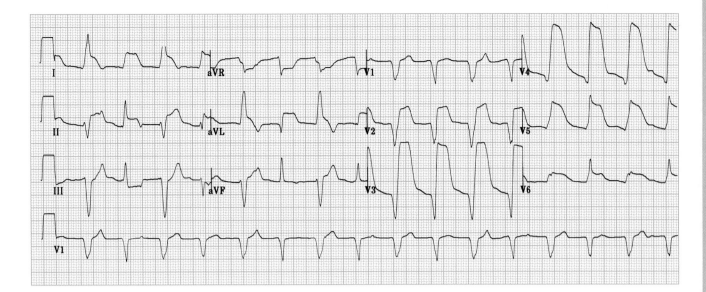

131

1. Rate: _____
4. PR Interval: _____
+2. ST depression: _____

2. Rhythm: _____
5. QRS complex: _____
+3. Pathologic Q waves: _____

3. P wave: _____
+1. ST elevation: _____
Interpretation: _____

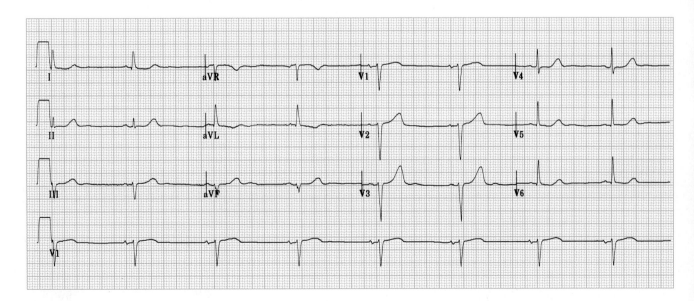

132

1. Rate: _____
4. PR Interval: _____
+2. ST depression: _____

2. Rhythm: _____
5. QRS complex: _____
+3. Pathologic Q waves: _____

3. P wave: _____
+1. ST elevation: _____
Interpretation: _____

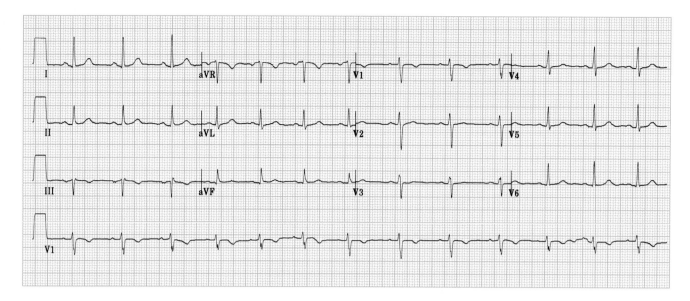

133

1. Rate: _____   2. Rhythm: _____   3. P wave: _____
4. PR Interval: _____   5. QRS complex: _____   +1. ST elevation: _____
+2. ST depression: _____   +3. Pathologic Q waves: _____   Interpretation: _____

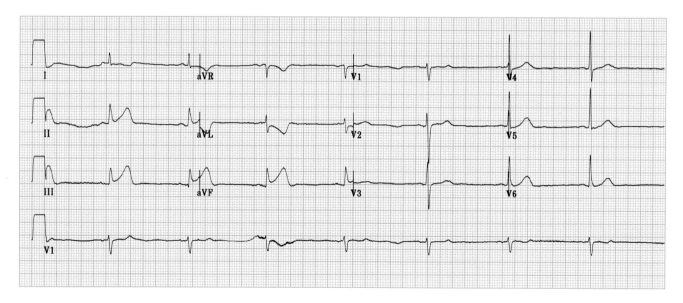

134

1. Rate: _____   2. Rhythm: _____   3. P wave: _____
4. PR Interval: _____   5. QRS complex: _____   +1. ST elevation: _____
+2. ST depression: _____   +3. Pathologic Q waves: _____   Interpretation: _____

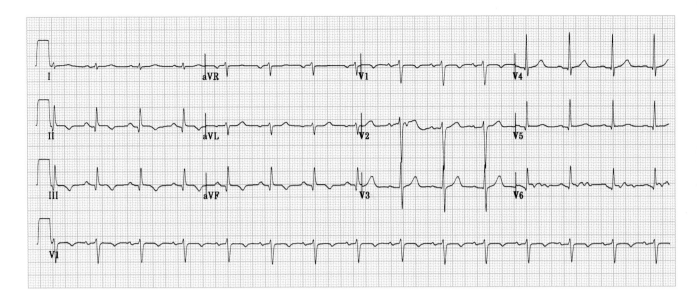

135

1. Rate: _____
4. PR Interval: _____
+2. ST depression: _____

2. Rhythm: _____
5. QRS complex: _____
+3. Pathologic Q waves: _____

3. P wave: _____
+1. ST elevation: _____
Interpretation: _____

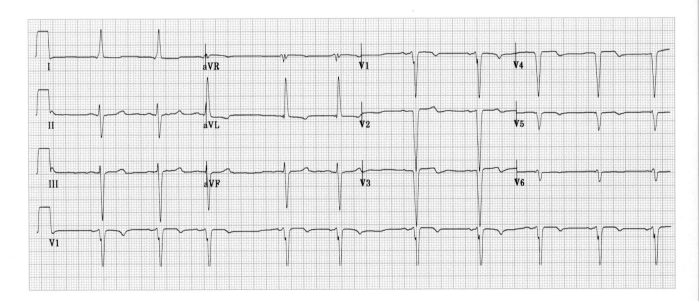

136

1. Rate: _____
4. PR Interval: _____
+2. ST depression: _____

2. Rhythm: _____
5. QRS complex: _____
+3. Pathologic Q waves: _____

3. P wave: _____
+1. ST elevation: _____
Interpretation: _____

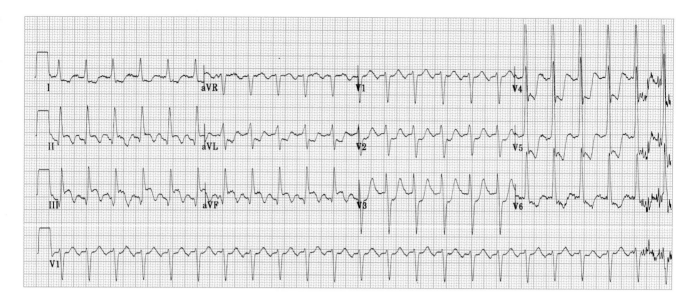

137

1. Rate: _____
4. PR Interval: _____
+2. ST depression: _____

2. Rhythm: _____
5. QRS complex: _____
+3. Pathologic Q waves: _____

3. P wave: _____
+1. ST elevation: _____
Interpretation: _____

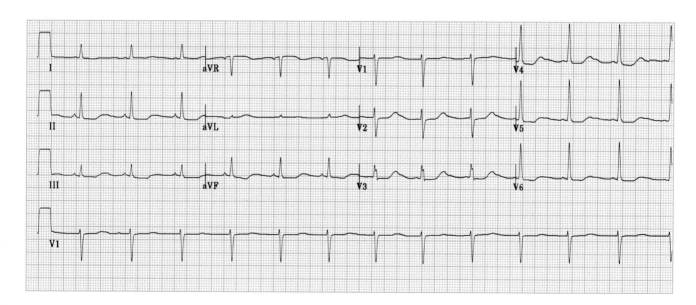

138

1. Rate: _____
4. PR Interval: _____
+2. ST depression: _____

2. Rhythm: _____
5. QRS complex: _____
+3. Pathologic Q waves: _____

3. P wave: _____
+1. ST elevation: _____
Interpretation: _____

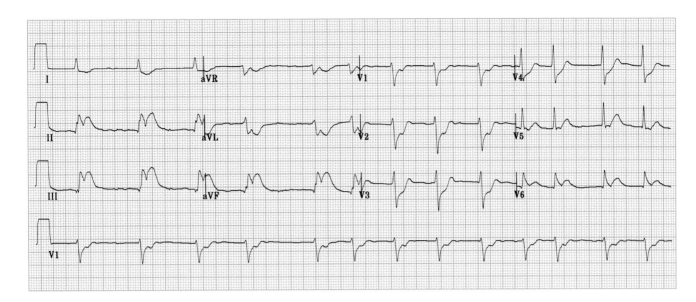

139

1. Rate: _____
4. PR Interval: _____
+2. ST depression: _____

2. Rhythm: _____
5. QRS complex: _____
+3. Pathologic Q waves: _____

3. P wave: _____
+1. ST elevation: _____
Interpretation: _____

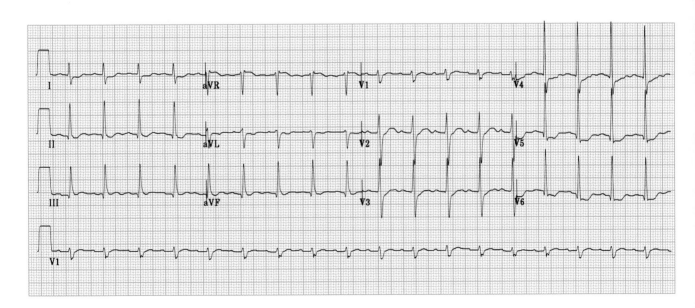

140

1. Rate: _____
4. PR Interval: _____
+2. ST depression: _____

2. Rhythm: _____
5. QRS complex: _____
+3. Pathologic Q waves: _____

3. P wave: _____
+1. ST elevation: _____
Interpretation: _____

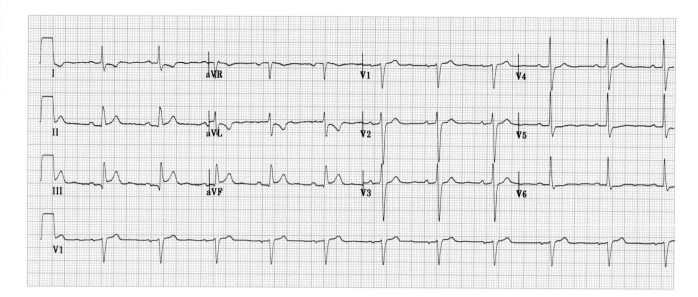

141

1. Rate: _____   2. Rhythm: _____   3. P wave: _____
4. PR Interval: _____   5. QRS complex: _____   +1. ST elevation: _____
+2. ST depression: _____   +3. Pathologic Q waves: _____   Interpretation: _____

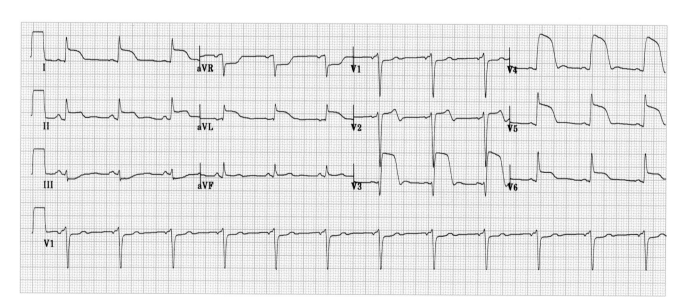

142

1. Rate: _____   2. Rhythm: _____   3. P wave: _____
4. PR Interval: _____   5. QRS complex: _____   +1. ST elevation: _____
+2. ST depression: _____   +3. Pathologic Q waves: _____   Interpretation: _____

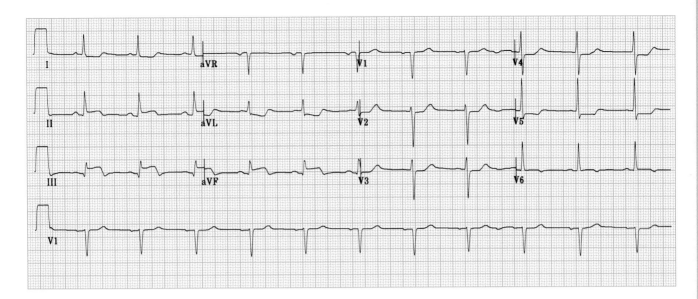

143

1. Rate: _____
4. PR Interval: _____
+2. ST depression: _____

2. Rhythm: _____
5. QRS complex: _____
+3. Pathologic Q waves: _____

3. P wave: _____
+1. ST elevation: _____
Interpretation: _____

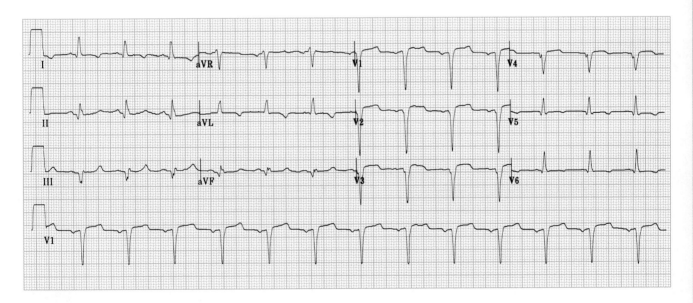

144

1. Rate: _____
4. PR Interval: _____
+2. ST depression: _____

2. Rhythm: _____
5. QRS complex: _____
+3. Pathologic Q waves: _____

3. P wave: _____
+1. ST elevation: _____
Interpretation: _____

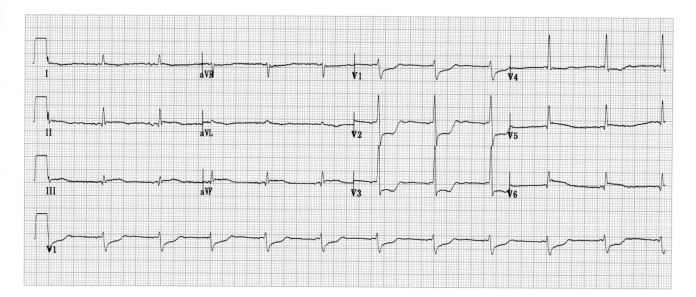

145

1. Rate: _____
2. Rhythm: _____
3. P wave: _____
4. PR Interval: _____
5. QRS complex: _____
+1. ST elevation: _____
+2. ST depression: _____
+3. Pathologic Q waves: _____
Interpretation: _____

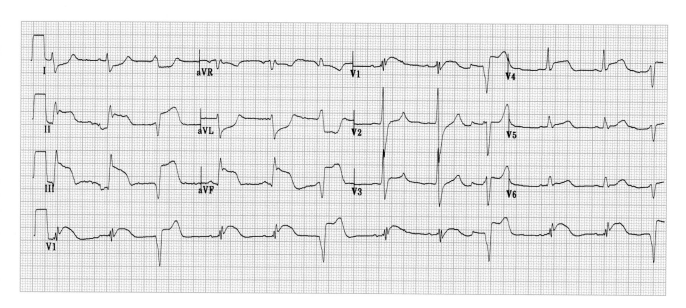

146

1. Rate: _____
2. Rhythm: _____
3. P wave: _____
4. PR Interval: _____
5. QRS complex: _____
+1. ST elevation: _____
+2. ST depression: _____
+3. Pathologic Q waves: _____
Interpretation: _____

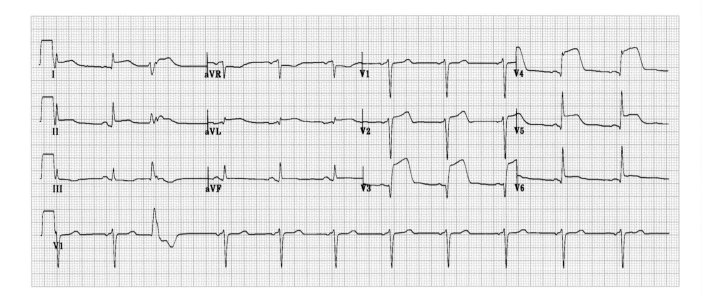

147

1. Rate: _____
2. Rhythm: _____
3. P wave: _____
4. PR Interval: _____
5. QRS complex: _____
+1. ST elevation: _____
+2. ST depression: _____
+3. Pathologic Q waves: _____
Interpretation: _____

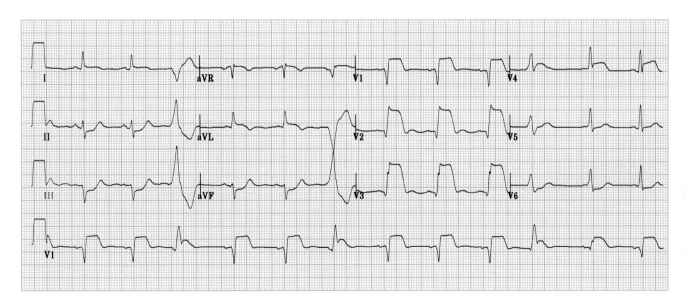

148

1. Rate: _____
2. Rhythm: _____
3. P wave: _____
4. PR Interval: _____
5. QRS complex: _____
+1. ST elevation: _____
+2. ST depression: _____
+3. Pathologic Q waves: _____
Interpretation: _____

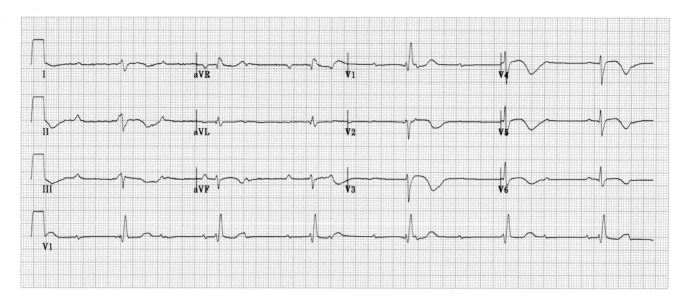

149

1. Rate: _____   2. Rhythm: _____   3. P wave: _____
4. PR Interval: _____   5. QRS complex: _____   +1. ST elevation: _____
+2. ST depression: _____   +3. Pathologic Q waves: _____   Interpretation: _____

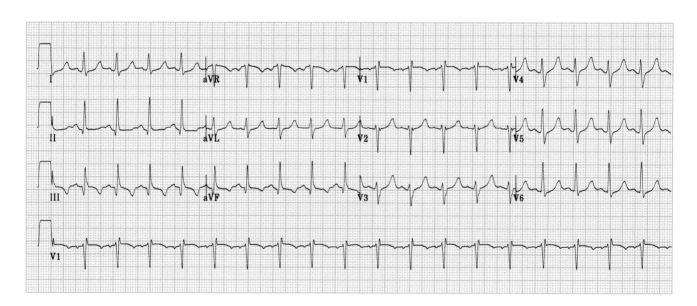

150

1. Rate: _____   2. Rhythm: _____   3. P wave: _____
4. PR Interval: _____   5. QRS complex: _____   +1. ST elevation: _____
+2. ST depression: _____   +3. Pathologic Q waves: _____   Interpretation: _____

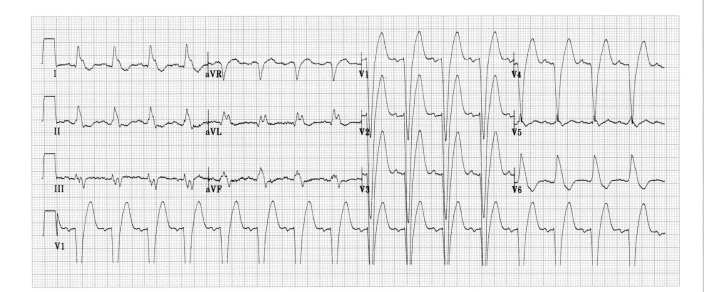

151

1. Rate: _____
2. Rhythm: _____
3. P wave: _____
4. PR Interval: _____
5. QRS complex: _____
+1. ST elevation: _____
+2. ST depression: _____
+3. Pathologic Q waves: _____
Interpretation: _____

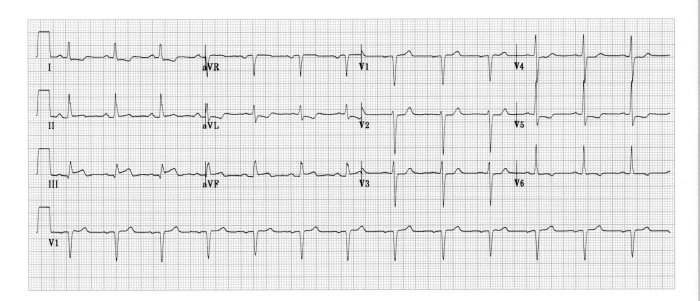

152

1. Rate: _____
2. Rhythm: _____
3. P wave: _____
4. PR Interval: _____
5. QRS complex: _____
+1. ST elevation: _____
+2. ST depression: _____
+3. Pathologic Q waves: _____
Interpretation: _____

Appendix 1

ANSWERS TO REVIEW QUESTIONS

CHAPTERS 1–17

CHAPTER 1

1. c
2. b
3. a
4. c
5. a
6. b
7. d
8. c
9. c
10. c
11. d
12. b
13. d
14. b
15. c

CHAPTER 2

1. b
2. b
3. b
4. d
5. a
6. c
7. b
8. d
9. a
10. b
11. c
12. b
13. a
14. b
15. b

CHAPTER 3

1. c
2. a
3. c
4. d
5. a
6. b
7. b
8. a
9. b
10. a
11. b
12. b
13. a
14. b
15. a

CHAPTER 4

1. a
2. d
3. d
4. c
5. c
6. b
7. b
8. c

9. a
10. d
11. d
12. a
13. b
14. b
15. c

CHAPTER 5

1. b
2. c
3. d
4. b
5. d
6. b
7. a
8. c

9. d
10. a
11. d
12. d
13. b
14. a
15. a

CHAPTER 6

1. a
2. d
3. c
4. b
5. d
6. b
7. a
8. d

9. b
10. c
11. a
12. d
13. a
14. c
15. d

CHAPTER 7

1. c
2. a
3. b
4. d
5. c
6. d
7. b
8. c

9. a
10. d
11. a
12. b
13. b
14. b
15. c

CHAPTER 8

1. a
2. d
3. c
4. c

5. b
6. a
7. a
8. a

9. d
10. b
11. b
12. a

13. b
14. b
15. a

CHAPTER 9

1. c
2. d
3. a
4. b
5. c
6. b
7. a
8. c

9. d
10. c
11. c
12. a
13. d
14. a
15. b

Rate: 50
Rhythm: Regular
P wave: Present, upright and rounded
PR Interval: 0.28 sec
QRS complex: 0.08 sec
ST elevation: Leads II, III, aVF
ST depression: Lead I, aVL, V_1, V_2
Pathologic Q waves: None
Interpretation: Sinus bradycardia, first-degree block with acute inferior MI

CHAPTER 10

1. b
2. a
3. c
4. d
5. a
6. a
7. c
8. c

9. b
10. d
11. b
12. a
13. d
14. b
15. b

Rate: 90
Rhythm: Irregular
P wave: Present, upright and rounded
PR Interval: 0.16 sec
QRS complex: 0.04 sec
ST elevation: Leads V_2, V_3, V_4, V_5
ST depression: None
Pathologic Q waves: None
Interpretation: Sinus rhythm, occasional PJCs and PVCs; acute anterior MI

CHAPTER 11

1. b
2. a
3. c

4. d
5. c
6. a

7. b   12. a
8. d   13. c
9. a   14. b
10. b   15. d
11. b

Rate: 76
Rhythm: Regular
P wave: Present, upright
PR Interval: 0.16 sec
QRS complex: 0.04 sec
ST elevation: V_1, V_2, V_3
ST depression: None
Pathologic Q waves: None
Interpretation: Sinus rhythm with acute septal MI

CHAPTER 12

1. d   9. d
2. a   10. b
3. d   11. a
4. a   12. b
5. a   13. b
6. a   14. b
7. c   15. a
8. a

Rate: 80
Rhythm: Regular
P wave: Present, upright
PR Interval: 0.16 sec
QRS complex: 0.6 sec
ST elevation: Lead 1, aVL, V_5, V_6,
ST depression: None
Pathologic Q waves: None
Interpretation: Sinus rhythm with acute lateral MI

CHAPTER 13

1. c   9. b
2. a   10. c
3. d   11. b
4. d   12. b
5. c   13. a
6. c   14. b
7. b   15. c
8. c

CHAPTER 14

1. b   4. a
2. d   5. c
3. c   6. b

7. b
8. b
9. a

10. a
11. b
12. b

CHAPTER 15

1. b
2. c
3. b
4. d
5. c
6. b
7. b
8. a

9. a
10. a
11. b
12. b
13. b
14. a
15. a

CHAPTER 16

1. b
2. c
3. a
4. d
5. b
6. c
7. c
8. a

9. b
10. b
11. d
12. c
13. b
14. a
15. c

CHAPTER 17

1. a
2. c
3. b
4. b
5. a
6. c
7. a
8. c
9. d
10. c
11. c
12. a
13. a
14. b
15. d
16. d
17. d
18. a
19. a
20. c
21. c
22. d
23. a
24. d

25. d
26. a
27. d
28. a
29. b
30. c
31. c
32. c
33. d
34. a
35. a
36. d
37. b
38. a
39. c
40. d
41. d
42. d
43. d
44. b
45. c
46. a
47. a
48. a

49.	d	100.	b
50.	a	101.	b
51.	d	102.	c
52.	a	103.	a
53.	a	104.	d
54.	a	105.	c
55.	c	106.	a
56.	a	107.	a
57.	b	108.	a
58.	c	109.	b
59.	b	110.	b
60.	c	111.	c
61.	c	112.	a
62.	c	113.	a
63.	a	114.	c
64.	a	115.	b
65.	b	116.	a
66.	c	117.	c
67.	d	118.	a
68.	c	119.	b
69.	c	120.	c
70.	d	121.	a
71.	a	122.	d
72.	b	123.	c
73.	c	124.	d
74.	b	125.	a
75.	c	126.	b
76.	d	127.	d
77.	c	128.	c
78.	a	129.	b
79.	b	130.	b
80.	a	131.	a
81.	c	132.	b
82.	c	133.	c
83.	a	134.	d
84.	a	135.	c
85.	b	136.	a
86.	a	137.	b
87.	a	138.	d
88.	a	139.	c
89.	c	140.	a
90.	b	141.	d
91.	d	142.	b
92.	a	143.	b
93.	d	144.	b
94.	a	145.	b
95.	b	146.	c
96.	a	147.	b
97.	b	148.	b
98.	a	149.	a
99.	a	150.	c

Appendix 2

ANSWERS TO REVIEW STRIPS

CHAPTER 18

1. Rate: 66
   Rhythm: Regular
   P wave: Present, upright (II)
   PR Interval: 0.18 sec
   QRS complex: 0.08 sec
   ST elevation: V_1, V_2, V_3, V_4 with inversion of T wave
   ST depression: None
   Pathologic Q waves: None
   Interpretation: Normal sinus rhythm with anterior/lateral MI

2. Rate: 107
   Rhythm: Irregular
   P wave: Present, upright (II)
   PR Interval: 0.16 sec
   QRS complex: 0.13 sec
   ST elevation: II, III, aVF
   ST depression: None
   Pathologic Q waves: None
   Interpretation: Sinus tachycardia with frequent PVCs, inferior injury

3. Rate: 88
   Rhythm: Regular
   P wave: Present, notched (II)
   PR Interval: 0.20 sec
   QRS complex: 0.12 sec
   ST elevation: None
   ST depression: None
   Pathologic Q waves: None
   Interpretation: Normal sinus rhythm, left axis deviation, left bundle branch block

4. Rate: 74
   Rhythm: Regular
   P wave: Inverted (III)
   PR Interval: 0.20 sec
   QRS complex: 0.14 sec
   ST elevation: None
   ST depression: I, aVL
   Pathologic Q waves: II, III, aVF
   Interpretation: Junctional rhythm, inferior infarct, anterior ischemia

5. Rate: 55
   Rhythm: Irregular
   P wave: None present
   PR Interval: 0
   QRS complex: 0.16 sec
   ST elevation: None
   ST depression: None
   Pathologic Q waves: None
   Interpretation: Atrial fibrillation with junctional escape, right bundle branch block

6. Rate: 93
   Rhythm: Regular
   P wave: Present, upright (II)
   PR Interval: 0.15 sec
   QRS complex: 0.13 sec
   ST elevation: II, III, aVF
   ST depression: V_5, V_6
   Pathologic Q waves: II, aVF
   Interpretation: Normal sinus rhythm, inferior infarct, lateral ischemia, incomplete bundle branch block

7. Rate: 73
   Rhythm: Regular
   P wave: Present, notched (II)
   PR Interval: 0.14 sec
   QRS complex: 0.08 sec
   ST elevation: None
   ST depression: None
   Pathologic Q waves: None
   Interpretation: Normal sinus rhythm, left axis deviation

8. Rate: 99
   Rhythm: Irregular
   P wave: Present, upright (II)
   PR Interval: 0.14 sec
   QRS complex: 0.08 sec
   ST elevation: II, III, aVF
   ST depression: None
   Pathologic Q waves: II, III, aVF
   Interpretation: Normal sinus rhythm with sinus dysrhythmia, inferior infarct pattern

9. Rate: 200
   Rhythm: Regular
   P wave: Not present
   PR Interval: 0
   QRS complex: 0.07 sec
   ST elevation: None
   ST depression: None
   Pathologic Q waves: None
   Interpretation: Supraventricular tachycardia

10. Rate: 60
    Rhythm: Regular
    P wave: Present, upright (II)
    PR Interval: 0.17 sec
    QRS complex: 0.10 sec
    ST elevation: V_1, V_2, V_3, V_4 with T wave inversion
    ST depression: None
    Pathologic Q waves: None
    Interpretation: Normal sinus rhythm, anterior/lateral injury

11. Rate: 68
    Rhythm: Regular
    P wave: Present (II)
    PR Interval: 0.12 sec
    QRS complex: 0.06 sec
    ST elevation: II, III, aVF, V_5, V_6
    ST depression: None
    Pathologic Q waves: None
    Interpretation: Normal sinus rhythm, inferolateral infarct

12. Rate: 94
    Rhythm: Regular
    P wave: Present (II)
    PR Interval: 0.12 sec
    QRS complex: 0.08 sec
    ST elevation: II, III, aVF
    ST depression: V_1, V_2, V_3, V_4
    Pathologic Q waves: None
    Interpretation: Normal sinus rhythm, acute inferior infarct

13. Rate: 75
    Rhythm: Regular
    P wave: Present, notched (II)
    PR Interval: 0.20 sec
    QRS complex: 0.08 sec
    ST elevation: V_1, V_2, V_3, V_4, V_5, V_6
    ST depression: None
    Pathologic Q waves: None
    Interpretation: Normal sinus rhythm, anterolateral infarct pattern

14. Rate: >200
    Rhythm: Irregular
    P wave: None present
    PR Interval: 0
    QRS complex: 0.16 sec
    ST elevation: None
    ST depression: None
    Pathologic Q waves: None
    Interpretation: Ventricular tachycardia

15. Rate: 78
    Rhythm: Regular
    P wave: Present
    PR Interval: 0.12 sec
    QRS complex: 0.08 sec
    ST elevation: Slight in II, III, aVF with T wave inversion
    ST depression: None
    Pathologic Q waves: None
    Interpretation: Normal sinus rhythm, inferior ischemia

16. Rate: 74
    Rhythm: Regular
    P wave: Present
    PR Interval: 0.22 sec
    QRS complex: 0.08 sec
    ST elevation: V_1, V_2, V_3, V_4 with poor R wave progression
    ST depression: None
    Pathologic Q waves: None
    Interpretation: Sinus rhythm with first-degree block, anteroseptal infarct

17. Rate: 60
    Rhythm: Regular
    P wave: Present
    PR Interval: 0.26 sec
    QRS complex: 0.08 sec
    ST elevation: None
    ST depression: None
    Pathologic Q waves: None
    Interpretation: Normal sinus rhythm with first-degree block

18. Rate: 74
    Rhythm: Regular
    P wave: Present, upright (II)
    PR Interval: 0.18 sec
    QRS complex: 0.08 sec
    ST elevation: V_1, V_2, V_3, V_4 with T wave inversion
    ST depression: None
    Pathologic Q waves: None
    Interpretation: Normal sinus rhythm, left axis deviation, anteroseptal infarct

19. Rate: 88
    Rhythm: Regular
    P wave: Present, upright (II)
    PR Interval: 0.14 sec
    QRS complex: 0.08 sec
    ST elevation: II, III, aVF
    ST depression: I, aVL
    Pathologic Q waves: None
    Interpretation: Normal sinus rhythm, right axis deviation, inferior infarct

20. Rate: 87
    Rhythm: Regular
    P wave: Present, upright (II)
    PR Interval: 0.16 sec
    QRS complex: 0.08 sec
    ST elevation: V_1, V_2, V_3, V_4, V_5, V_6
    ST depression: None
    Pathologic Q waves: None
    Interpretation: Normal sinus rhythm, anterolateral infarct

21. Rate: 71
    Rhythm: Regular
    P wave: None
    PR Interval: 0
    QRS complex: 0.14 sec
    ST elevation: None
    ST depression: None
    Pathologic Q waves: None
    Interpretation: Pacer rhythm

22. Rate: 74
    Rhythm: Regular
    P wave: Present, upright (II)
    PR Interval: 0.16 sec
    QRS complex: 0.08 sec
    ST elevation: I, aVL, V_2, V_3, V_4, V_5, V_6
    ST depression: III, aVF
    Pathologic Q waves: None
    Interpretation: Normal sinus rhythm, anterolateral infarct

23. Rate: 98
    Rhythm: Irregular
    P wave: None
    PR Interval: 0
    QRS complex: 0.12 sec
    ST elevation: I, II, III, aVL, aVF, V_1, V_2, V_3, V_4, V_5, V_6
    ST depression: aVR
    Pathologic Q waves: None
    Interpretation: Junctional rhythm with bigeminy PVCs, anteroseptal,
                                 inferolateral infarct

24. Rate: 68
    Rhythm: Regular
    P wave: Present, upright (II)
    PR Interval: 0.11 sec
    QRS complex: 0.04 sec
    ST elevation: None
    ST depression: None
    Pathologic Q waves: None
    Interpretation: Normal sinus rhythm

25. Rate: 67
    Rhythm: Irregular
    P wave: Present, upright (II)
    PR Interval: 0.16 sec
    QRS complex: 0.06 sec
    ST elevation: I, aVL, V_1, V_2, V_3, V_4
    ST depression: III, aVF
    Pathologic Q waves: None
    Interpretation: Normal sinus rhythm with sinus dysrhythmia,
                        anteroseptal infarct

26. Rate: 108
    Rhythm: Irregular
    P wave: None
    PR Interval: 0
    QRS complex: 0.08 sec
    ST elevation: None
    ST depression: V_2, V_3, V_4
    Pathologic Q waves: III, aVF
    Interpretation: Atrial fibrillation with rapid ventricular response,
                        inferior MI

27. Rate: 104
    Rhythm: Irregular
    P wave: Present, upright (II)
    PR Interval: 0.12 sec
    QRS complex: 0.08 sec
    ST elevation: None
    ST depression: None
    Pathologic Q waves: None
    Interpretation: Normal sinus rhythm with bigeminy PVCs

28. Rate: 55
    Rhythm: Regular
    P wave: Present, upright (II)
    PR Interval: 0.10 sec
    QRS complex: 0.08 sec
    ST elevation: None
    ST depression: None
    Pathologic Q waves: None
    Interpretation: Sinus bradycardia

29. Rate: 96
    Rhythm: Regular
    P wave: Present, upright (II)
    PR Interval: 0.14 sec
    QRS complex: 0.08 sec
    ST elevation: II, III, aVF, V_1, V_2, V_3
    ST depression: I, aVL
    Pathologic Q waves: III, aVF
    Interpretation: Normal sinus rhythm, inferior-anterior MI

30. Rate: 79
    Rhythm: Regular
    P wave: Present, upright (II)
    PR Interval: 0.16 sec
    QRS complex: 0.08 sec
    ST elevation: I, aVL, V_1, V_2, V_3, V_4, V_5
    ST depression: None
    Pathologic Q waves: None
    Interpretation: Normal sinus rhythm, anterior MI

31. Rate: 70
    Rhythm: Regular
    P wave: None
    PR Interval: 0
    QRS complex: 0.18 sec
    ST elevation: None
    ST depression: None
    Pathologic Q waves: None
    Interpretation: Pacer rhythm

32. Rate: 90
    Rhythm: Irregular
    P wave: Present, upright (II)
    PR Interval: 0.16 sec
    QRS complex: 0.12 sec
    ST elevation: None
    ST depression: II, III, aVF
    Pathologic Q waves: None
    Interpretation: Normal sinus rhythm going into V-tach/V-fib with
                         inferior ischemia

33. Rate: 50
    Rhythm: Regular
    P wave: Present, upright (II)
    PR Interval: 0.32 sec
    QRS complex: 0.12 sec
    ST elevation: II, III, aVF
    ST depression: I, aVL, V_2, V_3
    Pathologic Q waves: None
    Interpretation: Second-degree block Type II, inferior MI, posterior MI

34. Rate: 69
    Rhythm: Regular
    P wave: Present, upright (II); delta waves
    PR Interval: 0.08 sec
    QRS complex: 0.08 sec
    ST elevation: None
    ST depression: None
    Pathologic Q waves: None
    Interpretation: Normal sinus rhythm with sinus dysrhythmia, Wolfe-
                               Parkinson-White syndrome

35. Rate: 55
    Rhythm: Regular
    P wave: Present, upright (II)
    PR Interval: 0.22 sec
    QRS complex: 0.08 sec
    ST elevation: II, III, aVF
    ST depression: I, aVL, V_1, V_2, V_3, V_4
    Pathologic Q waves: None
    Interpretation: Sinus bradycardia with first-degree block, inferior MI

36. Rate: 57
    Rhythm: Irregular
    P wave: None
    PR Interval: 0
    QRS complex: 0.08 sec
    ST elevation: V_5, V_6
    ST depression: None
    Pathologic Q waves: None
    Interpretation: Atrial flutter, lateral infarct

37. Rate: 99
    Rhythm: Regular
    P wave: Present, upright (II)
    PR Interval: 0.17 sec
    QRS complex: 0.08 sec
    ST elevation: II, aVF
    ST depression: I, aVL, V_2, V_3
    Pathologic Q waves: III, aVF
    Interpretation: Normal sinus rhythm, inferior MI, anterior ischemia

38. Rate: 70
    Rhythm: Regular
    P wave: Present (II)
    PR Interval: 0.12 sec
    QRS complex: 0.08 sec
    ST elevation: I, II, III, aVL, V_3, V_4, V_5, V_6
    ST depression: None
    Pathologic Q waves: None
    Interpretation: Normal sinus rhythm, anterior/inferolateral MI

39. Rate: 64
    Rhythm: Regular
    P wave: Present, notched (II)
    PR Interval: 0.20 sec
    QRS complex: 0.12 sec
    ST elevation: II, III, aVF
    ST depression: aVR, aVL, V_1, V_2, V_3
    Pathologic Q waves: None
    Interpretation: Normal sinus rhythm, inferior MI, septal ischemia

40. Rate: 55
    Rhythm: Regular
    P wave: Present, upright (II)
    PR Interval: 0.16 sec
    QRS complex: 0.08 sec
    ST elevation: V_1, V_2, V_3, V_4, V_5, V_6 with T wave inversion
    ST depression: None
    Pathologic Q waves: None
    Interpretation: Sinus bradycardia, anterolateral MI

41. Rate: 50
    Rhythm: Regular
    P wave: Present, upright (II)
    PR Interval: Variable
    QRS complex: 0.10 sec
    ST elevation: II, III, aVF, V_5, V_6
    ST depression: I, aVL, V_1, V_2
    Pathologic Q waves: None
    Interpretation: Third-degree block, right axis deviation, inferolateral MI

42. Rate: 88
    Rhythm: Regular
    P wave: Present, upright (II)
    PR Interval: 0.16 sec
    QRS complex: 0.10 sec
    ST elevation: I, II, III, aVF, V_1, V_2, V_3, V_4, V_5, V_6
    ST depression: None
    Pathologic Q waves: None
    Interpretation: Normal sinus rhythm, anterolateral MI, inferior MI

43. Rate: 67
    Rhythm: Regular
    P wave: Present, upright (II)
    PR Interval: 0.12 sec
    QRS complex: 0.08 sec
    ST elevation: I, aVL, V_1, V_2, V_3, V_4
    ST depression: II, III, aVF
    Pathologic Q waves: None
    Interpretation: Normal sinus rhythm, anteroseptal MI

44. Rate: 70
    Rhythm: Regular
    P wave: Present, upright (II)
    PR Interval: 0.16 sec
    QRS complex: 0.08 sec
    ST elevation: V_1, V_2, V_3, V_4, V_5, V_6 with T wave inversion
    ST depression: None
    Pathologic Q waves: None
    Interpretation: Normal sinus rhythm, anterolateral MI

45. Rate: 82
    Rhythm: Regular
    P wave: Present, upright (II)
    PR Interval: 0.16 sec
    QRS complex: 0.08 sec
    ST elevation: None
    ST depression: None
    Pathologic Q waves: None
    Interpretation: Normal sinus rhythm

46. Rate: 69
    Rhythm: Regular
    P wave: Present, notched (II)
    PR Interval: 0.24 sec
    QRS complex: 0.08 sec
    ST elevation: None
    ST depression: None
    Pathologic Q waves: None
    Interpretation: Normal sinus rhythm with first-degree block

47. Rate: 75
    Rhythm: Regular
    P wave: Present, notched (II)
    PR Interval: 0.16 sec
    QRS complex: 0.08 sec
    ST elevation: Slight in I, aVL, V_1, V_2, V_3, V_4, V_5 with T wave
                             inversion
    ST depression: None
    Pathologic Q waves: None
    Interpretation: Normal sinus rhythm, left axis deviation, anterolateral
                             ischemia

48. Rate: 79
    Rhythm: Regular
    P wave: Present, upright (II)
    PR Interval: 0.18 sec
    QRS complex: 0.08 sec
    ST elevation: II, III, aVF
    ST depression: I, aVL, V_1, V_2, V_3, V_4, V_5
    Pathologic Q waves: II, III, aVF
    Interpretation: Normal sinus rhythm, inferior MI

49. Rate: 74
    Rhythm: Regular
    P wave: Present, upright (II)
    PR Interval: 0.20 sec
    QRS complex: 0.08 sec
    ST elevation: V_1, V_2, V_3, V_4
    ST depression: None
    Pathologic Q waves: None
    Interpretation: Normal sinus rhythm, anteroseptal MI

50. Rate: 71
    Rhythm: Irregular
    P wave: Present, upright (II)
    PR Interval: Varies
    QRS complex: 0.08 sec
    ST elevation: None
    ST depression: None
    Pathologic Q waves: II, aVF
    Interpretation: Normal sinus rhythm with second-degree block Mobitz
                             Type I, left axis deviation, consider old inferior MI

51. Rate: 150
    Rhythm: Regular
    P wave: If present, hidden in QRS complex
    PR Interval: 0
    QRS complex: 0.16 sec
    ST elevation: I, aVL, V_1, V_2, V_3, V_4, V_5, V_6
    ST depression: None
    Pathologic Q waves: None
    Interpretation: Wide complex tachycardia, left axis deviation,
                             anterolateral/septal MI

52. Rate: 90
    Rhythm: Irregular
    P wave: Absent
    PR Interval: 0
    QRS complex: 0.08 sec
    ST elevation: None
    ST depression: None
    Pathologic Q waves: None
    Interpretation: Accelerated junctional rhythm with bigeminy PVCs and
                             couplet PVCs

53. Rate: 84
    Rhythm: Regular
    P wave: Present, upright (II)
    PR Interval: 0.16 sec
    QRS complex: 0.08 sec
    ST elevation: II, III, aVF
    ST depression: I, aVL, V_2, V_3, V_4, V_5
    Pathologic Q waves: None
    Interpretation: Normal sinus rhythm, inferior MI

54. Rate: 138
    Rhythm: Regular
    P wave: Absent or hidden in QRS complex
    PR Interval: 0
    QRS complex: 0.16 sec
    ST elevation: I, aVL, V_1, V_2, V_3, V_4, V_5, V_6
    ST depression: None
    Pathologic Q waves: None
    Interpretation: Wide complex tachycardia, anteroseptal-lateral MI

55. Rate: 128
    Rhythm: Regular
    P wave: Present, upright (II)
    PR Interval: 0.16 sec
    QRS complex: 0.08 sec
    ST elevation: None
    ST depression: V_4, V_5, V_6
    Pathologic Q waves: None
    Interpretation: Normal sinus rhythm, lateral ischemia

56. Rate: 121
    Rhythm: Regular
    P wave: Present, upright (II)
    PR Interval: 0.16 sec
    QRS complex: 0.08 sec
    ST elevation: None
    ST depression: None
    Pathologic Q waves: None
    Interpretation: Sinus tachycardia

57. Rate: 35
    Rhythm: Irregular
    P wave: Absent
    PR Interval: 0
    QRS complex: 0.08 sec
    ST elevation: None
    ST depression: V_2, V_3, V_4, V_5, V_6
    Pathologic Q waves: None
    Interpretation: Junctional bradycardia with PJCs, anterolateral ischemia

58. Rate: 124
    Rhythm: Regular
    P wave: Present, upright (II)
    PR Interval: 0.18 sec
    QRS complex: 0.08 sec
    ST elevation: V_1, V_2
    ST depression: None
    Pathologic Q waves: None
    Interpretation: Sinus tachycardia, septal MI

59. Rate: 96
    Rhythm: Regular
    P wave: Present, upright (II)
    PR Interval: 0.16 sec
    QRS complex: 0.12 sec
    ST elevation: None
    ST depression: None
    Pathologic Q waves: None
    Interpretation: Normal sinus rhythm, left bundle branch block

60. Rate: 59
    Rhythm: Regular
    P wave: Absent
    PR Interval: 0
    QRS complex: 0.14 sec
    ST elevation: None
    ST depression: None
    Pathologic Q waves: None
    Interpretation: Ventricular pacemaker rhythm

61. Rate: 70
    Rhythm: Regular
    P wave: Flutter waves
    PR Interval: 0
    QRS complex: 0.08 sec
    ST elevation: None
    ST depression: None
    Pathologic Q waves: None
    Interpretation: Atrial flutter

62. Rate: 68
    Rhythm: Irregular
    P wave: Present, upright (II)
    PR Interval: 0.12 sec
    QRS complex: 0.08 sec
    ST elevation: II, III, aVF
    ST depression: I, aVL, V_3, V_4, V_5, V_6
    Pathologic Q waves: II, aVF
    Interpretation: Sinus dysrhythmia, inferior MI

63. Rate: 96
    Rhythm: Regular
    P wave: Present, upright (II)
    PR Interval: 0.12 sec
    QRS complex: 0.08 sec
    ST elevation: II, III, aVF, V_2, V_3, V_4
    ST depression: None
    Pathologic Q waves: None
    Interpretation: Normal sinus rhythm, inferior/anterior MI

64. Rate: 86
    Rhythm: Irregular
    P wave: Absent
    PR Interval: 0
    QRS complex: 0.04 sec
    ST elevation: None
    ST depression: None
    Pathologic Q waves: None
    Interpretation: Junctional rhythm with run of V-tach

65. Rate: 43
    Rhythm: Regular
    P wave: Present, upright (II)
    PR Interval: 0.22 sec
    QRS complex: 0.08 sec
    ST elevation: II, III, aVF, V_3, V_4, V_5, V_6
    ST depression: I, aVL, V_1, V_2
    Pathologic Q waves: None
    Interpretation: Second-degree block Type II, anterior/inferolateral MI, right axis deviation

66. Rate: 88
    Rhythm: Regular
    P wave: Present, upright (II)
    PR Interval: 0.16 sec
    QRS complex: 0.08 sec
    ST elevation: I, aVL, V_1, V_2, V_3, V_4, V_5, V_6
    ST depression: III, aVR
    Pathologic Q waves: None
    Interpretation: Normal sinus rhythm, anterolateral MI

67. Rate: 67
    Rhythm: Regular
    P wave: Present, upright (II)
    PR Interval: 0.12 sec
    QRS complex: 0.04 sec
    ST elevation: I, aVL, V_1, V_2, V_3, V_4 (tombstones)
    ST depression: II, III, aVF
    Pathologic Q waves: None
    Interpretation: Normal sinus rhythm, anteroseptal MI

68. Rate: 96
    Rhythm: Irregular
    P wave: Present, notched (II)
    PR Interval: 0.32 sec
    QRS complex: 0.11 sec
    ST elevation: I, II, III, aVL, aVF, V_1, V_2, V_3, V_4, V_5, V_6
    ST depression: None
    Pathologic Q waves: None
    Interpretation: Sinus rhythm with first-degree block and run of bigeminy PVCs, anteroseptal MI, inferolateral MI

69. Rate: 85
    Rhythm: Regular
    P wave: Present, upright (II)
    PR Interval: 0.16 sec
    QRS complex: 0.04 sec
    ST elevation: II, III, aVF
    ST depression: None
    Pathologic Q waves: III, aVF
    Interpretation: Normal sinus rhythm, inferior MI

70. Rate: 117
    Rhythm: Regular
    P wave: Present, upright (II)
    PR Interval: 0.16 sec
    QRS complex: 0.04 sec
    ST elevation: None
    ST depression: None
    Pathologic Q waves: None
    Interpretation: Sinus tachycardia rhythm

71. Rate: 146
    Rhythm: Regular
    P wave: Absent
    PR Interval: 0
    QRS complex: 0.12 sec
    ST elevation: None
    ST depression: V_4, V_5, V_6
    Pathologic Q waves: None
    Interpretation: Supraventricular rhythm with run of V-tach, lateral
                        ischemia

72. Rate: 115
    Rhythm: Regular
    P wave: Present, upright (II)
    PR Interval: 0.16 sec
    QRS complex: 0.08 sec
    ST elevation: II, III, aVF
    ST depression: I, aVL, V_1, V_2, V_3, V_4, V_5, V_6
    Pathologic Q waves: III, aVF
    Interpretation: Sinus tachycardia, inferior MI, anterior ischemia

73. Rate: 74
    Rhythm: Regular
    P wave: Present, upright (II)
    PR Interval: 0.16 sec
    QRS complex: 0.08 sec
    ST elevation: II, III, aVF
    ST depression: I, aVL
    Pathologic Q waves: None
    Interpretation: Normal sinus rhythm, inferior MI

74. Rate: 93
    Rhythm: Irregular
    P wave: Present, upright (II)
    PR Interval: 0.16 sec
    QRS complex: 0.08 sec
    ST elevation: None
    ST depression: V_4, V_5, V_6
    Pathologic Q waves: None
    Interpretation: Normal sinus rhythm with PJCs, lateral ischemia

75. Rate: 128
    Rhythm: Regular
    P wave: Absent
    PR Interval: 0
    QRS complex: 0.10 sec
    ST elevation: II, III, aVF
    ST depression: None
    Pathologic Q waves: None
    Interpretation: Supraventricular tachycardia, left axis deviation, right bundle branch block, inferior MI

76. Rate: 88
    Rhythm: Irregular
    P wave: Present, upright (II)
    PR Interval: 0.16 sec
    QRS complex: 0.08 sec
    ST elevation: None
    ST depression: None
    Pathologic Q waves: Poor R wave progression, V_1, V_2, V_3
    Interpretation: Sinus rhythm with occasional PACs, consider old septal MI

77. Rate: 123
    Rhythm: Irregular
    P wave: Absent
    PR Interval: 0
    QRS complex: 0.10 sec
    ST elevation: None
    ST depression: None
    Pathologic Q waves: II, III, aVF
    Interpretation: Atrial fibrillation with rapid ventricular response, left axis deviation, left bundle branch block, consider inferior MI (old), right bundle branch block, demand pacemaker firing twice

78. Rate: 86
    Rhythm: Regular
    P wave: Present, upright (II)
    PR Interval: 0.16 sec
    QRS complex: 0.08 sec

ST elevation:	II, aVF, V$_2$, V$_3$, V$_4$
ST depression:	I, aVL
Pathologic Q waves:	III, aVF
Interpretation:	Normal sinus rhythm, inferior MI, anterior MI

79. Rate: 70

Rhythm:	Regular
P wave:	Present, upright (II)
PR Interval:	0.16 sec
QRS complex:	0.06 sec
ST elevation:	II, III, aVF, V$_5$, V$_6$
ST depression:	None
Pathologic Q waves:	None
Interpretation:	Normal sinus rhythm, inferolateral MI

80. Rate: 64

Rhythm:	Irregular
P wave:	Present, upright (II)
PR Interval:	0.14 sec
QRS complex:	0.12 sec
ST elevation:	None
ST depression:	None
Pathologic Q waves:	None
Interpretation:	Sinus rhythm with premature ventricular complexes

81. Rate: 86

Rhythm:	Regular
P wave:	Present, upright (II)
PR Interval:	0.16 sec
QRS complex:	0.08 sec
ST elevation:	II, III, aVF
ST depression:	aVL, V$_1$, V$_2$, V$_3$, V$_4$
Pathologic Q waves:	None
Interpretation:	Normal sinus rhythm, inferior MI

82. Rate: 60

Rhythm:	Regular
P wave:	Present, upright (II)
PR Interval:	0.18 sec
QRS complex:	0.08 sec
ST elevation:	V$_1$, V$_2$, V$_3$, V$_4$, V$_5$, with T wave inversion
ST depression:	T wave inversion in I, aVL
Pathologic Q waves:	None
Interpretation:	Normal sinus rhythm, anterolateral MI

83. Rate: 72

Rhythm:	Irregular
P wave:	Present, upright (II)
PR Interval:	0.18 sec
QRS complex:	0.14 sec

ST elevation:	None
ST depression:	None
Pathologic Q waves:	None
Interpretation:	Sinus rhythm with occasional PVCs, left axis deviation, left bundle branch block

84.

Rate:	74
Rhythm:	Irregular
P wave:	Absent
PR Interval:	0
QRS complex:	0.14 sec
ST elevation:	II, III, aVF
ST depression:	None
Pathologic Q waves:	None
Interpretation:	Junctional rhythm with PJCs, right bundle branch block, inferior MI

85.

Rate:	80
Rhythm:	Regular
P wave:	Present, upright (II)
PR Interval:	0.16 sec
QRS complex:	0.08 sec
ST elevation:	II, III, aVF
ST depression:	None
Pathologic Q waves:	III, aVF
Interpretation:	Normal sinus rhythm, incomplete right bundle branch block, inferior MI

86.

Rate:	98
Rhythm:	Regular
P wave:	Present, upright (II)
PR Interval:	0.16 sec
QRS complex:	0.08 sec
ST elevation:	I, aVL, V_2, V_3, V_4, V_5, V_6
ST depression:	None
Pathologic Q waves:	None
Interpretation:	Normal sinus rhythm, anterolateral MI

87.

Rate:	130
Rhythm:	Irregular
P wave:	Absent
PR Interval:	0
QRS complex:	0.06 sec
ST elevation:	None
ST depression:	None
Pathologic Q waves:	Poor R wave progression
Interpretation:	Atrial fibrillation with rapid ventricular response, consider anteroseptal injury

88. Rate: 118
    Rhythm: Irregular
    P wave: Absent
    PR Interval: 0
    QRS complex: 0.08 sec
    ST elevation: None
    ST depression: None
    Pathologic Q waves: Poor R wave progression
    Interpretation: Atrial fibrillation with rapid ventricular response

89. Rate: 84
    Rhythm: Regular
    P wave: Present, upright (II)
    PR Interval: 0.16 sec
    QRS complex: 0.04 sec
    ST elevation: V_5, V_6
    ST depression: aVR, V_1, V_2, V_3
    Pathologic Q waves: None
    Interpretation: Normal sinus rhythm, lateral MI

90. Rate: 88
    Rhythm: Regular
    P wave: Present, upright (II)
    PR Interval: 0.14 sec
    QRS complex: 0.08 sec
    ST elevation: II, III, aVF
    ST depression: I, aVR, aVL
    Pathologic Q waves: None
    Interpretation: Normal sinus rhythm, right axis deviation, inferior MI

91. Rate: 68
    Rhythm: Irregular
    P wave: Present, upright (II)
    PR Interval: 0.12 sec
    QRS complex: 0.06 sec
    ST elevation: I, aVL, V_2, V_3, V_4, V_5, V_6
    ST depression: None
    Pathologic Q waves: None
    Interpretation: Sinus rhythm with occasional PVCs, anterior/lateral MI

92. Rate: 80
    Rhythm: Irregular
    P wave: Present, upright (II)
    PR Interval: 0.12 sec
    QRS complex: 0.6 sec
    ST elevation: I, aVL, V_1, V_2, V_3, V_4, V_5, V_6
    ST depression: II, III, aVF
    Pathologic Q waves: None
    Interpretation: Sinus rhythm with occasional PVCs, anterolateral MI

93. Rate: 92
    Rhythm: Irregular
    P wave: Present, upright (II)
    PR Interval: 0.22 sec
    QRS complex: 0.08 sec
    ST elevation: None
    ST depression: None
    Pathologic Q waves: Poor R wave progression
    Interpretation: Sinus rhythm with first-degree block with PVCs

94. Rate: 69
    Rhythm: Regular
    P wave: Present, upright (II)
    PR Interval: 0.08 sec
    QRS complex: 0.11 sec
    ST elevation: None
    ST depression: None
    Pathologic Q waves: None
    Interpretation: Normal sinus rhythm with sinus dysrhythmia, Wolfe-Parkinson-White syndrome (delta waves)

95. Rate: 74
    Rhythm: Irregular
    P wave: Present, upright (II)
    PR Interval: 0.16 sec
    QRS complex: 0.08 sec
    ST elevation: I, aVL, V_1, V_2, V_3, V_4
    ST depression: V_5, V_6, II, III, aVF
    Pathologic Q waves: None
    Interpretation: Sinus rhythm with frequent PVCs, anteroseptal MI, lateral ischemia

96. Rate: 67
    Rhythm: Regular
    P wave: Present, upright (II)
    PR Interval: 0.16 sec
    QRS complex: 0.08 sec
    ST elevation: I, aVL, V_1, V_2, V_3, V_4
    ST depression: II, III, aVF
    Pathologic Q waves: None
    Interpretation: Normal sinus rhythm, anterior MI (tombstones)

97. Rate: 128
    Rhythm: Irregular
    P wave: Present, upright (II)
    PR Interval: 0.16 sec
    QRS complex: 0.06 sec
    ST elevation: V_1, V_2, V_3, V_4, V_5
    ST depression: None

Pathologic Q waves:	Poor R wave progression
Interpretation:	Sinus tachycardia with occasional PJCs, consider anterior MI

98. Rate: 77

Rhythm:	Irregular
P wave:	Present, upright (II)
PR Interval:	0.16 sec
QRS complex:	0.08 sec
ST elevation:	I, aVL, V_1, V_2, V_3, V_4, V_5
ST depression:	II, III, aVF
Pathologic Q waves:	None
Interpretation:	Sinus rhythm with sinus dysrhythmia, anterolateral MI

99. Rate: 38

Rhythm:	Regular
P wave:	Present
PR Interval:	Variable
QRS complex:	0.08 sec
ST elevation:	II, III, aVF, V_4, V_5, V_6
ST depression:	I, aVL, V_1, V_2, V_3
Pathologic Q waves:	None
Interpretation:	Third-degree block, right axis deviation, inferolateral MI

100. Rate: 54

Rhythm:	Regular
P wave:	Present, upright (II)
PR Interval:	0.18 sec
QRS complex:	0.08 sec
ST elevation:	II, III, aVF
ST depression:	aVL, V_2
Pathologic Q waves:	None
Interpretation:	Sinus bradycardia, inferior MI

101. Rate: 98

Rhythm:	Regular
P wave:	Present, upright (II)
PR Interval:	0.16 sec
QRS complex:	0.08 sec
ST elevation:	II, III, aVF
ST depression:	I, aVL, V_1, V_2
Pathologic Q waves:	None
Interpretation:	Normal sinus rhythm, inferior MI

102. Rate: 60

Rhythm:	Regular
P wave:	Present, upright (II)
PR Interval:	0.16 sec

QRS complex:	0.08 sec
ST elevation:	I, aVL, V$_1$, V$_2$, V$_3$, V$_4$
ST depression:	None
Pathologic Q waves:	None
Interpretation:	Normal sinus rhythm, anterior MI, lateral ischemia (T wave inversion)

103.

Rate:	88
Rhythm:	Regular
P wave:	Present, upright (II)
PR Interval:	0.16 sec
QRS complex:	0.06 sec
ST elevation:	None
ST depression:	None
Pathologic Q waves:	None
Interpretation:	Normal sinus rhythm

104.

Rate:	62
Rhythm:	Irregular
P wave:	Present, upright (II)
PR Interval:	0.08 sec
QRS complex:	0.08 sec
ST elevation:	II, III, aVF
ST depression:	I, aVL, V$_2$, V$_3$, V$_4$, V$_5$
Pathologic Q waves:	II, III, aVF
Interpretation:	Sinus rhythm with sinus dysrhythmia with short PR Interval, inferior MI, consider also posterior MI

105.

Rate:	44
Rhythm:	Regular
P wave:	Present, inverted (II)
PR Interval:	0.16 sec
QRS complex:	0.08 sec
ST elevation:	None
ST depression:	I, aVL, V$_1$, V$_2$, V$_3$, V$_4$, V$_5$, V$_6$
Pathologic Q waves:	None
Interpretation:	Junctional rhythm, septal MI (inverted T waves), lateral ischemia, right bundle branch block

106.

Rate:	86
Rhythm:	Regular
P wave:	Present, upright (II)
PR Interval:	0.16 sec
QRS complex:	0.08 sec
ST elevation:	None
ST depression:	None
Pathologic Q waves:	None
Interpretation:	Normal sinus rhythm

107. Rate: 88
      Rhythm: Regular
      P wave: Present, upright (II)
      PR Interval: 0.16 sec
      QRS complex: 0.08 sec
      ST elevation: I, II, III, aVF, V_1, V_2, V_3, V_4, V_5, V_6
      ST depression: None
      Pathologic Q waves: Poor R wave progression
      Interpretation: Normal sinus rhythm, anterolateral MI, inferior MI

108. Rate: 78
      Rhythm: Irregular
      P wave: Present, upright (II)
      PR Interval: 0.12 sec
      QRS complex: 0.08 sec
      ST elevation: I, aVL, V_2, V_3, V_4, V_5, V_6
      ST depression: III, aVF
      Pathologic Q waves: None
      Interpretation: Sinus rhythm with sinus dysrhythmia, anterolateral MI

109. Rate: 74
      Rhythm: Regular
      P wave: Present, upright (II)
      PR Interval: 0.16 sec
      QRS complex: 0.08 sec
      ST elevation: I, aVL, V_1, V_2, V_3, V_4
      ST depression: III, aVF
      Pathologic Q waves: None
      Interpretation: Normal sinus rhythm, anterior MI

110. Rate: 89
      Rhythm: Regular
      P wave: Present, upright (II)
      PR Interval: 0.12 sec
      QRS complex: 0.06 sec
      ST elevation: II, III, aVF
      ST depression: I, aVL, V_2, V_3
      Pathologic Q waves: None
      Interpretation: Normal sinus rhythm, right axis deviation, inferior MI

111. Rate: 112
      Rhythm: Regular
      P wave: Absent
      PR Interval: 0
      QRS complex: 0.18 sec
      ST elevation: None
      ST depression: None
      Pathologic Q waves: None
      Interpretation: AV sequential or dual-chamber electronic pacemaker

112. Rate: 55
     Rhythm: Regular
     P wave: Present, upright (II)
     PR Interval: 0.14 sec
     QRS complex: 0.06 sec
     ST elevation: V_1, V_2
     ST depression: None
     Pathologic Q waves: None
     Interpretation: Sinus bradycardia, consider septal MI

113. Rate: 69
     Rhythm: Irregular
     P wave: Present, upright (II)
     PR Interval: 0.12 sec
     QRS complex: 0.08 sec
     ST elevation: I, II, aVL, aVF, V_1, V_2, V_3, V_4, V_5, V_6
     ST depression: None
     Pathologic Q waves: None
     Interpretation: Sinus rhythm with occasional PVC, anterior MI, inferolateral MI

114. Rate: 62
     Rhythm: Regular
     P wave: Present, upright (II)
     PR Interval: 0.18 sec
     QRS complex: 0.08 sec
     ST elevation: None
     ST depression: V_1, V_2, V_3, V_4
     Pathologic Q waves: II, III, aVF
     Interpretation: Normal sinus rhythm, inferior MI (old), right bundle branch block

115. Rate: 79
     Rhythm: Regular
     P wave: Present, upright (II)
     PR Interval: 0.12 sec
     QRS complex: 0.11 sec
     ST elevation: II, III, aVF, V_5, V_6
     ST depression: I, aVL, V_1, V_2, V_3, V_4
     Pathologic Q waves: None
     Interpretation: Normal sinus rhythm, inferolateral MI

116. Rate: 62
     Rhythm: Regular
     P wave: Present, upright (II)
     PR Interval: 0.22 sec
     QRS complex: 0.08 sec
     ST elevation: II, III, aVF
     ST depression: I, aVL, V_1, V_2, V_3, V_4
     Pathologic Q waves: None
     Interpretation: Sinus rhythm with first-degree block, inferior MI

117. Rate: 77
     Rhythm: Regular
     P wave: Present, upright (II)
     PR Interval: 0.16 sec
     QRS complex: 0.12 sec
     ST elevation: V_1, V_2, V_3, V_4
     ST depression: II, III, aVF
     Pathologic Q waves: None
     Interpretation: Normal sinus rhythm, anteroseptal MI, right bundle
                               branch block

118. Rate: 200
     Rhythm: Regular
     P wave: Absent or hidden
     PR Interval: 0
     QRS complex: 0.06 sec
     ST elevation: None
     ST depression: None
     Pathologic Q waves: None
     Interpretation: Supraventricular tachycardia

119. Rate: 86
     Rhythm: Regular
     P wave: Present, upright (II)
     PR Interval: 0.16 sec
     QRS complex: 0.08 sec
     ST elevation: II, III, aVF
     ST depression: I, aVL
     Pathologic Q waves: II, III, aVF
     Interpretation: Normal sinus rhythm, left axis deviation, inferior MI

120. Rate: 70
     Rhythm: Regular
     P wave: Present, upright (II)
     PR Interval: 0.16 sec
     QRS complex: 0.08 sec
     ST elevation: None
     ST depression: I, aVL, V_2, V_3, V_4, V_5, V_6, T wave inversion in I, aVL,
                               V_2, V_3, V_4, V_5, V_6
     Pathologic Q waves: III, aVF
     Interpretation: Normal sinus rhythm, left axis deviation, inferior MI,
                               anterolateral ischemia

121. Rate: 76
     Rhythm: Irregular
     P wave: Present, upright (II)
     PR Interval: 0.18 sec
     QRS complex: 0.08 sec
     ST elevation: V_1, V_2, V_3, V_4
     ST depression: None

Pathologic Q waves:	None
Interpretation:	Sinus rhythm with frequent PJCs, anteroseptal MI, left axis deviation

122.
Rate:	66
Rhythm:	Irregular
P wave:	Present, upright (II)
PR Interval:	0.16 sec
QRS complex:	0.08 sec
ST elevation:	$V_1, V_2, V_3, V_4, V_5, V_6$
ST depression:	III, aVF
Pathologic Q waves:	None
Interpretation:	Sinus rhythm, anteroseptal MI

123.
Rate:	84
Rhythm:	Regular
P wave:	Present, upright (II)
PR Interval:	0.12 sec
QRS complex:	0.04 sec
ST elevation:	None
ST depression:	None
Pathologic Q waves:	None
Interpretation:	Normal sinus rhythm

124.
Rate:	91
Rhythm:	Irregular
P wave:	Present, upright (II)
PR Interval:	0.16 sec
QRS complex:	0.08 sec
ST elevation:	None
ST depression:	V_1, V_2, V_3, V_4
Pathologic Q waves:	None
Interpretation:	Sinus rhythm with occasional PJCs, posterior MI (artifact)

125.
Rate:	56
Rhythm:	Irregular
P wave:	Absent
PR Interval:	0
QRS complex:	0.08 sec
ST elevation:	I, II, aVF, aVL, V_2, V_3, V_4, V_5, V_6
ST depression:	None
Pathologic Q waves:	None
Interpretation:	Junctional rhythm with PVCs, anterior/inferolateral MI

126.
Rate:	80
Rhythm:	Regular
P wave:	Present, upright (II)
PR Interval:	0.12 sec
QRS complex:	0.08 sec

ST elevation:	V_1, V_2, V_3, V_4
ST depression:	None
Pathologic Q waves:	II, III, aVF
Interpretation:	Normal sinus rhythm, anterior MI, inferior MI

127. Rate: 70

Rhythm:	Regular
P wave:	Present, upright (II)
PR Interval:	0.16 sec
QRS complex:	0.08 sec
ST elevation:	None
ST depression:	None
Pathologic Q waves:	None
Interpretation:	Normal sinus rhythm

128. Rate: 72

Rhythm:	Irregular
P wave:	Present, upright (II)
PR Interval:	0.12 sec
QRS complex:	0.08 sec
ST elevation:	I, aVL, V_1, V_2, V_3, V_4
ST depression:	II, III, aVF, V_5, V_6
Pathologic Q waves:	None
Interpretation:	Normal sinus rhythm with frequent PVCs, anteroseptal MI, lateral ischemia, left axis deviation

129. Rate: 60

Rhythm:	Regular
P wave:	Present, upright (II)
PR Interval:	0.12 sec
QRS complex:	0.06 sec
ST elevation:	I, aVL, V_1, V_2, V_3, V_4, V_5, V_6
ST depression:	III, aVF
Pathologic Q waves:	None
Interpretation:	Normal sinus rhythm, anteroseptal lateral MI

130. Rate: 67

Rhythm:	Regular
P wave:	Present, upright (II)
PR Interval:	0.12 sec
QRS complex:	0.08 sec
ST elevation:	I, aVL, V_1, V_2, V_3, V_4
ST depression:	II, III, aVF
Pathologic Q waves:	None
Interpretation:	Normal sinus rhythm, anterior MI (tombstones in V_2, V_3)

131. Rate: 96

Rhythm:	Irregular
P wave:	Present, upright (II)
PR Interval:	0.28 sec

QRS complex:	0.10 sec
ST elevation:	I, II, III, aVL, aVF, V_1, V_2, V_3, V_4, V_5, V_6
ST depression:	None
Pathologic Q waves:	None
Interpretation:	Sinus rhythm with first-degree block, anteroseptal MI, inferolateral MI, PVCs

132.
Rate:	46
Rhythm:	Regular
P wave:	Present, upright (II)
PR Interval:	0.16 sec
QRS complex:	0.04 sec
ST elevation:	V_1, V_2, V_3
ST depression:	None
Pathologic Q waves:	None
Interpretation:	Sinus bradycardia rhythm, septal MI

133.
Rate:	78
Rhythm:	Regular
P wave:	Present, upright (II)
PR Interval:	0.16 sec
QRS complex:	0.08 sec
ST elevation:	None
ST depression:	None
Pathologic Q waves:	None
Interpretation:	Normal sinus rhythm

134.
Rate:	46
Rhythm:	Regular
P wave:	Present, upright (II)
PR Interval:	0.12 sec
QRS complex:	0.08 sec
ST elevation:	II, III, aVF
ST depression:	None
Pathologic Q waves:	None
Interpretation:	Marked sinus bradycardia rhythm, inferior MI

135.
Rate:	86
Rhythm:	Regular
P wave:	Present, upright (II)
PR Interval:	0.16 sec
QRS complex:	0.08 sec
ST elevation:	II, III, aVF, with T wave inversion
ST depression:	None
Pathologic Q waves:	II, III, aVF
Interpretation:	Normal sinus rhythm, inferior MI

136.
Rate:	60
Rhythm:	Irregular
P wave:	Present, upright (II)
PR Interval:	0.12 sec

QRS complex:	0.10 sec
ST elevation:	V_1, V_2, V_3, V_4, V_5
ST depression:	None
Pathologic Q waves:	None
Interpretation:	Sinus rhythm with sinus dysrhythmia, anteroseptal MI

137.

Rate:	134
Rhythm:	Regular
P wave:	Present, upright (II)
PR Interval:	0.16 sec
QRS complex:	0.10 sec
ST elevation:	II, III, aVF
ST depression:	I, aVL, V_2, V_3, V_4, V_5, V_6
Pathologic Q waves:	None
Interpretation:	Sinus tachycardia rhythm, inferior-posterior MI

138.

Rate:	75
Rhythm:	Regular
P wave:	Present, upright (II)
PR Interval:	0.12 sec
QRS complex:	0.08 sec
ST elevation:	None
ST depression:	III, aVF, V_2, V_3, V_4, V_5, V_6
Pathologic Q waves:	None
Interpretation:	Normal sinus rhythm, inferior/anterior ischemia

139.

Rate:	78
Rhythm:	Irregular
P wave:	Absent
PR Interval:	0
QRS complex:	0.14 sec
ST elevation:	II, III, aVF
ST depression:	I, aVL, V_1, V_2, V_3, V_4
Pathologic Q waves:	None
Interpretation:	Atrial fibrillation, inferior MI, nonspecific intraventricular block

140.

Rate:	110
Rhythm:	Regular
P wave:	Present, upright (II)
PR Interval:	0.18 sec
QRS complex:	0.08 sec
ST elevation:	None
ST depression:	I, aVL, V_3, V_4, V_5, V_6
Pathologic Q waves:	None
Interpretation:	Sinus tachycardia rhythm, consider anterolateral ischemia

141.

Rate:	66
Rhythm:	Regular
P wave:	Present, upright (II)
PR Interval:	0.18 sec

QRS complex:	0.08 sec
ST elevation:	II, III, aVF
ST depression:	I, aVL, V_2, V_3
Pathologic Q waves:	None
Interpretation:	Normal sinus rhythm, inferior MI

142.

Rate:	70
Rhythm:	Regular
P wave:	Present, upright (II)
PR Interval:	0.16 sec
QRS complex:	0.08 sec
ST elevation:	I, II, aVL, aVF, V_3, V_4, V_5, V_6
ST depression:	aVR, V_1
Pathologic Q waves:	None
Interpretation:	Normal sinus rhythm, anterior MI, inferolateral MI

143.

Rate:	67
Rhythm:	Regular
P wave:	Present, upright (II)
PR Interval:	0.16 sec
QRS complex:	0.08 sec
ST elevation:	II, III, aVF
ST depression:	I, aVL, V_2, V_3, V_4, V_5
Pathologic Q waves:	None
Interpretation:	Normal sinus rhythm, inferior MI

144.

Rate:	80
Rhythm:	Regular
P wave:	Present, upright (II)
PR Interval:	0.12 sec
QRS complex:	0.12 sec
ST elevation:	I, aVL, V_1, V_2, V_3, V_4
ST depression:	None
Pathologic Q waves:	II, III, aVF
Interpretation:	Normal sinus rhythm, anteroseptal MI, inferior MI (old)

145.

Rate:	66
Rhythm:	Regular
P wave:	Present, inverted (II)
PR Interval:	0.16 sec
QRS complex:	0.08 sec
ST elevation:	II, III, aVF, V_5, V_6
ST depression:	V_1, V_2, V_3
Pathologic Q waves:	None
Interpretation:	Junctional rhythm, inferolateral MI

146.

Rate:	74
Rhythm:	Irregular
P wave:	Present, upright (II)
PR Interval:	0.16 sec
QRS complex:	0.08 sec

ST elevation:	II, III, aVF, V_4, V_5, V_6
ST depression:	I, aVL, V_2, V_3
Pathologic Q waves:	None
Interpretation:	Sinus rhythm with trigeminy PVCs, inferolateral MI

147. Rate: 65

Rhythm:	Irregular
P wave:	Present, upright (II)
PR Interval:	0.16 sec
QRS complex:	0.08 sec
ST elevation:	I, II, III, aVF, aVL, V_2, V_3, V_4, V_5, V_6
ST depression:	aVR
Pathologic Q waves:	None
Interpretation:	Sinus rhythm with occasional PVCs, anterior MI, inferolateral MI

148. Rate: 72

Rhythm:	Irregular
P wave:	Present, upright (II)
PR Interval:	0.16 sec
QRS complex:	0.08 sec
ST elevation:	I, aVL, V_1, V_2, V_3
ST depression:	II, III, aVF, V_5, V_6
Pathologic Q waves:	None
Interpretation:	Sinus rhythm with frequent PVCs, anteroseptal MI, lateral ischemia

149. Rate: 38

Rhythm:	Regular
P wave:	Present, no relation with QRS complex
PR Interval:	Variable
QRS complex:	0.12 sec
ST elevation:	II, III, aVF, V_2, V_3, V_4, V_5, V_6
ST depression:	None
Pathologic Q waves:	None
Interpretation:	Third-degree block, inferolateral MI, anterior MI, right bundle branch block

150. Rate: 112

Rhythm:	Regular
P wave:	Present, upright (II)
PR Interval:	0.14 sec
QRS complex:	0.08 sec
ST elevation:	III, aVF
ST depression:	V_3, V_4, V_5
Pathologic Q waves:	II, III, aVF
Interpretation:	Sinus tachycardia, inferior MI

151. Rate: 98

Rhythm:	Regular
P wave:	Present, upright (II)

PR Interval: 0.16 sec
QRS complex: 0.16 sec
ST elevation: None
ST depression: None
Pathologic Q waves: None
Interpretation: Normal sinus rhythm, left bundle branch block

152. Rate: 78
     Rhythm: Regular
     P wave: Present, upright (II)
     PR Interval: 0.16 sec
     QRS complex: 0.08 sec
     ST elevation: II, III, aVF
     ST depression: I, aVL, V_2, V_3, V_4, V_5
     Pathologic Q waves: III
     Interpretation: Normal sinus rhythm, inferior MI

Glossary

A

absolute refractory period   stage of cell activity in which the cardiac cell cannot spontaneously depolarize.

acetylcholine   chemical neurotransmitter for the parasympathetic system.

ACLS   advanced cardiac life support.

action potential   a change in polarity; a five-phase cycle that produces changes in the cell membrane's electrical charge; caused by stimulation of myocardial cells that extends across the myocardium; propagated in an "all or none" fashion.

acute myocardial infarction (AMI)   condition that results from a prolonged lack of blood flow to a portion of the myocardial tissue, which leads to a lack of oxygen.

afterload   resistance against which the heart must pump.

alkaline agents   agents used to buffer the acids present in the body.

alkalinizing agent   an agent that causes blood to become alkaline; an agent utilized in the treatment of metabolic acidosis.

ALS   advanced life support.

AMI   acute myocardial infarction.

anaerobic metabolism   metabolism that occurs in the absence of oxygen.

analgesics   agents used to relieve or reduce pain.

anaphylaxis   severe allergic reaction.

anastomoses   communications between two or more vessels.

angina pectoris   pain that results from a reduction in blood supply to myocardial tissue.

angioplasty   procedure used to alter the structure of a vessel either surgically or by dilating it with a balloon inside the lumen.

anion   ion with a negative charge.

antagonist   an agent that prevents a response from occurring.

anterior apex placement   the negative electrode is placed to the right of the sternum just beneath the clavicle and the positive electrode is placed to the left of the nipple of the left thorax in the midaxillary position.

anterior MI   the interruption of blood supply to the anterior myocardial wall; primarily involves the left anterior descending artery.

anterior-posterior placement   the anterior or negative electrode is placed over the left precordium, with the posterior or positive electrode in the infrascapular space of the left scapula.

anterolateral MI   involves decreased blood supply to the lateral wall of the left ventricle in conjunction with proximal occlusion of the left anterior descending artery; illustrated by ST segment elevation in Leads V_3, V_4, V_5, V_6, I, and aVL.

anteroseptal MI   involves decreased blood supply to the interventricular septum and the anterior wall of the left ventricle; illustrated by ST segment elevation in Leads V_1, V_2, V3, and V_4.

antianginals   agents that relax smooth muscles.

anticoagulant   an agent that delays or prevents blood coagulation.

antidysrhythmics   agents that serve to remedy disturbances in the heart's electrical activity.

antiemetic agent   an agent that prevents or relieves nausea and vomiting.

aortic valve   semilunar valve located between the left ventricle and the trunk of the aorta.

arteries   thick-walled and muscular blood vessels that function under high pressure to convey blood from the heart out to the rest of the body.

atrioventricular (AV) node   located on the floor of the right atrium near the opening of the coronary sinus and just above the tricuspid valve; at the level of the AV node, the electrical activity is delayed approximately 0.05 second.

atrium   upper chamber of the heart.

augmented limb leads   Leads aVR, aVL, and aVF; current flows from the heart outward to the extremities. Also called unipolar leads.

automaticity   ability of cardiac pacemaker cells to generate their own electrical impulses spontaneously without external (or nervous) stimulation.

autonomic nervous system   regulates functions of the body that are involuntary or not under conscious control.

AV   atrioventricular.

AV junction   region where the AV node joins the bundle of His.

axis   the direction of the heart's electrical current from negative to positive.

axis deviation   occurs when the conduction pattern is altered due to disease or death of the muscle.

B

Bachmann's Bundle   subdivision of the anterior internodal tract; conducts electrical activity from the SA node to the left atrium.

baseline   straight line seen on an EKG strip; represents the beginning and end point of all waves. Also called isoelectric line.

beta blockers   agents that antagonize (oppose) adrenergic receptor sites.

biphasic defibrillator   a device with which energy is delivered to the heart via current traveling in one direction in the first phase of a shock and then reversing and traveling in the opposite direction.

bipolar leads   leads that have one positive electrode and one negative electrode.

BPM   beats per minute.

bradycardia   heart rate of less than 60 beats per minute.

bundle branches   two main branches, the right bundle branch and the left bundle branch, conduct electrical activity from the bundle of His down to the Purkinje's network.

bundle of His   conduction pathway that leads out of the AV node. Also called the common bundle.

C

calcium channel blockers   agents that relax vascular smooth muscle, cause vascular dilation, and consequently act to slow conduction through the AV node.

capillaries   tiny blood vessels that allow for the exchange of oxygen, nutrients, and waste products between the blood and body tissues; connectors between arteries and veins.

capnography   involves a device that measures the expiratory CO_2 partial pressures.

cardiac cycle   actual time sequence between ventricular contraction and ventricular relaxation.

cardiac glycosides   agents that increase the force of cardiac contraction, as well as cardiac output.

cardiac output   amount of blood pumped by the left ventricle in one minute.

cardiogenic shock   condition caused by inadequate cardiac output (pump failure).

cardiovascular pharmacological agents   drugs aimed at the specialized treatment of the heart and blood vessels.

cation   ion with a positive charge.

cc   cubic centimeters.

chest leads   Leads V_1 through V_6; unipolar leads. Also called precordial or vector leads.

chest pain   the most common presenting symptom of cardiac disease and the most common patient complaint.

CHF   congestive heart failure.

chordae tendineae   fine chords of dense connective tissue that attach to papillary muscles in the walls of the ventricles.

collateral circulation   allows for an alternate path of blood flow in event of vascular occlusion; a protective mechanism.

complete bundle branch block   one in which the width of the QRS complex will measure 0.12 second or greater.

conductivity   ability of cardiac cells to receive an electrical stimulus and then transmit it to other cardiac cells.

contractility   ability of cardiac cells to shorten and cause cardiac muscle contraction in response to an electrical stimulus. Also called rhythmicity.

contraindications   signs or symptoms that indicate an inappropriate response to a form of treatment.

COPD   chronic obstructive pulmonary disease.

coronary arteries   the two arteries—right and left—that supply blood to the myocardium.

coronary sinus   passage that receives deoxygenated blood from the major veins of the myocardium.

costrochondritis   inflammation of intercostal muscles.

D

defibrillation   therapeutic modality by virtue of its ability to terminate fibrillation by passing a current of electricity through the heart's critical mass.

depolarization   an electrical occurrence normally expected to result in myocardial contraction; involves the movement of ions across cardiac cell membranes resulting in positive polarity inside the cell membrane.

diagonal arteries   supply blood to the anterolateral wall of the left ventricle.

diaphoresis   profuse sweating.

diastole   synonymous with ventricular relaxation.

diuretics   agents that increase urine secretion.

dosages   determination of the amount, number, and frequency of medication for a patient.

drugs   agents used in the cure, treatment, or prevention of disease.

dyspnea   difficulty breathing.

dysrhythmia   abnormal rhythm.

E

ectopy   out of place.

EKG waveform   wave recorded on an EKG strip; refers to movement away from the baseline or isoelectric line and is represented as a positive deflection (above the isoelectric line) or as a negative deflection (below the isoelectric line).

electrocardiogram (EKG)   graphic representation of the electrical activity of the heart.

electrode   adhesive pad that contains conductive gel and is designed to be attached to the patient's skin.

electrolyte   substance or compound whose molecules dissociate into charged components when placed in water, producing positively and negatively charged ions.

endocardium   innermost layer of the heart; composed of thin connective tissue.

epicardium   smooth outer surface of the heart.

epistaxis   nosebleed.

excitability   ability of all cardiac cells to respond to an electrical stimulus. Also called irritability.

extreme right axis deviation   an axis deviation between −90 and + or −180 degrees. Also called indeterminate axis deviation.

F

facing leads   leads that "view" or "look at" specific areas of damaged myocardium.

fascicles   the two main divisions of the left bundle branch.

fibrinolytic therapy   the use of agents to activate enzymes that dissolve a thrombus.

15-lead EKG   method used to interpret posterior MIs using posterior Leads V₇, V₈, and V₉.

5 + 3 approach   a combination of the basic five steps to EKG interpretation plus analysis of the ST segment and Q wave.

frontal plane leads   bipolar limb leads and augmented limb leads (Leads I, II, III, aVR, aVL, and aVF).

G

gtt   drops.

H

half-life   the time required for the total amount of a drug in the body to diminish by one-half.

heart rate   number of contractions, or beats, per minute; number of electrical impulses conducted through the myocardium in 60 seconds.

heart rhythm   sequential beating of the heart as a result of the generation of electrical impulses.

hematuria   presence of blood in urine.

hemopneumothorax   the collection of blood and air within the pleural cavity.

hemothorax   the collection of blood within the pleural cavity.

hypersensitivity   abnormal sensitivity to a stimulus of any kind.

I

incomplete bundle branch block   one in which the width of the QRS complex measures between 0.10 and 0.11 second.

infarct   necrosis of tissue following loss of blood supply.

inferior vena cava   collects blood from the lower portion of the body.

inferior wall infarction   interruption of the supply of oxygen-rich blood to the inferior myocardial wall involved with the right coronary artery.

intercostal muscles   muscles located between the ribs.

internodal tracts   distribute the electrical impulse throughout the atria and transmit the impulse from the SA node to the AV node.

IV   intravenous.

J

J point   the point on the EKG strip where the QRS complex meets the ST segment.

joules   watt-seconds.

L

L   liters.

LAD   left anterior descending artery.

lead axis   the axis of a given lead.

leads   electrodes connected to the monitor or EKG machine by wires; also, may refer to a pair of electrodes.

left axis deviation   an axis deviation between 0 and −90 degrees.

lethal dysrhythmias   abnormalities in heart rhythms that if left untreated result in death.

LPM   liters per minute.

M

mA   milliamps.

malaise   generalized feeling of discomfort and fatigue.

mean QRS axis   refers to the normal QRS axis, which falls between 0 and +90 degrees.

mechanism of action   interaction at the cellular level between a drug and cellular components.

mediastinum   central section of the thorax (chest cavity).

min   minutes.

mirror test   method used to view posterior myocardial infarction EKG changes.

mitral valve   similar in structure to the tricuspid valve but has only two cusps; located between the left atrium and the left ventricle. Also called bicuspid valve.

mm   millimeters.

monophasic defibrillator   a device with which energy is delivered to the heart via current traveling in one direction.

mV   millivolts.

myocardial injury   damage to the myocardium; most commonly results from and follows myocardial ischemia.

myocardial ischemia   deprivation of oxygen and other nutrients to the myocardium; tendency to produce repolarization abnormalities.

myocardial necrosis   death of the myocardial tissue; myocardial infarction.

myocardial working cells   responsible for generating the physical contraction of the heart muscle.

myocardium   thick middle layer of the heart composed primarily of cardiac muscle cells; responsible for the heart's ability to contract.

N

negative inotropic agent   an agent that decreases contractility.

neuropathy   the inability to perceive pain due to destruction of nerve endings.

nitroglycerin   medication that causes blood vessel dilation, reducing the workload of the heart and the need for oxygen.

norepinephrine   chemical neurotransmitter for the sympathetic nervous system.

P

P wave   represents depolarization of the left and right atria.

pallor   paleness.

parasympathetic nervous system   regulates the calmer ("rest and digest") functions.

parasympatholytics   agents that block the effects of the parasympathetic nervous system.

pathologic Q wave   a Q wave that is equal or greater than 0.04 second (one small box) in width and has a depth of greater than one-third of the height of the succeeding R wave.

pericarditis   inflammation of the serous pericardium.

pericardium   closed, two-layered sac that surrounds the heart.

peripheral vascular resistance (PVR)   amount of opposition to blood flow offered by the arterioles.

pharmacology   the study of drugs and their effects on living organisms.

pleurisy   inflammation of the covering of the lungs.

pneumothorax   the collection of air within the pleural cavity.

polarized state   the resting state of a cardiac cell wherein the inside of the cell is electrically negative relative to the outside of the cell.

positive inotropic agent   an agent that increases contractility.

posterior MI   involves a decrease in oxygen-rich blood supply from the right coronary artery to the posterior wall of the left ventricle.

PR interval   represents the time interval needed for the impulse to travel from the SA node through the internodal pathways in the atria and downward to the ventricles; measures the time intervals from the onset of atrial contraction to the onset of ventricular contraction. Sometimes referred to as PRI.

precipitates   deposits formed as a result of reaction with a reagent.

precordial leads   chest leads (V_1, V_2, V_3, V_4, V_5, and V_6).

preload   pressure in the ventricles at the end of diastole.

PSVT   paroxysmal supraventricular tachycardia.

pulmonic valve   semilunar valve located between the right ventricle and the pulmonary artery.

pure septal MIs   recognized by the development of QS complexes in Leads V_1 and V_2.

Purkinje's network   network of fibers that carries electrical impulses directly to ventricular muscle cells.

PVCs   premature ventricular contractions.

PVR   peripheral vascular resistance.

Q

Q wave   in the QRS complex, the first negative or downward deflection; a small wave that precedes the R wave.

QRS axis   the largest of the axes and the most commonly measured.

QRS complex   consists of the Q, R, and S waves and represents the conduction of the electrical impulse from the bundle of His throughout the ventricular muscle, or ventricular depolarization; represents the depolarization (or contraction) of the ventricles.

R

R wave   in the QRS complex, the first upward or positive deflection following the P wave; in chest Lead II, the R wave is the tallest waveform noted.

reciprocal leads   leads that record electrical impulses in myocardial cells opposite involved myocardium.

relative refractory period   period when repolarization is almost complete, and the cardiac cell can be stimulated to contract prematurely if the stimulus is much stronger than normal.

reperfusion dysrhythmias   dysrhythmias that occur after a vessel is reopened and blood flow returned.

repolarization   process whereby the depolarized cell is polarized and positive charges are again on the outside and negative charges on the inside of the cell; a return to the resting state.

resting membrane potential   the state of a cardiac cell in which the inside of the cell membrane is negative when compared to the outside of the cell membrane; exists when cardiac cells are in the resting state.

rhythm strip   printed record of the electrical activity of the heart. Also called EKG strip.

right axis deviation   an axis deviation between +90 and + or −180 degrees.

right ventricular infarction (RVI)   a complication that occurs in approximately 40% of inferior MIs and indicates a larger infarction that most likely involves both ventricles.

RVI   right ventricular infarction.

S

S wave   in the QRS complex, the sharp, negative or downward deflection that follows the R wave.

SA   sinoatrial.

sec   seconds.

semilunar valves   prevent the backflow of blood into the ventricles; each valve contains three semilunar (or moon-shaped) cusps.

septal MIs   interruption of oxygen-rich blood supply to the interventricular septum.

septal perforating arteries   supply the anterior two-thirds of the interventricular septum.

side effects   undesirable effects of a drug.

sinoatrial (SA) node   commonly referred to as the primary pacemaker of the heart because it normally depolarizes more rapidly than any other part of the conduction system.

specialized pacemaker cells   responsible for controlling the rate and rhythm of the heart by coordinating regular depolarization; found in the electrical conduction system of the heart.

ST segment   time interval during which the ventricles are depolarized and ventricular depolarization begins.

ST segment depression   characterized by a dip below the isoelectric line of 1 to 2 millimeters or one to two small boxes on the EKG graph paper.

ST segment elevation   characterized by a rise above the isoelectric line of 1 to 2 millimeters or one to two small boxes on the EKG graph paper.

stacked shocks   three consecutive shocks that are delivered without pausing between each defibrillation.

standard limb leads   Leads I, II, and III; current flows from the limbs through the heart.

Starling's Law of the heart   the more the myocardial fibers are stretched, up to a certain point, the more forceful the subsequent contraction will be.

stroke volume   volume of blood pumped out of one ventricle of the heart in a single beat or contraction.

subendocardial infarction   involves only a portion of the ventricular wall, most commonly the subendocardial layer closest to the endocardium. Also called nontransmural infarction.

superior vena cava   drains blood from the heart and neck.

supraventricular   above the ventricles.

sympathetic nervous system   responsible for preparation of the body for physical activity ("fight or flight").

sympatholytics   agents that inhibit adrenergic nerve function; agents that antagonize or oppose adrenergic receptor sites.

sympathomimetics   agents that mimic the actions of the sympathetic nervous system.

synchronized cardioversion   the delivery of an electrical shock to the heart, synchronized so as to coincide with the R wave of the cardiac cycle.

syncytium   cardiac muscle cell groups that are connected together and function collectively as a unit.

systole   contraction of the chambers of the heart. Also called ventricular systole.

T

T wave   represents ventricular repolarization; follows the ST segment.

T wave inversion   negative deflection of the T wave below the isoelectric line.

tachycardia   heart rate greater than 100 beats per minute.

tachydysrhythmias   irregular rhythms in combination with a rapid heart rate.

TCP   transcutaneous cardiac pacing.

tension pneumothorax   air trapped in the thoracic cavity without an escape route; pressure builds and affects the lungs, heart, and other vital organs.

therapeutic level   refers to an optimum level of a medication in the blood.

threshold   refers to a point at which a stimulus will produce a cell response.

thrombus   stationary blood clots that can lead to vessel occlusion.

tinnitus   the sound of "ringing in the ears."

tolerance   progressive decrease in effectiveness of a drug.

transcutaneous cardiac pacing (TCP)   therapy performed via two large electrode pads placed in an anterior-posterior position on a patient's chest to conduct electrical impulses through the skin to the heart.

transmural infarction   involves the entire full thickness of the ventricular wall, extending from the endocardium to the epicardial surface.

transthoracic resistance   resistance to current flow across the chest.

tricuspid valve   named for its three cusps; located between the right atrium and right ventricle.

V

vasodilators   agents that cause dilation of blood vessels.

vector   a mark or symbol that can be used to describe any force having both magnitude and direction; the direction of electrical currents in cardiac cells that are generated by depolarization and repolarization of the atria and ventricles as the currents spread from the endocardium outward to the epicardium.

veins   blood vessels that carry blood back to the heart, operate under low pressure, and are relatively thin-walled.

ventricle   lower chamber of the heart.

V-fib ventricular fibrillation. Also called VF.

V-tach ventricular tachycardia. Also called VT.

W

widowmaker term used to illustrate the serious result of total occlusion of the left anterior descending artery.

Wolfe-Parkinson-White syndrome a cardiac rhythm disturbance that is characterized by a delta wave, or a slur of the R wave on a QRS complex.

Index